Women's Behavioral Health

Ardis Hanson • Bruce Lubotsky Levin

Editors

Women's Behavioral Health

A Public Health Perspective

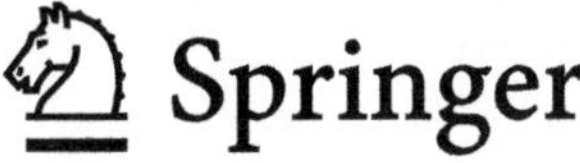 Springer

Editors
Ardis Hanson
USF Health Libraries and the College
of Public Health
University of South Florida
Tampa, FL, USA

Bruce Lubotsky Levin
College of Behavioral & Community
Sciences, College of Public Health
University of South Florida
Tampa, FL, USA

ISBN 978-3-031-58295-0   ISBN 978-3-031-58293-6   (eBook)
https://doi.org/10.1007/978-3-031-58293-6

Preface

National and global studies show that women are nearly twice as likely as men to suffer from mental and substance use disorders. However, despite the increased attention in the past two decades to women's behavioral health issues (alcohol, drug abuse, and mental disorders), few texts in the medical and/or behavioral health literature can be identified which offer an extensive examination of women's behavioral health problems from a *public health perspective* that did not focus primarily on a clinical perspective.

The 2016 workshop conducted by the National Academies of Sciences, Engineering, and Medicine, *Improving the Health of Women in the United States*, has drawn attention to the social, institutional, and economic determinants that result in service inequities for women with health and behavioral health disorders in the United States compared to women in other high-income countries. In addition, the framework for *Healthy People 2030* includes core objectives and developmental objectives targeted to improve behavioral health. Globally, the Sustainable Development Goals have a strong focus on women's health and behavioral health. This textbook responds to this gap in the literature, providing the current state of knowledge of women's behavioral health and examining the need for behavioral health services and the effect of behavioral health disorders upon women's daily lives.

The development and organization of *Women's Behavioral Health: A Public Health Perspective* has been influenced by our work and experiences as well as those of our colleagues in teaching, research, and community service. Our efforts culminated in the development of the Behavioral Health Concentration (BHC) at the University of South Florida (USF) College of Public Health (COPH), a collaborative teaching initiative between the USF COPH and the USF College of Behavioral & Community Sciences. The BHC is one of only a relatively few US accredited schools/colleges of public health offering a concentration or focus on alcohol, drug use, and mental disorders from a population or public health perspective.

Women's Behavioral Health: A Public Health Perspective examines major issues in the organization, financing, and provision of alcohol, drug abuse, and mental health services for women. The book incorporates the social determinants of behavioral health, an interprofessional as well as a population and public health perspective, including a global perspective. In order to accomplish these objectives, an editorial decision was made to include applied services research chapters, including quantitative, qualitative, and other empirically based chapters. In addition, an effort was made to have current working documents and reports (national and international) represented within relevant chapters.

The textbook contains 14 chapters organized into three content areas: (1) *Framing Women's Behavioral Health* (Chaps. 1, 2, 3, 4, and 5); (2) *Selected At-Risk Populations* (Chaps. 6, 7, and 8); and (3) *Services Delivery* (Chaps. 9, 10, 11, 12, 13, and 14). Each chapter closes with the unifying theme "Implications for Women's Behavioral Health," which discusses the significance of each chapter for the broader fields of women's behavioral health as well as public health.

Part I, *Framing Women's Behavioral Health*, introduces readers to women's behavioral health. In Chap. 1, "Overview and Global Issues in Women's Behavioral Health," Hanson and Levin examine women's behavioral health services from a public health and population health perspective. Using a global frame, the authors incorporate the social determinants of health (socio-structural factors) and the Sustainable Development Goals, as well as national initiatives in the United States (e.g., *Healthy People 2030*), to create an overview of significant issues affecting behavioral health services and policy for women throughout their lifespan.

Chapters 2, 3, and 4 examine the epidemiology of behavioral health disorders across the lifespan (girls, adult women, and older women). Mental health disorders are a public health emergency, yet they remain underdiagnosed, undertreated, and under-resourced despite their high prevalence and roles as leading causes of disability globally. As mental health disorders can begin in early life, the purpose of Chap. 2, "Epidemiology of Mental Health Disorders in Female Children and Adolescents," is to examine the behavioral health challenges for girls and boys. Leung et al. provide an overview of the epidemiology of mental health disorders in children and adolescents globally and its impact from the COVID-19 pandemic with particular emphasis on female differences regarding prevalence, presentation, disparities, trajectory across the lifespan, and implications for women's behavioral health. The chapter focuses on common mental disorders in children and adolescents and those with notable disproportionate disease burden in females including depressive disorders, anxiety disorders, post-traumatic stress disorder, schizophrenia-spectrum disorders, eating disorders, autism spectrum disorders, and attention-deficit/hyperactivity disorder.

In Chap. 3, "Epidemiology of Mental Disorders in Adult Women," Carpenter et al. address the epidemiology of mental disorders in adult women. It has been acknowledged that adult women experience a higher disease burden relative to adult men. Accordingly, a special effort is needed to identify causative factors for this difference and to adjust approaches to care when possible. The COVID-19 pandemic has led to both an exacerbation of this disparity and an increase in prevalence of mental health disorders in general.

In Chap. 4, "Epidemiology of Mental Health Conditions in Older Adult Women," Webb et al. examine the epidemiology of mental disorders in older adult women. Globally, women are two times more likely to experience a mental health condition compared with men. Older women are at increased risk for mental health conditions. This chapter focuses on the epidemiology of mental health conditions among women aged 65 years or older living in the United States and presents the etiology of mental health conditions, including risk and protective factors, and the estimated impact of the COVID-19 pandemic.

In Chap. 5, "Epidemiology of Substance Use Disorders in Women," Johnson discusses the history of research on SUDs in women, what is known about the biological and social determinants of SUD, and sex and gender differences in those determinants. It covers the prevention, screening, assessment, diagnosis, and treatment of SUDs and what is known and not known regarding efficacy for girls and women. The chapter also covers adaptations that have been made for women and identifies opportunities for new research and evaluation to better prevent and treat SUD in women.

Part II, *Selected At-Risk Populations*, examines special populations at-risk for behavioral health disorders. In Chap. 6, "Behavioral Health Disorders and HIV Incidence and Treatment Among Women," Lynn et al. examine women, behavioral health, and HIV/AIDS. The acquisition and transmission of HIV can be influenced by behavioral health conditions such as mental and substance use disorders. Women with these conditions have a higher risk of acquiring HIV and worse health outcomes than those without. Lynn et al. discuss the most prevalent conditions associated with HIV incidence and treatment among women as well as social determinants of health (SDOH) that affect the relationship between these conditions and HIV. The chapter also addresses the challenges and disparities faced by transgender women and the barriers that women with behavioral health conditions face in HIV prevention efforts. Overall, the chapter emphasizes the importance of prioritizing behavioral health screening and treatment in concert with HIV treatment and the need for further research to understand the implementation of HIV prevention strategies in mental health and community-based settings.

Although there are common characteristics that define rural communities, not all rural communities are the same. In Chap. 7, "Rural Behavioral Health Services," Levin and Hanson examine the most prevalent and significant behavioral health problems affecting women in rural and frontier communities. They also offer a comparison of rural frameworks, and contextualize challenges rural women face from the perspectives of availability, accessibility, affordability, and acceptability.

In Chap. 8, "Stereotypes, Stigma, and Social/Mass Media in Women's Behavioral Health," Levin and Hanson address the effects of stereotypes and stigma, examining the role social and mass media play in women's behavioral health. The role played by traditional media in ameliorating or exacerbating stigma, prejudice, discrimination, and trivialization of persons with behavioral health disorders continues new media forms in the twenty-first century. However, social/mass media can be powerful tools to reduce these misperceptions, promoting safe spaces for open discussion and treatment, and providing new pathways for health education and health promotion initiatives.

In Part III, *Services Delivery*, chapters focus on integration, insurance and financing of care, services implementation and evaluation, challenges in data collection, and reframing behavioral health disorders form a policy perspective. Most women with mental health and substance use concerns presented to primary or prenatal care rather than to specialty mental health care. Owing to unique barriers such as transportation, childcare, competing demands, and stigma, women also often prefer to receive mental health treatment from their obstetric or primary care provider. Given these considerations, integrated models of care are an important approach to increasing access to identification and treatment of women's behavioral health concerns. In Chap. 9, "Integration of Behavioral Health and Primary Care Services for Women," Koire et al. address how women's behavioral health care can be integrated into various settings including primary care, prenatal care, and community-based settings, with a focus on specific integrated care models including collaborative care, primary care behavioral health, and perinatal psychiatry access programs.

Financing and payment for behavioral health services influence the organization of services, access, and quality of care and are, therefore, essential to behavioral health services delivery for women. In Chap. 10, "Financing Behavioral Health Services: Influence on Access to and Quality of Behavioral Health Care," Stewart et al. examine how behavioral health care is financed with public and/or private dollars and is paid for primarily through health insurance. They look at efforts to improve access to and quality of care and how integration of behavioral health services with physical health depend on changes to financing and payment models.

Closing the research-to-practice gap is an ongoing problem. The field of implementation science attempts to address this problem through understanding adoption and use of evidence-based practices. In Chap. 11, "Implementation Science to Promote Equity in Women's Behavioral Health," Vroom and Sharp provide a broad lens of both implementation science and women's behavioral health, focusing on how women's behavioral health issues may be more equitably addressed through the consistent application of evidence-based practices guided by implementation science. They explore the history of inequities of women in scientific research, the emergence of women's issues in behavioral health over time, and the development of implementation science and identify global research.

Pharmacists are highly accessible health care professionals who play a critical role in providing comprehensive medication management and person-centered care to patients. An important part of interdisciplinary teams in various hospital and clinic settings, pharmacists are well-positioned to address the social determinants of health in their practice. In Chap. 12, "The Role of Pharmacists in the Intersection of Women's Health and Mental Health," Ott and Wartman discuss pharmacist practice settings outside of dispensing roles, treatment considerations for opioid use disorder in pregnancy, psychotropic medications and risks to women, and advocacy considerations for mental health in women. A women's health checklist from a pharmacist's perspective is provided.

In Chap. 13, "Behavioral Health Data: Addressing Women's Needs," Hanson, Levin, and Menendez identify gender data gaps in health, mental health, substance abuse, and other elements of the social determinants or socio-structural components of behavioral health. This chapter describes the effects of gender gap data in the provision of services, the planning of services, evaluation, and assessment, as well as addressing the lack of relevant data on women's well-being.

Behavioral health policymaking should address the many roles women have across the workplace, home, family, and community. In Chap. 14, "Policymaking Addressing Women and Behavioral Health," Hanson and Levin maintain effective and thoughtful policymaking can help to address the socio-structural or social determinants of health that adversely affect women and their behavioral health. They examine the public policymaking process and make recommendations on how it could be altered to improve the well-being of women with effective behavioral health treatment and support services.

It is impossible to include every possible topic area in a single textbook devoted to women's behavioral health services. Nevertheless, *Women's Behavioral Health: A Public Health Perspective* emphasizes the critical importance of using a transdisciplinary public health approach to understand women's behavioral health issues from a public health framework.

This text is particularly timely given the substantial ongoing changes in financing and services delivery of health and behavioral health services at state, national, and international levels. In addition, national legislation and policy are adopting global frameworks, such as the social determinants of health, burden of disease studies, DALYS, and the Sustainable Development Goals.

Designed for a variety of academic and professional audiences, these target audiences include undergraduate and graduate students in the social and behavioral sciences, public health, behavioral health, women's studies, medical anthropology, medical sociology, as well as graduate and postdoctoral students in public and population health and the health professions.

Accreditation requirements for undergraduate and graduate medical, health, and pharmacy education programs emphasize focal areas in underserved populations (e.g., women with HIV/AIDS, women living in rural areas, women with behavioral health problems and encountering stigma) at the intersection of health and behavioral health. Professionals currently employed in mental health and substance abuse programs in various healthcare organizations, including managed care organizations, women's health centers, hospitals, substance abuse clinics, and community mental health centers, will benefit from this type of overview that addresses issues of importance to the behavioral health and public health fields.

Finally, consumers, policymakers, advocates, and professionals involved in the fields of mental health and substance abuse services within local, state, and federal government will find this text of value when addressing changes to existing legislation and/or practice.

Throughout the development and preparation of this *Women's Behavioral Health: A Public Health Perspective* textbook, there have been a number of individuals who have provided sage advice, continued support, and significant encouragement. We would like to extend our deep appreciation to Ms. Janet Kim, Ms. Olivia Ramya Chitranjan, and Tessy Priya for their many helpful suggestions. We also thank the chapter authors for the many contributions to this book. We are ultimately grateful to our families for their continuing love and support during this very lengthy process of preparing this *Women's Behavioral Health: A Public Health Perspective* textbook.

Tampa, FL, USA   Ardis Hanson
Bruce Lubotsky Levin

Contents

About the Editors

Ardis Hanson, PhD, MLIS, AHIP, is the Assistant Director of Research and Education at the University of South Florida (USF) Health Libraries and holds affiliate faculty positions in the USF College of Public Health and in the Department of Child and Family Studies at the USF College of Behavioral & Community Sciences. She is a Co-Investigator for the National Institute on Drug Abuse grant *USF Institute for Translational Research in Adolescent Substance Use*. Dr. Hanson has over 30 years of experience as a research librarian and has published extensively in the areas of behavioral health services, health and behavioral health policy, and health services research. Her research focus also includes language and social interaction and how language is used in everyday practice to negotiate claims and identities, particularly in how behavioral health policy is created and developed.

Bruce Lubotsky Levin, DrPH, MPH, is an Associate Professor in the Department of Child and Family Studies at the University of South Florida (USF) College of Behavioral & Community Sciences. He is also an Associate Professor and Head of the *Behavioral Health Concentration (BHC)* at the USF College of Public Health. He is Co-Principal Investigator and Director of Curriculum at the *USF Institute for Translational Research in Adolescent Substance* Use. This grant has been refunded for a third consecutive 5-year period by the National Institutes of Health and National Institute on Drug Abuse. Dr. Levin also currently serves as Editor-in-Chief of the *Journal of Behavioral Health Services & Research (JBHS&R)*, a quarterly scholarly journal that publishes articles on the organization, financing, delivery, dissemination and implementation, and outcomes of behavioral health (including alcohol, drug use, and mental health) services. The *JBHS&R* is the official publication of the *National Council for Mental Wellbeing* and is published by Springer Nature. He is Senior Editor of numerous textbooks and textbook chapters, including *Foundations of Behavioral Health* (Springer, 2020); *Introduction to Public Health in Pharmacy, Second Edition* (Oxford University Press, 2018); and *Mental Health Services: A Public Health Perspective, Third Edition* (Oxford University Press, 2010). He is co-author (with Ardis Hanson) of *Mental Health Informatics* (Oxford University Press, 2013).

Contributors

Laren Alexander, MD, Department of Psychiatry, University of Florida College of Medicine – Jacksonville, Jacksonville, FL, USA

Juan Aparicio, MD, Department of Psychiatry and Behavioral Sciences, University of Washington, Seattle, WA, USA

Amritha Bhat, MD, MPH, Department of Psychiatry and Behavioral Sciences, University of Washington, Seattle, WA, USA

Michael Carpenter, MD, Department of Emergency Medicine, University of Florida, College of Medicine—Jacksonville, Jacksonville, FL, USA

Rachel Carpenter, MD, Department of Psychiatry, University of Florida College of Medicine—Jacksonville, Jacksonville, FL, USA

Koriann Cox, PhD, Department of Psychiatry and Behavioral Sciences, University of Washington, Seattle, WA, USA

Steven Cuffe, MD, Department of Psychiatry, University of Florida College of Medicine – Jacksonville, Jacksonville, FL, USA

Shelby Goicochea, MD, Department of Psychiatry, University of Florida College of Medicine – Jacksonville, Jacksonville, FL, USA

Ardis Hanson, PhD, MLIS, USF Health Libraries and the College of Public Health, University of South Florida, Tampa, FL, USA

Crystal Joerg University of South Florida, Tampa, FL, USA

Kimberly A. Johnson, PhD, Department of Mental Health Law and Policy, College of Behavioral and Community Sciences, University of South Florida, Tampa, FL, USA

Amanda Koire, MD, Department of Psychiatry, Brigham and Women's Hospital, Harvard Medical School, Boston, MA, USA

Anika Kumar Institute for Behavioral Health, The Heller School for Social Policy and Management, Brandeis University, Waltham, MA, USA

Kitty Leung, MD, Department of Psychiatry, University of Florida College of Medicine – Jacksonville, Jacksonville, FL, USA

Bruce Lubotsky Levin, DrPH, MPH, College of Behavioral & Community Sciences, College of Public Health, University of South Florida, Tampa, FL, USA

Vickie A. Lynn, PhD, MSW, MPH, University of South Florida, Tampa, FL, USA

Kimberly Menendez, MS, College of Behavioral and Community Sciences, University of South Florida, Tampa, FL, USA

Kayla Nembhard, MSPH, MA, University of South Florida, Tampa, FL, USA

Thuong Nong, MBA, MPP, Institute for Behavioral Health, The Heller School for Social Policy and Management, Brandeis University, Waltham, MA, USA

Carol A. Ott, PharmD, College of Pharmacy, Purdue University, West Lafayette, IN, USA

Elizabeth Richards, MD, Department of Psychiatry and Behavioral Sciences, University of Washington, Seattle, WA, USA

Amanda Sharp, PhD, MPH, Department of Psychiatry, Harvard Medical School, Boston, MA, USA

Maureen T. Stewart, PhD, Institute for Behavioral Health, The Heller School for Social Policy and Management, Brandeis University, Waltham, MA, USA

Phildra Swagger, PhD, MBA, Combined Expertise Inc., Tampa, FL, USA

Enya Vroom, PhD, MS, Department of Medicine, University of Texas Health Science Center at San Antonio, San Antonio, TX, USA

Carolanne C. Wartman, PharmD, College of Pharmacy, University of Arizona, Tucson, USA

Fern J. Webb, PhD, Department of Surgery, Center for Health Equity and Engagement Research (CHEER), University of Florida, Jacksonville, FL, USA

Selena Webster-Bass, DMin, MPH, Voices Institute LLC, Jacksonville, FL, USA

Part I
Framing Women's Behavioral Health

Chapter 1
Overview and Global Issues in Women's Behavioral Health

Ardis Hanson and Bruce Lubotsky Levin

Introduction

More than 20 years into the twenty-first century, behavioral health disorders remain significant and costly public health problems. Behavioral health disorders, defined as mental illnesses and substance use (alcohol/drug) disorders, are associated with a significant burden of morbidity and disability (Rehm & Shield, 2019) across the lifespan. Behavioral health disorders can be singular disorders or complex, comorbid disorders which can occur simultaneously or sequentially. The interaction between mental illnesses, substance use disorders, and/or somatic disorders affects not only the course of the disease(s) but also their diagnosis, treatment, and management (National Institute on Drug Abuse, 2021, April 13).

Persons with behavioral health disorders have a significant burden of disease, due to the increased morbidity and mortality rates often found within these populations. Common risk factors, such as environmental influences, the social determinants of health (SDOH), genetic vulnerability, brain abnormalities, and stress, trauma, and adverse childhood experiences, contribute to mental and substance use disorders. However, we would argue gender itself is a critical societal and social factor in behavioral health research, practice, and policy.

Gender interacts with the social, economic, and biological determinants that create different behavioral health outcomes for males and females. Gender plays a role

A. Hanson (✉)
USF Health Libraries and the College of Public Health, University of South Florida, Tampa, FL, USA
e-mail: hanson@usf.edu

B. L. Levin
College of Behavioral & Community Sciences, College of Public Health, University of South Florida, Tampa, FL, USA
e-mail: levin@usf.edu

in vulnerability to and the consequences of specific health conditions. Gender influences how policymakers conceive and implement health policies in response to specific populations. Gender affects health-seeking behavior and the ability to engage effectively with health care providers and to utilize health systems. Gender also affects society's response to stigmatizing disorders, such as mental illness, substance use, or HIV/AIDS. Simply stated, women are more marginalized by health and behavioral health service systems and by provider attitudes, and are more prone to misdiagnoses (or no diagnoses), which often result in poorer health outcomes.

This chapter examines women's behavioral health services from a public health and population health perspective. Using a global lens, we incorporate the social determinants of health (socio-structural factors), the Sustainable Development Goals, and national initiatives in the United States (e.g., Healthy People 2030) to create an overview of significant issues affecting behavioral health services and policy for women throughout their lifespan.

The Global Burden of Disease

The Global Burden of Disease (GBD) is a significant factor in the prevalence and incidence of behavioral health disorders (Murray & Lopez, 1996). GBD is based on three elements: DALYS, YLL, and YLD. DALYs (disability-adjusted life years) represent the sum of the years of life lost due to premature mortality (YLLs) and the years lived with a disability (YLDs) for a disease or health condition. YLL represents the number of years a disease will reduce average life expectancy while YLD represents the number of years with a lower quality of life. In 2019, the DALYs rank for mental illnesses rose to seventh in causes for global deaths (GBD 2019 Diseases and Injuries Collaborators, 2020). This indicates an increase in lifetime prevalence rates for behavioral health disorders (Degenhardt et al., 2019; Rehm & Shield, 2019).

Mental illnesses and substance use disorders affect more than 1 billion people globally, causing 7% of all GBD measured in DALYS and 19% of all YLDs (Rehm & Shield, 2019). Substance use disorders affect an estimated 150 million people, with alcohol use disorders the most prevalent, followed by cannabis dependence, and opioid dependence, with 99.2 million DALYs (4.2% of all DALYs) lost to alcohol use and 31.8 million DALYs (1.3% of all DALYs) lost to drug use (GBD 2016 Alcohol and Drug Use Collaborators, 2018). While the overall prevalence of mental or substance use disorders affects women and men to a similar degree, there are marked differences in age-adjusted rates for different diseases. Women have higher rates in all internalizing disorders, e.g., depressive, bipolar, anxiety, and eating disorders, while men have higher prevalence of externalizing disorders. The prevalence of schizophrenia was almost identical by gender (Rehm & Shield, 2019).

In addition, there is evidence the global COVID pandemic has not only increased the prevalence of major depressive and anxiety disorders (76.2 million and 53.2 million, respectively) but has exacerbated many determinants of poor mental health, with an overall increase in behavioral disorders (COVID-19 Mental Disorders

Collaborators, 2021). Further, with the increase of national conflicts globally, the United Nations Office for the Coordination of Humanitarian Affairs (2022) estimates 274 million people will require humanitarian assistance in 2022, an increase of 100 million from 2021 estimates.

In the United States, two of the most striking differences between men's and women's behavioral health are (1) the frequency and persistence of behavioral health disorders in women and (2) the higher rate of morbidity found in women with behavioral health disorders. From a lifespan or developmental perspective, these differences are shown clearly in the age of symptom onset, the frequency of symptoms, and the progression of disease, as well as in an individual's social adjustment, and their long-term outcomes. Women have higher prevalence and increased persistence of depression and anxiety disorders (Albert, 2015; Merikangas et al., 2007). For example, women are more than twice as likely to suffer from unipolar depression than men (Bromet et al., 2011; Kessler et al., 2003) and may be more likely to be misdiagnosed with bipolar depression (Rastelli et al., 2013). These differences are worsened with the diagnosis of complex comorbidity (3 or more comorbid disorders), which is diagnosed more often in women. Complex comorbidities, defined as any combination of mental, substance, or physical disorders, result in a greater burden of disease, longer duration of disability, and increased severity of disability.

Although the overall rates of behavioral health disorders are similar for women and men, there are significant gender differences in the patterns of mental illnesses and substance use disorders. Among comparable countries, the United States not only has the highest rate of death from mental and substance use disorders, but these disorders are the leading cause of disease burden for females and the third leading cause of disease burden for males (Tikkanen et al., 2020, May 21; Whiteford et al., 2013). It is clear from the data that behavioral health problems not only disproportionately affect women compared to men, but that factors affecting women's behavioral health change across their lifespan. Hence, issues women will face will be different depending upon where they are in their life course.

Sex/Gender Issues

It is difficult to examine any sex (biological) effect independent of gender (social-structural determinants), especially in diagnosis and treatment to ensure beneficial outcomes for girls and women across a life-course (developmental) view. Sex/gender differences not only affect presentation of symptoms, likelihood of disorders, risk factors, and disease progression and/or course but can be confounded or amplified over time. The biological model for depression, which addresses the activation of the amygdala and hypothalamic pituitary adrenal axis, and the neurosequential model, which examines childhood disruption of the stress response system and its dysregulation into adulthood, have been linked to social factors (Murphy et al., 2022). Early childhood traumas experienced by girls and women are suggested to play a key role in the long-term activity of these biological mechanisms (Kessler et al., 2010), and affect subsequent developmental responses across the lifespan.

Behavioral health disorders not only transform across developmental stages of an individual, but they also are affected over the life course with cumulative adverse life events, which may have additive, multiplicative, or curvilinear effects. Due to the changeable nature of behavioral health disorders, individuals often satisfy criteria for different diagnoses over time or present differentially within the same diagnosis across time. A "point-in-time" diagnosis does not mean that a diagnosis or the symptoms will be persistent or remain the same over time. Diagnosing behavioral health disorders is more difficult due to the complexity of the diagnostic tools needed for a formal diagnosis. The heterogeneity of symptoms that exist within a formal diagnosis across the *Diagnostic and Statistical Manual of Mental Disorders* (*DSM*) and/or the *International Classification of Diseases* (*ICD*), and the frequent co-occurrence of disorders may confound diagnoses or result in inaccurate diagnoses when applied to women.

A "transdiagnostic" approach, which focuses on underlying and fundamental processes embedded within multiple behavioral health conditions, seeks to cut across traditional diagnostic boundaries by reconceptualizing psychiatric taxa (e. g., *DSM*) with new classification schema (Dalgleish et al., 2020; Kotov et al., 2021). These processes are further complicated by comorbid disorders, which can result in latent trans-diagnostic domains, as in the case of mental illnesses and substance use disorders (Hasin & Grant, 2015). However, transdiagnostic risk factors, such as psychological stress (severity, coping styles), psychological inflexibility, and loneliness (perceived social isolation), may help to account for comorbidities and divergent trajectories of behavioral disorders across populations (Beutel et al., 2017; Carragher et al., 2015; Cohen et al., 2016; Dalgleish et al., 2020; Evans-Lacko et al., 2018; Levin et al., 2014; Ruisoto et al., 2022). Tied to current "predictive" work on heterogeneous treatment effects (Ruisoto et al., 2022) and the "process-oriented" focus of the Research Domain Criteria (RDoC) (Yücel et al., 2019), a transdiagnostic approach could better illustrate the biopsychosocial substrates of behavioral ill health, resulting in more accurate sex and gender-based diagnoses and treatment over a lifespan.

A look at how gender moderates associations between childhood adversity and types of substance use disorders (SUDs) is a good example (Evans et al., 2017). Gender differences are evident in SUD antecedents, correlates, and consequences (Greenfield et al., 2007). Women are much more likely than men to present with internalizing disorders and be diagnosed with co-occurring mood or anxiety disorders (Hasin & Grant, 2015). Women with depression are more at risk for alcohol use disorder (AUD) and a comorbid diagnosis of AUD and depression results in greater severity of symptoms and poorer prognosis than men (McHugh & Weiss, 2019). Further, impairment of stress-response coping mechanisms and the inability to emotionally regulate in childhood has been shown to increase women's risk of SUDs from a lifespan perspective (Myers et al., 2014), as well as an enhanced vulnerability to mental illnesses triggered by stressful life events as an adult (McLaughlin et al., 2010; Pfluger et al., 2022).

However, the long-term effects of biological or neurosequential mechanisms in concert with socio-structural determinants may or may not be factored into effective treatment programs for women with mental illnesses or substance use disorders. Effective treatment, which begins with finding care and using that care, is also affected by gender differences. There are gender patterns in help-seeking behaviors for behavioral health disorders (Lim et al., 2019). For example, women are more likely than men to seek help from primary care providers for mental health issues (Thompson et al., 2016). Studies have also shown that numerous factors, such as age, affordability of health care, socioeconomic status, illness prevention, trust in physicians, and chronic conditions, are predictors of women's mental health care-seeking behaviors (Evans-Lacko et al., 2018; Lim et al., 2019; Slaunwhite, 2015; Thompson et al., 2016).

Even though studies have found that women-focused treatment programs show better retention and improved outcomes, the data still shows inequities in serving women. Mental disorders and distress alone will have a dramatic effect on quality of life and productivity, accounting for the loss of an additional 16.1 trillion in US dollars by the year 2030 (Jan et al., 2018). For low- and middle-income countries, approximately 90% of people who need treatment do not receive it (Alonso et al., 2018; Docrat et al., 2019) This means implementing effective treatment for mental and substance use disorders will require significant capacity building and workforce expansion, including peer supports and trained lay health workers (Docrat et al., 2019; van Ginneken et al., 2021).

Data from the U. S. National Survey of Substance Abuse Treatment Services (SAMHSA, 2021b, July 14) shows 49% of substance abuse treatment facilities offered specially designed programs for adult women. In addition, 32% of facilities offered programs specifically for pregnant or post-partum women, and 24% offered programs for lesbian, gay, bisexual, transgender, or queer/questioning (LGBTQ) clients. The programs encompassed counseling, ancillary, and pre-treatment services; co-occurring disorders (55%); domestic violence- (30%) and trauma-related services (45%), pregnancy and postpartum services (26%), childcare (6%), and child live-in capacity (2%).

Sex/gender differences also need to be accounted for in data collection (please see Chap. 14 in this volume on behavioral health data). Almost a decade ago, the Institute of Medicine (IOM, 2013, 2014) recommended including a number of inter-sectional variables in electronic health records. In addition to gender, sex, and sexual orientation, the IOM (2013) recommended four domains, covering "sociodemographic" (e.g., food insecurity, financial resource strain), "behavioral" (e.g., childhood history, adverse childhood experiences, self-efficacy, social isolation, intimate partner violence), "individual-level social relationships and living conditions", and "neighborhoods and communities". Of particular interest is the relation of the IOM domains and subdomains to the SDOH, the behavioral determinants of health, and indicators across other national initiatives, such as *Healthy People*. Although the IOM domains/subdomains may not exactly mirror the domains as described in other initiatives, the indicators are similarly defined and could easily be crosswalked for comparison or data collection/analysis purposes. This would allow providers to assess risks associated with the patient's profile, which would then inform diagnosis, enabling more effective treatment plans that incorporate the patient's social context, behaviors, and psychosocial risks into the care plan.

However, issues of terminology and standardized data collection practices and guidelines need to be addressed to ensure sex/gender factors and socio-structural determinants affecting diagnosis, treatment, and research on women's behavioral health disorders are captured (Clark et al., 2019; Lau et al., 2020; Miller et al., 2015; Yılmaz et al., 2020). This becomes more critical as we look at the global effects of pandemics, wars, natural disasters, and humanitarian crises on behavioral health services and systems, as well as patient outcomes based on YLL and DALYS (Coelho et al., 2022; Diaz et al., 2021; Ramiz et al., 2021; St John & Walmsley, 2021).

In 2019, the global number of deaths attributable to noncommunicable diseases (NCDs), where behavioral health disorders are classed, increased from 61% in 2000 to almost 74% (World Health Organization, 2022d). The COVID-19 pandemic not only led to a rise in anxiety, depression, and substance use but also increased global demand for behavioral health services, which could no longer be delivered in person. However, as the need for mental health, substance use, and neurological services increased, the provision, access, and use of services decreased. Countries reported disruptions in one or more of their standard services (93%), life-saving and emergency services (35%), and supplies of medications (30%) (World Health Organization, 2022d). By the end of 2021, 44% of 71 countries still reported standard service disruptions and 30% reported life-saving and emergency services disruptions (World Health Organization, 2022c). Women, the elderly, and young children appeared to be more vulnerable to collective trauma, with increased depression symptoms and poorer self-rated physical health (Diaz et al., 2021; Ramiz et al., 2021).

Attention to associated inequalities in mortality and morbidity profiles between and within countries is essential to ensure women's behavioral health needs are met is essential (Coley & Baum, 2022; Côté et al., 2022; Papautsky et al., 2021). Standardized language, data elements, and reporting mechanisms are essential to track gaps in services tied to morbidity, mortality, and the behavioral and social determinants of health to better improve women's quality of life and behavioral health outcomes.

Women's Behavioral Health Systems

However, even with the ubiquitousness of behavioral health disorders globally, nationally, regionally, and locally, the underdiagnosis and misdiagnosis of these disorders continue. More than 20 years ago, a World Health Organization study found less than half of all individuals who met diagnostic criteria for behavioral health disorders were identified by primary care professionals (Sartorius et al., 1993). More recent studies still report similar underdiagnoses of mental and substance use disorders (Fekadu et al., 2022; Mitchell et al., 2009; Wang et al., 2007).

Further, behavioral health services delivery systems generally are not integrated, which makes it difficult to address complex and co-occurring disorders across the lifespan, and arduous to engage with and navigate from provider, patient, and caregiver perspectives (Levin & Hanson, 2020). Because there are so many siloed components involved (behavioral health and health facilities, social welfare, justice, safety net, and educational systems across both public and private sector services), communication within and across these sectors is equally difficult and often contributes to a lack of continuity of care. Treatment also varies based on diagnosis, access to and use of services, insurance coverage, and availability of services across the public/private sector divide.

The barriers to effective diagnosis and treatment result in substantial numbers of individuals with behavioral health disorders who have an unmet need for services (Hunt & Adams, 2021; Reinert et al., 2020) or are reluctant to seek services or continue treatment (Boerema et al., 2017; Fernández et al., 2020; Harris et al., 2020; Jones et al., 2018; Thornicroft et al., 2017; Yang et al., 2019). Globally, mental health service utilization ranged from 33% in high-income countries to 8% in low- and lower middle-income countries (Moitra et al., 2022). Minimally adequate treatment, according to evidence-based guidelines, ranged from 23% in high-income countries to 3% in low- and lower middle-income countries (Moitra et al., 2022). In the United States, approximately 30% (or 16.1 million people) reported an unmet need for services. The most common reasons for not receiving services were the cost of care, unfamiliarity with where to find treatment, concerns they would be involuntarily committed to a mental hospital or other mental health facility, the belief they can handle their illness without treatment, or the fear of taking medication (SAMHSA, 2021a).

System Models Different models identify different elements that play a role in the development and delivery of women's behavioral health services. Process-centered models, for example, identify mechanisms that link specific groups to health outcomes, while system-centered approaches identify how sex/gender are embedded in public policies and organizational/agency practices.

However, gendered life experiences have been shown to have material effects on the body (Bird & Rieker, 2008; Mays & Ghavami, 2018). The literature clearly illustrates the problematic task of distinguishing between sex (biological) and gender (social, cultural, and structural) in health and behavioral health practice, especially in the detection of differences. Researchers now propose using a composite term, "sex/gender", as a frame to examine the interactive effect of sex/gender on health outcomes (Kaiser et al., 2009; Springer et al., 2012). To address these effects, an intersectional approach, which examines how sex/gender interact at and across group, process, and structural levels, could be used to target interventions for modifiable factors, such as attitudes, beliefs, or structural constraints, or underlying social processes.

Behavioral Health System Costs Globally, in 2022, government behavioral health budgets are estimated to account for approximately 2% of total health budgets, with a median expenditure projection of $9.52 per capita in US dollars (Hasnain et al., 2022). Higher-income countries account for the largest proportion of spending; however, low-, lower-middle and upper-middle-income countries spending projections are estimated at $0.08 (US), $0.37 (US), and $3.29 (US), respectively (Hasnain et al., 2022). Increasing the global coverage of essential mental health services by 50% could be accomplished by 2030 with an increase of $0.20 (US) more per person each year (Hasnain et al., 2022) In 2019, the United States spent $225 billion on mental health, which was nearly 5.5% of all US health spending (OPEN MINDS, 2020, May 6). Most spending, $149.5 billion, was from public payers (62.7%) while $88.9 billion was from private payers (37.3%). From 2009 to 2019, spending for the US mental health market increased by 52.1% (Amri et al., 2021) (see Chap. 10 in this volume for more information on insurance and financing).

Health Equity and Behavioral Health

The lack of equitable access to behavioral health care leads to significant human and financial costs, affects access to and use of services, and contributes to poorer outcomes and decreased quality of life for individuals with mental and/or substance use disorders. Equitable access to care can be affected by many factors, some of which can be described as health disparities. Disparities are defined as health differences "closely linked with social, economic, and/or environmental disadvantage" (U.S. Department of Health and Human Services, 2008, October 28, p. 7). These differences may be attributed to "race or ethnicity, skin color, religion, or nationality; socioeconomic resources or position (e.g., income, education, or occupation); gender, sexual orientation, or gender identity; age, geography, mental health; cognitive, sensory, or physical disability or illness; political or other affiliation; or other characteristics associated with discrimination or marginalization" (Braveman et al. 2011, p. S149).

Health equity requires removing obstacles to health care and treatment so that everyone has "a fair and just opportunity to be as healthy as possible" (Braveman et al., 2017, p. 2). To do so requires society, governments, and individuals to address structural drivers (inequities in power, money, and resources), and conditions of daily living (social determinants of health) that constrain persons from having equity in care (Commission of the Pan American Health Organization on Equity and Health Inequalities in the Americas, 2019). It also requires a global commitment by both public and private behavioral health and health sectors to reduce health inequities, monitor progress, and increase health systems and government accountability (Barros et al., 2018). Metrics to assess health and behavioral health equity include traditional measures of health outcomes and health states; measures relating to structural and systemic factors; measures that examine infrastructure (housing, transportation, etc.); and measures of underlying structural social inequities (National Academies of Sciences et al., 2020). These measures may disaggregate data by race, ethnicity, or other populations of interest, be derived from needs assessments, or use formal instruments to assess inequities (Saha et al., 2020; Shah et al., 2014).

Global Responses

The push toward health and behavioral health equity is sustained by the foundational notion that health is a basic human right. In 1946, the Constitution of the World Health Organization (1946) declared that every human being had a fundamental right to the highest attainable standard of health. This right was reaffirmed by the United Nations (UN) General Assembly (1966, December 16) in the 1966 International Covenant on Economic, Social and Cultural Rights. A rights-based approach to health is again echoed in the 2030 Agenda for Sustainable Development and Universal Health Coverage (United Nations, 2015, October 21).

Since 2015, there has been international recognition that mental health is one of the essential bundles of human rights (Pūras, 2015, April 2). In 2016, the 73 States of the UN issued a joint statement that adopted a human rights perspective on mental health as part of the right to health. The UN Human Rights Council Resolution (A/HRC/RES/32/18) recognized the need to fully integrate a human rights perspective into mental health (Human Rights Council, 2016, July 1). Building upon the Special Rapporteur's 2015 reports (A/HRC/29/33), which recommended the mainstreaming of mental health in the SDGs to reduce the marginalization of mental health within health (Pūras, 2015, April 2), the 2019 Special Rapporteur's report (A/HRC/41/34) emphasized the critical role of the social determinants of mental health (Pūras, 2019, April 12).

Human rights not only provide all persons' fundamental rights and freedoms, but they also place duties on a government to respect them (Gostin & Gable, 2004). The 2020 Rapporteur's report (A/HRC/44/48) again reiterates the need for a human rights-based global agenda for mental health (Pūras, 2020a, April 20). Resolution A/HRC/RES/43/13 (July 2020) requested "harmonization of national mental health laws, policies, and practices with the norms of the Convention on the Rights of Persons with Disabilities" (Human Rights Council, 2020, June 19). The Special Rapporteur's final report (A/75/163) reiterated that the right to health is not just a social and economic right, but also encompasses civil and political rights (Pūras, 2020b, July 16). Hence, behavioral health equity, in concert with international human rights laws, ensures equitable access to high-quality behavioral health care and reduces disparities in health outcomes for all populations, regardless of identity, affiliation, ability, geography, or socioeconomic status.

US Responses

In the United States it wasn't until the early 1990s that women and minority groups were mandated to be included in all National Institutes of Health (NIH)-funded clinical research. The NIH Revitalization Act of 1993 (NIH, 1993) not only required women to be included in NIH-funded clinical research, but required researchers to determine if women were affected differently than other trial participants by variables in a clinical study (NIH, 1993). Subsequent legislation started the restructuring of service systems to prioritize equity, quality, and effectiveness. This is shown by language in the Patient Protection and Affordable Care Act (PPACA, 2010) and the Health Care and Education Reconciliation Act of 2010 (both Acts comprise the Affordable Care Act [ACA]). The twenty-first Century Cures Act (2016, P. L. 114–255) and the Evidence-based Policymaking Act of 2018 (P. L. 115–435) also mandated valid analyses by sex/gender in the design of clinical trials.

During the preparation of this chapter, President Biden signed two Executive Orders that strengthened basic civil rights provisions for women. The first Executive Order addressed discrimination on the basis of gender identity or sexual orientation (Biden, 2021). The second, "Protecting Access to Reproductive Healthcare Services", was a response to the recent overturning of *Roe v. Wade* by the Supreme Court (Biden, 2022). Both Orders directly affect access to, utilization of, and provision of behavioral health services for women. Both Orders also illustrate judicial, societal, and systemic challenges to ensure equitable care for women. The continued legislative emphasis on the inclusion of women as subjects in behavioral and clinical health research, as well as the effectiveness of treatments tailored to women, should eventually improve services delivery and treatment systems addressing women's behavioral health.

Frames for Practice and Policy in Women's Behavioral Health

The social contexts of women's health and behavioral health are bounded by the conditions in which they work and live. Multiple factors, such as poverty, social exclusion, unemployment, poor working conditions, and unequal gender relations, have a profound influence on patterns of health and illness. Diverse structures of inequality, shaped by gender, race, ethnicity, sexual orientation and identity, age, and stage in the life cycle, compound the disadvantages, discrimination, and stigmas that women continue to face. Stigma and discrimination also affect the ability of women with behavioral health disorders to seek and obtain treatment as well as to be integrated fully in their lives, in their work, and in their communities.

To address the implications of the social and structural determinants that affect behavioral health, we offer the framework of availability, accessibility, affordability, and acceptability (Table 1.1), first developed by Bushy (1997), still relevant today (Wilson et al., 2015, February), and mirrored by the WHO (World Health

Table 1.1 Availability, accessibility, affordability, and acceptability framework

Availability	Staffing or service shortages
Accessibility	Coordination of services
Affordability	Costs of care
Acceptability	Discrimination, perception, and stigma

Bushy (1997) and Wilson et al. (2015, February)

Organization, 2017, December 29). Each of these elements affects receipt of services, direct and indirect costs, insurance coverage of services, and the implicit or explicit discrimination, perception, and stigma attached to the receipt of or need for behavioral health services.

These four elements address the intersectionality of societal, economic, cultural, and infrastructural elements. These elements are addressed in socio-structural analyses that examine the influences gender plays in disparities and inequities experienced by women with behavioral health disorders. This framework also overlays well with larger global and national frames. It is exemplified in regional and national strategies to improve population health, including the Social Determinants of Health, the United Nations' Sustainable Development Goals, Health in All Policies, and the U.S. Healthy People 2030.

The social determinants of health (SDOH) are defined as "the non-medical factors that influence health outcomes. They are the conditions in which people are born, grow, work, live, and age, and the wider set of forces and systems shaping the conditions of daily life" (World Health Organization, 2022b). These factors not only result in inequities to and discrimination toward marginalized populations but affect and drive environmental, socioeconomic, political, sociocultural, and infrastructure policies and systems. The SDOH framework has been incorporated into an evidence-base of best practices, global assessment measures, and a global consensus (Alegría et al., 2018; Commission on Social Determinants of Health, 2008; Ewart et al., 2017; Langlois et al., 2020; Pera et al., 2021; Weil, 2020). More importantly, the SDOH framework has also been key in addressing women's health and behavioral health issues in the context of their lifespan and life experiences.

The United Nations' Sustainable Development Goals (SDGs) are considered a transformative development agenda, linking development, sustainability, and climate change agenda, with social justice, health, and behavioral health foci (Morton et al., 2017; Onabola et al., 2022). Linking the SDG domains to the SDOH can illuminate how societal factors simultaneously affect risk of, and protection from, mental illnesses and substance use disorders, especially for women (Lund et al., 2018). This data could effectively address trajectories into mental health systems, inform interventions from a contextual perspective (e.g., environmental or social factors), and create better outcomes for women across the lifespan, especially from a public health services delivery perspective.

The incorporation of the SDGs and SDOHs into global and national health policies and practices is an ongoing process, at the global, regional, national, and municipal levels. Globally, the World Health Organization (2019) *Special Initiative for Mental Health (2019–2023): Universal Health Coverage for Mental Health*

(UHC-MH) intends to implement quality and affordable behavioral health care services in 12 priority countries, covering 100 million people. The UHC-MH initiative incorporates two SDG indicators and two WHO 13th General Programme of Work (GPW) targets. The SDG and GPW12 indicators focus on reducing suicide mortality and increasing treatment coverage for severe mental health conditions, including substance use disorders, and other factors unique to the needs of women with behavioral health disorders. Building upon its 2001 *Mental Health—New Understanding, New Hope* report, WHO launched the *World Mental Health Report: Transforming Mental Health for All* (WHO, 2022a). *Transforming Mental Health for All* attempts to provide global values and normative standards to public and private sector decision-makers in behavioral health policy and services delivery, with the hope these recommendations are contextually relevant for each of its Member States.

At a national level, Health in All Policies (HiAP) takes an intersectoral responsibility approach which promotes health and equity goals into any public policy. HiAP focuses on the health implications in any public decision-making process to improve population health and health equity. It accomplishes this by addressing the SDOH as key drivers of health outcomes and health inequities in the governance process. Integrating municipal (county or city) planning and management systems into public health policies requires formal and sustained governance structures and mechanisms across health and non-health sectors. Such an intersectoral governance approach can maximize positive effects and minimize negative effects on population health. The use of HiAP is increasing in the literature, with narrative evidence supporting implementation of HiAP at municipal and national levels (Damari et al., 2020; Guglielmin et al., 2018; Khayatzadeh-Mahani et al., 2019; Shankardass et al., 2018; Van Vliet-Brown et al., 2018).

Since its introduction in 1979, the *Healthy People* initiative in the United States has established national goals and objectives for health promotion and disease prevention. Setting 10-year targets and objectives associated with specific metrics and measures, the *Healthy People 2030* has four overarching objectives: 1) Closing Gaps, 2) Cultivating Healthier Environments, 3) Increasing Knowledge and Action, and 4) Health and Well-Being Across the Lifespan (National Academies of Sciences et al., 2020). With the reorganization of the Healthy People framework in 2020 to include the phrase "well-being", indicators and measures now focus on the SDOHs, health equity, health literacy, and other indicators of subjective well-being (National Academies of Sciences et al., 2020).

These frames are important. Each of them, singly but more importantly in concert with each other, brings us closer to understanding the sex/gender differences, biological and neurosequential mechanisms, and societal and behavioral determinants of health, and their effects on women's behavioral health. Actionable data, evidence-based interventions, and strategic use of resources help us to create healthier environments, close the gaps to ensure equity to care and decrease disparities, and ensure multisectoral governance and action through evidence-informed laws, policies, and practices.

Implications for Women's Behavioral Health

As presented in this overview of global issues in women's behavioral health, mental and substance use disorders remain a significant public health problem for women in the United States, as well as across the world. This is true whether we are looking at mental and substance use disorders from individual, system, or societal perspectives. Women-focused treatment, practice, and research continues to be an emphasis in the research literature and within public and private sector service systems to address the health disadvantages women face daily.

A number of factors affect women's behavioral health, including institutional, socioeconomic, and behavioral health factors. Institutional factors affect women's access to health care, services delivery, and quality of care. Socioeconomic and behavioral health factors also influence differences in morbidity and mortality for women. Geographical influences, socioeconomic status, stigma, education, and employment affect the timely diagnosis of behavioral health disorders. These factors compound challenges in the delivery, treatment, and utilization of behavioral health services across women overall, as well as addressing issues common to distinct groups of women. This is particularly true when examining the relationships between the effects of socioeconomic status and the assessment of health policy, and assessments of delivery systems. It is also true when understanding the variation of services delivery within health plans in different geographic areas. The continued fragmentation of health and behavioral health systems has significant consequences for women, especially over a woman's lifespan.

Finally, interdisciplinary research and training is essential to better understand the effects of public health policies on women's behavioral health. Public health policies inevitably have intended and unintended consequences; the unintended consequences disproportionately affect women. This chapter has focused on the challenges women face in accessing behavioral health services and care in the United States and globally. The challenges also affect practitioners, policymakers, researchers, and health care systems. Acknowledging these challenges would help in the development and evaluation of effective interventions based on the differences men and women present in the manifestation of disorders and their responses to treatment.

References

Albert, P. R. (2015). Why is depression more prevalent in women? *Journal of Psychiatry and Neuroscience, 40*(4), 219–221. https://doi.org/10.1503/jpn.150205

Alegría, M., NeMoyer, A., Falgàs Bagué, I., Wang, Y., & Alvarez, K. (2018). Social determinants of mental health: Where we are and where we need to go. *Current Psychiatry Reports, 20*(11), 95. https://doi.org/10.1007/s11920-018-0969-9

Alonso, J., Liu, Z., Evans-Lacko, S., Sadikova, E., Sampson, N., Chatterji, S., Abdulmalik, J., Aguilar-Gaxiola, S., Al-Hamzawi, A., Andrade, L. H., Bruffaerts, R., Cardoso, G., Cia, A., Florescu, S., de Girolamo, G., Gureje, O., Haro, J. M., He, Y., de Jonge, P., Karam, E. G.,

Kawakami, N., Kovess-Masfety, V., Lee, S., Levinson, D., Medina-Mora, M. E., Navarro-Mateu, F., Pennell, B. E., Piazza, M., Posada-Villa, J., Ten Have, M., Zarkov, Z., Kessler, R. C., & Thornicroft, G. (2018). Treatment gap for anxiety disorders is global: Results of the World Mental Health Surveys in 21 countries. *Depression and Anxiety, 35*(3), 195–208. https://doi.org/10.1002/da.22711

Amri, M. M., Jessiman-Perreault, G., Siddiqi, A., O'Campo, P., Enright, T., & Di Ruggiero, E. (2021). Scoping review of the World Health Organization's underlying equity discourses: Apparent ambiguities, inadequacy, and contradictions. *International Journal for Equity in Health, 20*(1), 70. https://doi.org/10.1186/s12939-021-01400-x

Barros, A., Boutayeb, A., Brown, C., Dean, H. D., Di Ruggiero, E., Ferrelli, R. M., Frenz, P., Glover, J., Herel, M., Humuza, J., Kirigia, D., O'Campo, P., Pega, F., Reddy, S., Stankiewicz, A., Torgesen, T., Valentine, N. B., Villar, E., & Working Group for Monitoring Action on the Social Determinants of Health. (2018). Towards a global monitoring system for implementing the Rio Political Declaration on Social Determinants of Health: Developing a core set of indicators for government action on the social determinants of health to improve health equity. *International Journal for Equity in Health, 17*(1), 136. https://doi.org/10.1186/s12939-018-0836-7

Beutel, M. E., Klein, E. M., Brahler, E., Reiner, I., Junger, C., Michal, M., Wiltink, J., Wild, P. S., Munzel, T., Lackner, K. J., & Tibubos, A. N. (2017). Loneliness in the general population: Prevalence, determinants and relations to mental health. *BMC Psychiatry, 17*(7), 97. https://doi.org/10.1186/s12888-017-1262-x

Biden, J. R., Jr. (2021). Preventing and combating discrimination on the basis of gender identity or sexual orientation [Executive Order 13988 of January 20, 2021]. *Federal Register, 86*(14), 7023–7025. https://www.govinfo.gov/content/pkg/FR-2021-01-25/pdf/2021-01761.pdf

Biden, J. R., Jr. (2022). Protecting access to reproductive healthcare services [Executive Order 14076 of July 8, 2022]. *Federal Register*, 42053–42055. https://www.govinfo.gov/content/pkg/FR-2022-07-13/pdf/2022-15138.pdf

Bird, C. E., & Rieker, P. P. (2008). *Gender and health: The effects of constrained choices and social policies*. Cambridge University Press.

Boerema, A. M., Ten Have, M., Kleiboer, A., de Graaf, R., Nuyen, J., Cuijpers, P., & Beekman, A. T. F. (2017). Demographic and need factors of early, delayed and no mental health care use in major depression: A prospective study. *BMC Psychiatry, 17*(1), 367. https://doi.org/10.1186/s12888-017-1531-8

Braveman, P. A., Kumanyika, S., Fielding, J., Laveist, T., Borrell, L. N., Manderscheid, R., & Troutman, A. (2011). Health disparities and health equity: The issue is justice. *American Journal of Public Health, 101*, S149–S155. https://doi.org/10.2105/ajph.2010.300062

Braveman, P., Arkin, E., Orleans, T., Proctor, D., & Plough, A. (2017). *What is health equity? And what difference does a definition make?* https://www.rwjf.org/en/library/research/2017/05/what-is-health-equity-.html

Bromet, E., Andrade, L. H., Hwang, I., Sampson, N. A., Alonso, J., de Girolamo, G., de Graaf, R., Demyttenaere, K., Hu, C., Iwata, N., Karam, A. N., Kaur, J., Kostyuchenko, S., Lépine, J. P., Levinson, D., Matschinger, H., Mora, M. E., Browne, M. O., Posada-Villa, J., Viana, M. C., Williams, D. R., & Kessler, R. C. (2011). Cross-national epidemiology of DSM-IV major depressive episode. *BMC Medicine, 9*, 90. https://doi.org/10.1186/1741-7015-9-90

Bushy, A. (1997). Mental health and substance abuse: Challenges in providing services to rural clients. In Center for Substance Abuse Treatment (Ed.), *Bringing excellence to substance abuse services in rural and frontier America* (HHS Publication No. [SMA] 97-3134; TAP Series 20, pp. 45–54). U.S. Department of Health and Human Services, Rural Information Center Health Service. http://adaiclearinghouse.net/downloads/TAP-20-Bringing-Excellence-to-Substance-Abuse-Services-in-Rural-and-Frontier-America-110.pdf

Carragher, N., Krueger, R. F., Eaton, N. R., & Slade, T. (2015). Disorders without borders: Current and future directions in the meta-structure of mental disorders. *Social Psychiatry and Psychiatric Epidemiology, 50*(3), 339–350. https://doi.org/10.1007/s00127-014-1004-z

Clark, C. J., Wetzel, M., Renner, L. M., & Logeais, M. E. (2019). Linking partner violence survivors to supportive services: Impact of the M Health Community Network project on healthcare utilization. *BMC Health Services Research, 19*(1), 479. https://doi.org/10.1186/s12913-019-4313-9

Coelho, A., de Bienassis, K., Klazinga, N., Santo, S., Frade, P., Costa, A., & Gaspar, T. (2022). Mental health patient-reported outcomes and experiences assessment in Portugal. *International Journal of Environmental Research and Public Health, 19*(18). https://doi.org/10.3390/ijerph191811153

Cohen, S., Gianaros, P. J., & Manuck, S. B. (2016). A stage model of stress and disease. *Perspectives on Psychological Science, 11*(4), 456–463. https://doi.org/10.1177/1745691616646305

Coley, R. L., & Baum, C. F. (2022). Trends in mental health symptoms, service use, and unmet need for services among US adults through the first 8 months of the COVID-19 pandemic. *Translational Behavioral Medicine, 12*(2), 273–283. https://doi.org/10.1093/tbm/ibab133

Commission of the Pan American Health Organization on Equity and Health Inequalities in the Americas. (2019). *Just societies: Health equity and dignified lives: Report of the Commission of the Pan American Health Organization on Equity and Health Inequalities in the Americas.* https://iris.paho.org/handle/10665.2/51571

Commission on Social Determinants of Health. (2008). *Closing the gap in a generation: Health equity through action on the social determinants of health.* Final Report of the Commission on Social Determinants of Health. https://apps.who.int/iris/bitstream/handle/10665/43943/9789241563703_eng.pdf;jsessionid=C6A1E2BF60B19CB4949796A7511E2F41?sequence=1

Côté, S. M., Geoffroy, M. C., Haeck, C., Ouellet-Morin, I., Larose, S., Chadi, N., Zinszer, K., Gauvin, L., & Mâsse, B. (2022). Understanding and attenuating pandemic-related disruptions: A plan to reduce inequalities in child development. *Canadian Journal of Public Health, 113*(1), 23–35. https://doi.org/10.17269/s41997-021-00584-7

COVID-19 Mental Disorders Collaborators. (2021). Global prevalence and burden of depressive and anxiety disorders in 204 countries and territories in 2020 due to the COVID-19 pandemic. *Lancet, 398*(10312), 1700–1712. https://doi.org/10.1016/s0140-6736(21)02143-7

Dalgleish, T., Black, M., Johnston, D., & Bevan, A. (2020). Transdiagnostic approaches to mental health problems: Current status and future directions. *Journal of Consulting and Clinical Psychology, 88*(3), 179–195. https://doi.org/10.1037/ccp0000482

Damari, B., Heidari, A., Rahbari Bonab, M., & Vosoogh Moghadam, A. (2020). Designing a toolkit for the assessment of Health in All Policies at a national scale in Iran. *Health Promotion Perspective, 10*(3), 244–249. https://doi.org/10.34172/hpp.2020.38

Degenhardt, L., Bharat, C., Glantz, M. D., Sampson, N. A., Scott, K., Lim, C. C. W., Aguilar-Gaxiola, S., Al-Hamzawi, A., Alonso, J., Andrade, L. H., Bromet, E. J., Bruffaerts, R., Bunting, B., de Girolamo, G., Gureje, O., Haro, J. M., Harris, M. G., He, Y., de Jonge, P., Karam, E. G., Karam, G. E., Kiejna, A., Lee, S., Lepine, J. P., Levinson, D., Makanjuola, V., Medina-Mora, M. E., Mneimneh, Z., Navarro-Mateu, F., Posada-Villa, J., Stein, D. J., Tachimori, H., Torres, Y., Zarkov, Z., Chatterji, S., & Kessler, R. C. (2019). The epidemiology of drug use disorders cross-nationally: Findings from the WHO's World Mental Health Surveys. *The International Journal on Drug Policy, 71*, 103–112. https://doi.org/10.1016/j.drugpo.2019.03.002

Diaz, A., Baweja, R., Bonatakis, J. K., & Baweja, R. (2021). Global health disparities in vulnerable populations of psychiatric patients during the COVID-19 pandemic. *World Journal of Psychiatry, 11*(4), 94–108. https://doi.org/10.5498/wjp.v11.i4.94

Docrat, S., Besada, D., Cleary, S., Daviaud, E., & Lund, C. (2019). Mental health system costs, resources and constraints in South Africa: A national survey. *Health Policy and Planning, 34*(9), 706–719. https://doi.org/10.1093/heapol/czz085

Evans, E. A., Grella, C. E., & Upchurch, D. M. (2017). Gender differences in the effects of childhood adversity on alcohol, drug, and polysubstance-related disorders. *Social Psychiatry and Psychiatric Epidemiology, 52*(7), 901–912. https://doi.org/10.1007/s00127-017-1355-3

Evans-Lacko, S., Aguilar-Gaxiola, S., Al-Hamzawi, A., Alonso, J., Benjet, C., Bruffaerts, R., Chiu, W. T., Florescu, S., de Girolamo, G., Gureje, O., Haro, J. M., He, Y., Hu, C., Karam, E. G., Kawakami, N., Lee, S., Lund, C., Kovess-Masfety, V., Levinson, D., Navarro-Mateu, F., Pennell, B. E., Sampson, N. A., Scott, K. M., Tachimori, H., Ten Have, M., Viana, M. C., Williams, D. R., Wojtyniak, B. J., Zarkov, Z., Kessler, R. C., Chatterji, S., & Thornicroft, G. (2018). Socio-economic variations in the mental health treatment gap for people with anxiety, mood, and substance use disorders: Results from the WHO World Mental Health (WMH) surveys. *Psychological Medicine, 48*(9), 1560–1571. https://doi.org/10.1017/s0033291717003336

Ewart, S. B., Happell, B., Bocking, J., Platania-Phung, C., Stanton, R., & Scholz, B. (2017). Social and material aspects of life and their impact on the physical health of people diagnosed with mental illness. *Health Expectations, 20*(5), 984–991. https://doi.org/10.1111/hex.12539

Fekadu, A., Demissie, M., Birhane, R., Medhin, G., Bitew, T., Hailemariam, M., Minaye, A., Habtamu, K., Milkias, B., Petersen, I., Patel, V., Cleare, A. J., Mayston, R., Thornicroft, G., Alem, A., Hanlon, C., & Prince, M. (2022). Under detection of depression in primary care settings in low and middle-income countries: A systematic review and meta-analysis. *Systematic Reviews, 11*(1), 21. https://doi.org/10.1186/s13643-022-01893-9

Fernández, D., Vigo, D., Sampson, N. A., Hwang, I., Aguilar-Gaxiola, S., Al-Hamzawi, A. O., Alonso, J., Andrade, L. H., Bromet, E. J., de Girolamo, G., de Jonge, P., Florescu, S., Gureje, O., Hinkov, H., Hu, C., Karam, E. G., Karam, G., Kawakami, N., Kiejna, A., Kovess-Masfety, V., Medina-Mora, M. E., Navarro-Mateu, F., Ojagbemi, A., O'Neill, S., Piazza, M., Posada-Villa, J., Rapsey, C., Williams, D. R., Xavier, M., Ziv, Y., Kessler, R. C., & Haro, J. M. (2020). Patterns of care and dropout rates from outpatient mental healthcare in low-, middle- and high-income countries from the World Health Organization's World Mental Health Survey Initiative. *Psychological Medicine,* 1–13. https://doi.org/10.1017/s0033291720000884

GBD 2016 Alcohol and Drug Use Collaborators. (2018). The global burden of disease attributable to alcohol and drug use in 195 countries and territories, 1990-2016: A systematic analysis for the Global Burden of Disease Study 2016. *Lancet Psychiatry, 5*(12), 987–1012. https://doi.org/10.1016/s2215-0366(18)30337-7

GBD 2019 Diseases and Injuries Collaborators. (2020). Global burden of 369 diseases and injuries in 204 countries and territories, 1990-2019: A systematic analysis for the Global Burden of Disease Study 2019. *Lancet, 396*(10258), 1204–1222. https://doi.org/10.1016/s0140-6736(20)30925-9

Gostin, L. O., & Gable, L. (2004). The human rights of persons with mental disabilities: A global perspective on the application of human rights principles to mental health. *Maryland Law Review, 63*(1), 20–121.

Greenfield, S. F., Brooks, A. J., Gordon, S. M., Green, C. A., Kropp, F., McHugh, R. K., Lincoln, M., Hien, D., & Miele, G. M. (2007). Substance abuse treatment entry, retention, and outcome in women: A review of the literature. *Drug and Alcohol Dependence, 86*(1), 1–21. https://doi.org/10.1016/j.drugalcdep.2006.05.012

Guglielmin, M., Muntaner, C., O'Campo, P., & Shankardass, K. (2018). A scoping review of the implementation of health in all policies at the local level. *Health Policy, 122*(3), 284–292. https://doi.org/10.1016/j.healthpol.2017.12.005

Harris, M. G., Kazdin, A. E., Chiu, W. T., Sampson, N. A., Aguilar-Gaxiola, S., Al-Hamzawi, A., Alonso, J., Altwaijri, Y., Andrade, L. H., Cardoso, G., Cía, A., Florescu, S., Gureje, O., Hu, C., Karam, E. G., Karam, G., Mneimneh, Z., Navarro-Mateu, F., Oladeji, B. D., O'Neill, S., Scott, K., Slade, T., Torres, Y., Vigo, D., Wojtyniak, B., Zarkov, Z., Ziv, Y., & Kessler, R. C. (2020). Findings from world mental health surveys of the perceived helpfulness of treatment for patients with major depressive disorder. *JAMA Psychiatry, 77*(8), 830–841. https://doi.org/10.1001/jamapsychiatry.2020.1107

Hasin, D. S., & Grant, B. F. (2015). The National Epidemiologic Survey on Alcohol and Related Conditions (NESARC) Waves 1 and 2: Review and summary of findings. *Social Psychiatry and Psychiatric Epidemiology, 50*(11), 1609–1640. https://doi.org/10.1007/s00127-015-1088-0

Hasnain, A., Sale, J., & Kline, S. (2022). *Financing mental health for all* [Report]. United for Global Mental Health. https://unitedgmh.org/sites/default/files/2022-03/UNITEDGMH%20 UHC%20Policy%20Brief%202022%20-%2028%20March%202022_0.pdf?utm_ campaign=0322UHC&utm_medium=website&utm_source=article&utm_content=0322UHC

Human Rights Council. (2016, July 1). *Resolution adopted by the Human Rights Council on 1 July 2016: 32/18. Mental health and human rights* [Resolution; A/HRC/RES/32/18]. United Nations. https://documents-dds-ny.un.org/doc/UNDOC/GEN/G16/156/38/PDF/G1615638. pdf?OpenElement

Human Rights Council. (2020, June 19). *Resolution adopted by the Human Rights Council on 19 June 2020* [Resolution; A/HRC/RES/43/13]. United Nations General Assembly.

Hunt, A. D., & Adams, L. M. (2021). Perception of unmet need after seeking treatment for a past year major depressive episode: Results from the 2018 National Survey of Drug Use and Health. *Psychiatric Quarterly, 92*(3), 1271–1281. https://doi.org/10.1007/s11126-021-09913-y

Institute of Medicine. (2013). *Toward quality measures for population health and the leading health indicators*. The National Academies Press. https://doi.org/10.17226/18339

Institute of Medicine. (2014). *Capturing social and behavioral domains in electronic health records: Phase 1*. The National Academies Press. https://doi.org/10.17226/18709

Jan, S., Laba, T. L., Essue, B. M., Gheorghe, A., Muhunthan, J., Engelgau, M., Mahal, A., Griffiths, U., McIntyre, D., Meng, Q., Nugent, R., & Atun, R. (2018). Action to address the household economic burden of non-communicable diseases. *Lancet, 391*(10134), 2047–2058. https://doi. org/10.1016/s0140-6736(18)30323-4

Jones, J. M., Ali, M. M., Mutter, R., Mosher Henke, R., Gokhale, M., Marder, W., & Mark, T. (2018). Factors that affect choice of mental health provider and receipt of outpatient mental health treatment. *Journal of Behavioral Health Services and Research, 45*(4), 614–626. https:// doi.org/10.1007/s11414-017-9575-6

Kaiser, A., Haller, S., Schmitz, S., & Nitsch, C. (2009). On sex/gender related similarities and differences in fMRI language research. *Brain Research Reviews, 61*(2), 49–59. https://doi. org/10.1016/j.brainresrev.2009.03.005

Kessler, R. C., Berglund, P., Demler, O., Jin, R., Koretz, D., Merikangas, K. R., Rush, A. J., Walters, E. E., & Wang, P. S. (2003). The epidemiology of major depressive disorder: Results from the National Comorbidity Survey Replication (NCS-R). *JAMA, 289*(23), 3095–3105. https://doi. org/10.1001/jama.289.23.3095

Kessler, R. C., McLaughlin, K. A., Green, J. G., Gruber, M. J., Sampson, N. A., Zaslavsky, A. M., Aguilar-Gaxiola, S., Alhamzawi, A. O., Alonso, J., Angermeyer, M., Benjet, C., Bromet, E., Chatterji, S., de Girolamo, G., Demyttenaere, K., Fayyad, J., Florescu, S., Gal, G., Gureje, O., Haro, J. M., Hu, C. Y., Karam, E. G., Kawakami, N., Lee, S., Lépine, J. P., Ormel, J., Posada-Villa, J., Sagar, R., Tsang, A., Üstün, T. B., Vassilev, S., Viana, M. C., & Williams, D. R. (2010). Childhood adversities and adult psychopathology in the WHO World Mental Health Surveys. *British Journal of Psychiatry, 197*(5), 378–385. https://doi.org/10.1192/bjp.bp.110.080499

Khayatzadeh-Mahani, A., Ruckert, A., Labonté, R., Kenis, P., & Akbari-Javar, M. R. (2019). Health in All Policies (HiAP) governance: Lessons from network governance. *Health Promotion International, 34*(4), 779–791. https://doi.org/10.1093/heapro/day032

Kotov, R., Krueger, R. F., Watson, D., Cicero, D. C., Conway, C. C., DeYoung, C. G., Eaton, N. R., Forbes, M. K., Hallquist, M. N., Latzman, R. D., Mullins-Sweatt, S. N., Ruggero, C. J., Simms, L. J., Waldman, I. D., Waszczuk, M. A., & Wright, A. G. C. (2021). The Hierarchical Taxonomy of Psychopathology (HiTOP): A quantitative nosology based on consensus of evidence. *Annual Review of Clinical Psychology, 17*, 83–108. https://doi.org/10.1146/ annurev-clinpsy-081219-093304

Langlois, S., Zern, A., Anderson, S., Ashekun, O., Ellis, S., Graves, J., & Compton, M. T. (2020). Subjective social status, objective social status, and substance use among individuals with serious mental illnesses. *Psychiatry Research, 293*, 113352. https://doi.org/10.1016/j. psychres.2020.113352

Lau, F., Antonio, M., Davison, K., Queen, R., & Devor, A. (2020). A rapid review of gender, sex, and sexual orientation documentation in electronic health records. *Journal of the American Medical Informatics Association, 27*(11), 1774–1783. https://doi.org/10.1093/jamia/ocaa158

Levin, B. L., & Hanson, A. (2020). Population-based behavioral health. In B. L. Levin & A. Hanson (Eds.), *Foundations of behavioral health* (pp. 1–13). Springer.

Levin, M. E., MacLane, C., Daflos, S., Seeley, J., Hayes, S. C., Biglan, A., & Pistorello, J. (2014). Examining psychological inflexibility as a transdiagnostic process across psychological disorders. *Journal of Contextual Behavioral Science, 3*(3), 155–163. https://doi.org/10.1016/j.jcbs.2014.06.003

Lim, M. T., Lim, Y. M. F., Tong, S. F., & Sivasampu, S. (2019). Age, sex and primary care setting differences in patients' perception of community healthcare seeking behaviour towards health services. *PLoS One, 14*(10), e0224260. https://doi.org/10.1371/journal.pone.0224260

Lund, C., Brooke-Sumner, C., Baingana, F., Baron, E. C., Breuer, E., Chandra, P., Haushofer, J., Herrman, H., Jordans, M., Kieling, C., Medina-Mora, M. E., Morgan, E., Omigbodun, O., Tol, W., Patel, V., & Saxena, S. (2018). Social determinants of mental disorders and the Sustainable Development Goals: A systematic review of reviews. *Lancet Psychiatry, 5*(4), 357–369. https://doi.org/10.1016/s2215-0366(18)30060-9

Mays, V. M., & Ghavami, N. (2018). History, aspirations, and transformations of intersectionality: Focusing on gender. In C. B. Travis, J. W. White, A. Rutherford, W. S. Williams, S. L. Cook, & K. F. Wyche (Eds.), *APA handbook of the psychology of women: History, theory, and battlegrounds* (Vol. 1, pp. 541–566). American Psychological Association.

McHugh, R. K., & Weiss, R. D. (2019). Alcohol use disorder and depressive disorders. *Alcohol Research: Current Reviews, 40*(1), e1–e8[pdf]. https://doi.org/10.35946/arcr.v40.1.01

McLaughlin, K. A., Conron, K. J., Koenen, K. C., & Gilman, S. E. (2010). Childhood adversity, adult stressful life events, and risk of past-year psychiatric disorder: A test of the stress sensitization hypothesis in a population-based sample of adults. *Psychological Medicine, 40*(10), 1647–1658. https://doi.org/10.1017/s0033291709992121

Merikangas, K. R., Akiskal, H. S., Angst, J., Greenberg, P. E., Hirschfeld, R. M., Petukhova, M., & Kessler, R. C. (2007). Lifetime and 12-month prevalence of bipolar spectrum disorder in the National Comorbidity Survey replication. *Archives of General Psychiatry, 64*(5), 543–552. https://doi.org/10.1001/archpsyc.64.5.543

Miller, E., McCaw, B., Humphreys, B. L., & Mitchell, C. (2015). Integrating intimate partner violence assessment and intervention into healthcare in the United States: A systems approach. *Journal of Womens Health, 24*(1), 92–99. https://doi.org/10.1089/jwh.2014.4870

Mitchell, A. J., Vaze, A., & Rao, S. (2009). Clinical diagnosis of depression in primary care: A meta-analysis. *Lancet, 374*(9690), 609–619. https://doi.org/10.1016/s0140-6736(09)60879-5

Moitra, M., Santomauro, D., Collins, P. Y., Vos, T., Whiteford, H., Saxena, S., & Ferrari, A. J. (2022). The global gap in treatment coverage for major depressive disorder in 84 countries from 2000-2019: A systematic review and Bayesian meta-regression analysis. *PLoS Medicine, 19*(2), e1003901. https://doi.org/10.1371/journal.pmed.1003901

Morton, S., Pencheon, D., & Squires, N. (2017). Sustainable Development Goals (SDGs), and their implementation: A national global framework for health, development and equity needs a systems approach at every level. *British Medical Bulletin, 124*(1), 81–90. https://doi.org/10.1093/bmb/ldx031

Murphy, F., Nasa, A., Cullinane, D., Raajakesary, K., Gazzaz, A., Sooknarine, V., Haines, M., Roman, E., Kelly, L., O'Neill, A., Cannon, M., & Roddy, D. W. (2022). Childhood trauma, the HPA Axis and psychiatric illnesses: A targeted literature synthesis. *Frontiers in Psychiatry, 13*, 748372. https://doi.org/10.3389/fpsyt.2022.748372

Murray, C. J. L., & Lopez, A. D. (1996). *The global burden of disease: A comprehensive assessment of mortality and disability from diseases, injuries, and risk factors in 1990 and projected to 2020* [Book]. Harvard School of Public Health on behalf of the World Health Organization and the World Bank. https://apps.who.int/iris/handle/10665/41864

Myers, B., McLaughlin, K. A., Wang, S., Blanco, C., & Stein, D. J. (2014). Associations between childhood adversity, adult stressful life events, and past-year drug use disorders in the National Epidemiological Study of Alcohol and Related Conditions (NESARC). *Psychology of Addictive Behaviors, 28*(4), 1117–1126. https://doi.org/10.1037/a0037459

National Academies of Sciences, Engineering, & Medicine. (2020). *Leading health indicators 2030: Advancing health, equity, and well-being.* The National Academies Press. https://doi.org/10.17226/25682

National Institute on Drug Abuse. (2021, April 13). *Common comorbidities with substance use disorders research report.* NIDA. https://www.drugabuse.gov/publications/research-reports/common-comorbidities-substance-use-disorders/introduction

National Institutes of Health Revitalization Act [Women and Minorities as Subjects in Clinical Research], Pub. L. No. 103-43. (1993). https://www.govinfo.gov/content/pkg/STATUTE-107/pdf/STATUTE-107-Pg122.pdf

Onabola, C. O., Andrews, N., Gislason, M. K., Harder, H. G., & Parkes, M. W. (2022). Exploring cross-sectoral implications of the sustainable development goals: Towards a framework for integrating health equity perspectives with the land-water-energy nexus. *Public Health Reviews, 43*, 1604362. https://doi.org/10.3389/phrs.2022.1604362

OPEN MINDS. (2020, May 6). *The U.S. mental health market: $225.1 billion in spending in 2019: An OPEN MINDS Market Intelligence Report.* https://openminds.com/intelligence-report/the-u-s-mental-health-market-225-1-billion-in-spending-in-2019-an-open-minds-market-intelligence-report/

Papautsky, E. L., Rice, D. R., Ghoneima, H., McKowen, A. L. W., Anderson, N., Wootton, A. R., & Veldhuis, C. (2021). Characterizing health care delays and interruptions in the United States during the COVID-19 pandemic: Internet-based, cross-sectional survey study. *Journal of Medical Internet Research, 23*(5), e25446. https://doi.org/10.2196/25446

Patient Protection and Affordable Care Act, Pub. L. No. 111–148, U.S.C. 42 §18001. (2010). https://www.congress.gov/111/plaws/publ148/PLAW-111publ148.pdf

Pera, M. F., Cain, M. M., Emerick, A., Katz, S., Hirsch, N. A., Sherman, B. W., & Bravata, D. M. (2021). Social determinants of health challenges are prevalent among commercially insured populations. *Journal of Primary Care & Community Health, 12*, 1–10. https://doi.org/10.1177/21501327211025162

Pfluger, V., Rohner, S. L., Eising, C. M., Maercker, A., & Thoma, M. V. (2022). Associations between complex trauma exposure in childhood/adolescence and psychopathology in older age: The role of stress coping and coping self-perception. *Journal of Child & Adolescent Trauma, 15*(3), 539–551. https://doi.org/10.1007/s40653-021-00419-0

Pūras, D. (2015, April 2). *Report of the Special Rapporteur on the right of everyone to the enjoyment of the highest attainable standard of physical and mental health, Dainius Pūras* [Report; A/HRC/29/33]. United Nations.

Pūras, D. (2019, April 12). *Report of the Special Rapporteur on the right of everyone to the enjoyment of the highest attainable standard of physical and mental health* [Report; A/HRC/41/34]. United Nations. https://documents-dds-ny.un.org/doc/UNDOC/GEN/G19/105/97/PDF/G1910597.pdf?OpenElement

Pūras, D. (2020a, April 20). *Report of the Special Rapporteur on the right of everyone to the enjoyment of the highest attainable standard of physical and mental health* [Report; A/HRC/44/48]. United Nations General Assembly.

Pūras, D. (2020b, July 16). *Final report of the Special Rapporteur on the right of everyone to the enjoyment of the highest attainable standard of physical and mental health, Dainius Pūras* [Report; A/75/163]. U. Nations. https://documents-dds-ny.un.org/doc/UNDOC/GEN/N20/185/48/PDF/N2018548.pdf?OpenElement

Ramiz, L., Contrand, B., Rojas Castro, M. Y., Dupuy, M., Lu, L., Sztal-Kutas, C., & Lagarde, E. (2021). A longitudinal study of mental health before and during COVID-19 lockdown in the French population. *Globalization and Health, 17*(1), 29. https://doi.org/10.1186/s12992-021-00682-8

Rastelli, C. P., Cheng, Y., Weingarden, J., Frank, E., & Swartz, H. A. (2013). Differences between unipolar depression and bipolar II depression in women. *Journal of Affective Disorders, 150*(3), 1120–1124. https://doi.org/10.1016/j.jad.2013.05.003

Rehm, J., & Shield, K. D. (2019). Global burden of disease and the impact of mental and addictive disorders. *Current Psychiatry Reports, 21*(2), 10. https://doi.org/10.1007/s11920-019-0997-0

Reinert, M., Nguyen, T., & Fritze, D. (2020). *2021: The state of mental health in America* [Report]. Mental Health America. https://mhanational.org/sites/default/files/2021%20State%20of%20 Mental%20Health%20in%20America_0.pdf

Ruisoto, P., Lopez-Guerra, V. M., Lopez-Nunez, C., Sanchez-Puertas, R., Paladines-Costa, M. B., & Pineda-Cabrera, N. J. (2022). Transdiagnostic model of psychological factors and sex differences in depression in a large sample of Ecuador [Article]. *International Journal of Clinical and Health Psychology, 22*(3), 8, Article 100322. https://doi.org/10.1016/j.ijchp.2022.100322

Saha, S., Cohen, B. B., Nagy, J., Mc, P. M., & Phillips, R. (2020). Well-being in the nation: A living library of measures to drive multi-sector population health improvement and address social determinants. *Milbank Quarterly, 98*(3), 641–663. https://doi.org/10.1111/1468-0009.12477

Sartorius, N., Üstün, T. B., Costa e Silva, J.-A., Goldberg, D., Lecrubier, Y., Ormel, J., Von Korff, M., & Wittchen, H.-U. (1993). An International Study of Psychological Problems in Primary Care: Preliminary report from the World Health Organization collaborative project on 'Psychological Problems in General Health Care'. *Archives of General Psychiatry, 50*(10), 819–824. https://doi.org/10.1001/archpsyc.1993.01820220075008

Shah, S. N., Russo, E. T., Earl, T. R., & Kuo, T. (2014). Measuring and monitoring progress toward health equity: Local challenges for public health. *Preventing Chronic Disease, 11*, E159. https://doi.org/10.5888/pcd11.130440

Shankardass, K., Muntaner, C., Kokkinen, L., Shahidi, F. V., Freiler, A., Oneka, G., Bayoumi, A. M., & O'Campo, P. (2018). The implementation of Health in All Policies initiatives: A systems framework for government action. *Health Research Policy and Systems, 16*(1), 26. https://doi.org/10.1186/s12961-018-0295-z

Slaunwhite, A. K. (2015). The role of gender and income in predicting barriers to mental health care in Canada. *Community Mental Health Journal, 51*(5), 621–627. https://doi.org/10.1007/s10597-014-9814-8

Springer, K. W., Mager Stellman, J., & Jordan-Young, R. M. (2012). Beyond a catalogue of differences: A theoretical frame and good practice guidelines for researching sex/gender in human health. *Social Science and Medicine, 74*(11), 1817–1824. https://doi.org/10.1016/j. socscimed.2011.05.033

St John, L., & Walmsley, R. (2021). The latest treatment interventions improving mental health outcomes for women, following gender-based violence in low-and-middle-income countries: A mini review. *Frontiers in Global Women's Health, 2*, 792399. https://doi.org/10.3389/ fgwh.2021.792399

Substance Abuse and Mental Health Services Administration. (2021a). *Key substance use and mental health indicators in the United States: Results from the 2020 National Survey on Drug Use and Health* (HHS Publication No. PEP21-07-01-003, NSDUH Series H-56). https://www. samhsa.gov/data/sites/default/files/reports/rpt35325/NSDUHFFRPDFWHTMLFiles2020/202 0NSDUHFFR1PDFW102121.pdf

Substance Abuse and Mental Health Services Administration. (2021b, July 14). *National Survey Of Substance Abuse Treatment Services (N-SSATS): 2020, data on substance abuse treatment facilities.* Author. https://www.samhsa.gov/data/sites/default/files/reports/rpt35313/2020_ NSSATS_FINAL.pdf

Thompson, A. E., Anisimowicz, Y., Miedema, B., Hogg, W., Wodchis, W. P., & Aubrey-Bassler, K. (2016). The influence of gender and other patient characteristics on health care-seeking behaviour: A QUALICOPC study. *BMC Family Practice, 17*, 38. https://doi.org/10.1186/s12875-016-0440-0

Thornicroft, G., Chatterji, S., Evans-Lacko, S., Gruber, M., Sampson, N., Aguilar-Gaxiola, S., Al-Hamzawi, A., Alonso, J., Andrade, L., Borges, G., Bruffaerts, R., Bunting, B., de Almeida,

J. M., Florescu, S., de Girolamo, G., Gureje, O., Haro, J. M., He, Y., Hinkov, H., Karam, E., Kawakami, N., Lee, S., Navarro-Mateu, F., Piazza, M., Posada-Villa, J., de Galvis, Y. T., & Kessler, R. C. (2017). Undertreatment of people with major depressive disorder in 21 countries. *British Journal of Psychiatry, 210*(2), 119–124. https://doi.org/10.1192/bjp.bp.116.188078

Tikkanen, R., Fields, K., Williams II, R. D., & Abrams, M. K. (2020, May 21). *Mental health conditions and substance use: Comparing U.S. Needs and treatment capacity with those in other high-income countries* [Issue Brief].

U.S. Department of Health and Human Services. (2008, October 28). *The Secretary's Advisory Committee on National Health Promotion and Disease Prevention Objectives for 2020. Phase I report: Recommendations for the framework and format of Healthy People 2020.* http://www.healthypeople.gov/sites/default/files/PhaseI_0.pdf

United Nations. (2015, October 21). *Transforming our world: the 2030 Agenda for Sustainable Development* [Report; A/RES/70/1]. United Nations. https://sdgs.un.org/sites/default/files/publications/21252030%20Agenda%20for%20Sustainable%20Development%20web.pdf

United Nations General Assembly. (1966, December 16). *International covenant on economic, social and cultural rights.* [Web page, General Assembly resolution 2200A (XXI)]. United Nations.

United Nations Office for the Coordination of Humanitarian Affairs. (2022). *Global humanitarian overview 2021.* [Web page]. UNOCHA. https://gho.unocha.org/

van Ginneken, N., Chin, W. Y., Lim, Y. C., Ussif, A., Singh, R., Shahmalak, U., Purgato, M., Rojas-García, A., Uphoff, E., McMullen, S., Foss, H. S., Thapa Pachya, A., Rashidian, L., Borghesani, A., Henschke, N., Chong, L. Y., & Lewin, S. (2021). Primary-level worker interventions for the care of people living with mental disorders and distress in low- and middle-income countries. *Cochrane Database of Systematic Reviews, 8*(8), Cd009149. https://doi.org/10.1002/14651858.CD009149.pub3

Van Vliet-Brown, C. E., Shahram, S., & Oelke, N. D. (2018). Health in All Policies utilization by municipal governments: Scoping review. *Health Promotion International, 33*(4), 713–722. https://doi.org/10.1093/heapro/dax008

Wang, P. S., Aguilar-Gaxiola, S., Alonso, J., Angermeyer, M. C., Borges, G., Bromet, E. J., Bruffaerts, R., de Girolamo, G., de Graaf, R., Gureje, O., Haro, J. M., Karam, E. G., Kessler, R. C., Kovess, V., Lane, M. C., Lee, S., Levinson, D., Ono, Y., Petukhova, M., Posada-Villa, J., Seedat, S., & Wells, J. E. (2007). Use of mental health services for anxiety, mood, and substance disorders in 17 countries in the WHO world mental health surveys. *Lancet, 370*(9590), 841–850. https://doi.org/10.1016/s0140-6736(07)61414-7

Weil, A. R. (2020). Tackling social determinants of health around the globe. *Health Affairs, 39*(7), 1118–1121. https://doi.org/10.1377/hlthaff.2020.00691

Whiteford, H. A., Degenhardt, L., Rehm, J., Baxter, A. J., Ferrari, A. J., Erskine, H. E., Charlson, F. J., Norman, R. E., Flaxman, A. D., Johns, N., Burstein, R., Murray, C. J., & Vos, T. (2013). Global burden of disease attributable to mental and substance use disorders: Findings from the Global Burden of Disease Study 2010. *Lancet, 382*(9904), 1575–1586. https://doi.org/10.1016/s0140-6736(13)61611-6

Wilson, W., Bangs, A., & Hatting, T. (2015, February). *Future of rural behavioral health* (National Rural Health Association Policy Brief). National Rural Health Association. https://www.ruralhealthweb.org/NRHA/media/Emerge_NRHA/Advocacy/Policy%20documents/The-Future-of-Rural-Behavioral-Health_Feb-2015.pdf

World Health Organization. (2017, December 29). *Human rights and health.* [Web page]. WHO. https://www.who.int/news-room/fact-sheets/detail/human-rights-and-health

World Health Organization. (2019). *The WHO special initiative for mental health (2019–2023): Universal health coverage for mental health* [Report; WHO/MSD/19.1]. Author. https://apps.who.int/iris/handle/10665/310981

World Health Organization. (2022a, June 16). *World mental health report: Transforming mental health for all* [Report]. Author [WHO]. https://apps.who.int/iris/rest/bitstreams/1433523/retrieve

World Health Organization. (2022b). *Social determinants of health*. [Web page]. WHO. https://www.who.int/health-topics/social-determinants-of-health#tab=tab_1

World Health Organization. (2022c). *Third round of the global pulse survey on continuity of essential health services during the COVID-19 pandemic: November—December Interim report* [Report]. Author. https://www.who.int/publications-detail-redirect/WHO-2019-nCoV-EHS_continuity-survey-2022.1

World Health Organization. (2022d). *World health statistics 2022: Monitoring health for the SDGs* [Report]. Author. https://apps.who.int/iris/rest/bitstreams/1435584/retrieve

Yang, J. C., Roman-Urrestarazu, A., McKee, M., & Brayne, C. (2019). Demographic, socioeconomic, and health correlates of unmet need for mental health treatment in the United States, 2002-16: Evidence from the National Surveys on Drug Use and Health. *International Journal for Equity in Health, 18*(1), 122. https://doi.org/10.1186/s12939-019-1026-y

Yılmaz, S., Alghamdi, B., Singuri, S., Hacialiefendioglu, A. M., Özcan, T., Koyutürk, M., & Karakurt, G. (2020). Identifying health correlates of intimate partner violence against pregnant women. *Health Information Science and Systems, 8*(1), 36. https://doi.org/10.1007/s13755-020-00124-6

Yücel, M., Oldenhof, E., Ahmed, S. H., Belin, D., Billieux, J., Bowden-Jones, H., Carter, A., Chamberlain, S. R., Clark, L., Connor, J., Daglish, M., Dom, G., Dannon, P., Duka, T., Fernandez-Serrano, M. J., Field, M., Franken, I., Goldstein, R. Z., Gonzalez, R., Goudriaan, A. E., Grant, J. E., Gullo, M. J., Hester, R., Hodgins, D. C., Le Foll, B., Lee, R. S. C., Lingford-Hughes, A., Lorenzetti, V., Moeller, S. J., Munafò, M. R., Odlaug, B., Potenza, M. N., Segrave, R., Sjoerds, Z., Solowij, N., van den Brink, W., van Holst, R. J., Voon, V., Wiers, R., Fontenelle, L. F., & Verdejo-Garcia, A. (2019). A transdiagnostic dimensional approach towards a neuropsychological assessment for addiction: An international Delphi consensus study. *Addiction, 114*(6), 1095–1109. https://doi.org/10.1111/add.14424

Chapter 2
Epidemiology of Mental Health Disorders in Female Children and Adolescents

Kitty Leung, Laren Alexander, Shelby Goicochea, and Steven Cuffe

Introduction

An individual's mental health develops from a myriad of determinants, including biological, social, and psychological factors, and is shaped by life experiences that affect all aspects of the individual. Mental health is a vital component of one's health and well-being. The 2021 *Advisory* from the U. S. Office of the Surgeon General (2021) urges the recognition and prioritization of mental health as an essential part of overall health.

This chapter broadly discusses the epidemiology of mental health disorders in children and adolescents prior to exploring the prevalence of psychiatric disorders in female youth, gender differences in the presentation of psychiatric disorders, trajectory changes across the lifespan, impacts from the COVID-19 pandemic, and mental health disparities among females. This chapter will focus on the following psychiatric disorders emphasizing those with the highest prevalence, morbidity, and disproportionate disease distribution among female children and adolescents: attention-deficit/hyperactivity disorder (ADHD), anxiety disorders, mood disorders, post-traumatic stress disorder (PTSD), schizophrenia-spectrum disorders, autism spectrum disorders (ASD), and eating disorders. Suicide was also given an independent section in this chapter given its severity and prevalence amongst teens for both attempts and completion.

K. Leung (✉) · L. Alexander · S. Goicochea · S. Cuffe
Department of Psychiatry, University of Florida College of Medicine – Jacksonville, Jacksonville, FL, USA
e-mail: Kitty.leung@jax.ufl.edu; Laren.alexander@jax.ufl.edu; Shelby.goicochea@gmail.com; Steven.cuffe@jax.ufl.edu

A. Hanson, B. L. Levin (eds.), *Women's Behavioral Health*,
https://doi.org/10.1007/978-3-031-58293-6_2

25

National and Global Epidemiology

Mental disorders are highly prevalent and are the leading cause of living with a disability (World Health Organization (WHO), 2022). In the United States, 1 in 5 (20%) of children and adolescents ages 10–19 have a mental health condition (United Nations Children's Fund (UNICEF), 2021, October 21). Only approximately 10% of U. S. youth were reported to have received mental health care based on national surveys spanning from 2013 to 2019 (Bitsko et al., 2022). The prevalence of mental health conditions differs between females and males; females had increased prevalence of depression (4.8% vs 4.0% in males), suicidal ideation (24.1% vs 13.3% in males), and attempts (11.0% vs 6.6% in males), while males had increased prevalence of ADHD (13.3% vs 6.1% in females) and ASD (4.8% vs 1.3% in females). Unlike past studies, there was no gender difference in the prevalence of anxiety (9.4%). With increasing age, youth mental health disorder estimates for depression, anxiety, ADHD, and ASD increased overall as did reports of youth having received mental health services (Bitsko et al., 2022). Children and adolescents with at least one mental health disorder had significantly increased all-cause medical costs, approximately triple the costs compared to age- and gender-matched peers without these disorders (Tkacz & Brady, 2021).

There are limited studies on the global prevalence of mental disorders in children and adolescents. An epidemiological meta-analysis of the global prevalence of mental disorders in 18,000 young children revealed this population is overlooked and neglected (Vasileva et al., 2021). A meta-analysis of 41 studies in 27 countries estimated the worldwide-pooled prevalence of mental health disorders in children and adolescents was 13.4% and global prevalence of anxiety disorders (6.5%), ADHD (3.4%), and depressive disorders (2.6%) (Polanczyk et al., 2015). A systematic analysis for the Global Burden of Disease study 2019 database of 204 countries and territories estimated the mean prevalence of mental health disorders in children and adolescents globally was 8.8%. The overall incidence of global mental health disorders in children and adolescents increased by 6.8% from 1990 to 2019. The specific disorders observed to have the highest increased incidence were eating disorders (increased by 22.9%), major depressive disorder (by 8.7%), and conduct disorder (by 6.5%). From 1990 to 2019, there were observed increases in the prevalence of depression (by 10.9%), conduct disorder (by 8.2%), and anxiety disorders (by 1.6%). The total disease burden measured by disability-adjusted-life-years in this same three-decade time span increased by 14.9% (Piao et al., 2022).

A Danish study, using population-based medical databases, provides a unique and robust report on the international prevalence of child and adolescent mental health disorders. A nationwide population-based cohort study of all children born in Denmark from 1995 to 2016 found that 15.0% of children and adolescents (14.6% females and 15.5% males) were diagnosed with a mental disorder by age 18. Similar to results from the United States, females were more likely to be diagnosed with anxiety, while the most common diagnosis for males was ADHD. Interestingly, the incidence of ADHD peaked in males at age 8 while the peak age in females was 17 years old. Despite the current understanding that ADHD has an early age of onset based on diagnostic criteria, this finding suggests delayed identification of ADHD in females, which often goes undiagnosed. Similarly, neurodevelopmental disorders, including ASD, were diagnosed in late adolescence for females, peak age 16, compared to the peak age of 5 in males (Dalsgaard et al., 2020).

Delayed diagnosis of female children and adolescents may be in part associated with trends showing an increase in internalizing symptoms (i.e., inner-directed problems causing psychological distress) over the last century. A systematic review of studies from 12 countries compared the trend of males presenting with externalizing symptoms (i.e., outward problematic behavior) (Bor et al., 2014). Early identification of mental health disorders is especially important for improving prognosis. A cross-national comparison of over a half million adolescents across 73 countries found females have poorer mental health outcomes compared to males, highlighting a gender gap in adolescent mental health (Campbell et al., 2021).

The most recent report to date on global prevalence estimated that 166 million (89 million males and 77 million females) or 1 in 7 (14%) children and adolescents ages 10–19 had a mental health condition (United Nations Children's Fund, 2021), with the peak age of onset of 14.5 years old and median age of onset 18 years old (Solmi et al., 2022). However, the prevalence of mental health disorders is likely higher than the reported estimates as these conditions are often not diagnosed due to an individual's fear of mental health stigma, insufficient knowledge of mental health disorders, and difficulty accessing mental health services (Cheung et al., 2017). Identification of psychiatric symptoms is essential to begin early intervention, yet mental health is often underdiagnosed, undertreated, and under-resourced, resulting in significant morbidity and mortality (Bitsko et al., 2022; Hayes et al., 2023; Piao et al., 2022; Whitney & Peterson, 2019) Studying the epidemiology of mental health disorders can help promote recognition, diagnosis, treatment, and prioritize resources to better improve mental well-being.

As highlighted above, mental health disorders significantly affect females of all ages on a global level. In the following sections, we will further explore specific mental health disorders affecting female children and adolescents, examine the impact of the COVID-19 pandemic, and review mental health disparities affecting females and the subsequent implications for women's behavioral health.

Psychiatric Disorders in Girls and Female Adolescents

This section of the chapter delves into specific mental health disorders that commonly affect female children and adolescents, and it further highlights the epidemiological differences between female and male youth.

Depressive Disorders

Depressive disorders are defined by periods of loss of interest or pleasure in most activities or persistent sadness that causes functional impairment. In children and adolescents, irritable mood can be used as a diagnostic criterion in lieu of depressed mood (American Psychiatric Association (APA), 2022). In comparison to adults, since depressed youth often present with irritability, emotional reactivity, somatic symptoms, and behavioral disturbances, the diagnosis of depression may be missed (Thapar et al., 2012).

Bitsko et al. (2022) correlated prevalence data across a series of national studies on children and adolescents. Findings from the 2016 to 2019 National Survey of Children's Health (NSCH) revealed that 4.4% of youth ages 3–17 had a previous diagnosis of depression and 3.4% were reported by parents to be currently experiencing depression at the time of the survey. Prevalence of depression increases with age, particularly during adolescence. Lifetime prevalence of depression increased from 0.1% in children ages 3–5 to 2.3% in children ages 6–11 and increased to 8.6% in adolescents ages 12–17 based on parent-report of their child having been diagnosed with depression. Prevalence of depression in adolescents was higher on self-report from the 2018 to 2019 National Survey on Drug Use and Health (NSDUH) data with 20.9% of adolescents ages 12–17 reporting a lifetime episode of major depression and 15.1% reporting a major depressive episode in the last year. In the same adolescent age group, the 2013–2018 National Health and Nutrition Examination Survey (NHANES) found 5.8% of adolescents self-reported major depression within the last 2 weeks. Across all surveys and associated measures of depression, female youth had a higher prevalence of depression, which increases to nearly double that of males in adolescence based on self-report (Bitsko et al., 2022). This gender difference persists into adulthood (Merikangas et al., 2009).

Aside from gender and age differences in prevalence, depression is more likely to occur in children and adolescents who have special health care needs, have public (rather than private) insurance coverage, are living with a caregiver who has mental health issues, and have been a victim of or witnessed neighborhood violence (Figas et al., 2023). Mixed data regarding other risk factors for depression in youth, such as race, ethnicity, household income, and geographic location, are likely a consequence of differences in study samples and designs (Bitsko et al., 2022). Of the most common mental health disorders affecting children and adolescents, depressive disorder is the most likely to have a co-occurring mental health disorder, such as anxiety (73.8%) and a behavioral problem (47.2%) (Ghandour et al., 2019). In addition, Melton et al. (2016) found comorbid depression and anxiety in youth is associated with increased severity and treatment resistance compared to having either disorder alone.

The U.S. Preventive Services Task Force (USPSTF) recommends depression screenings in adolescents ages 12–18 years old (USPSTF et al., 2022a). Given that early identification of depression and intervention is vital for well-being, it is important to collect self-reported data when assessing adolescent mental health separately from and in addition to parent-reported information regarding depression (Cantwell et al., 1997).

Disruptive Mood Dysregulation Disorder (DMDD)

DMDD is a relatively new mood disorder characterized by persistent irritability and recurrent anger outbursts. The diagnosis is unique to childhood. Symptoms must present before age 10 and the disorder should only be diagnosed between ages 6 and 18 (APA, 2022). As DMDD is a newer diagnosis added to the *Diagnostic and Statistical Manual of Mental Disorders, Fifth Edition* (*DSM-5*) "Depressive Disorders" chapter, there is limited prevalence data.

A study based on data collected from Swedish twins examined factors influencing irritability in childhood. There was a higher genetic influence on irritability for females early in childhood, but this influence decreased with age. Additionally, there was less environmental influence on irritability in females when compared to genetic factors (Roberson-Nay et al., 2015). Based on a retrospective review of 3 earlier studies, Copeland et al. (2013) found the prevalence of DMDD ranged from 0.8% to 3.3%, with higher rates of DMDD in preschool-age youth. Prevalence appeared to decrease with age. Although there was no significant difference in prevalence between genders, the sample size of youth with DMDD was small. A more recent systematic review and meta-analysis of 41 studies found the prevalence of DMDD was around 1.60% (Spoelma et al., 2023). Similar to previous findings, there were no significant differences between genders; however, there is limited data available for DMDD (Spoelma et al., 2023).

Bipolar Disorder

Bipolar-spectrum disorders are characterized by fluctuations in mood from depressive to elevated or irritable states (APA, 2022). In comparison to depressive disorders, bipolar-spectrum disorders are less common in childhood.

In one recent mental health surveillance report, there was not enough data collected to provide estimates on the prevalence of bipolar-spectrum disorders (Bitsko et al., 2022). Previous studies indicate the prevalence of bipolar disorder varying from 0.0% to 2.1% in youth without significant differences in prevalence rate between genders (Merikangas et al., 2009). The 2001–2004 National Comorbidity Survey—Adolescent Supplement (NCS-A) study found the lifetime prevalence of bipolar I and bipolar II disorder collectively in adolescents aged 13–17 was 3.0% (3.1% for females and 2.8% for males, respectively). Bipolar I disorder was less prevalent (0.3% in females vs 0.1% in males) than bipolar II disorder (2.8% in females vs 2.8% in males). Consistent with previous studies, there was no significant difference in prevalence rates between genders (Kessler et al., 2012).

A recent cohort study in Denmark revealed a similar cumulative incidence of bipolar disorder between females (0.10%) and males (0.06%) (Dalsgaard et al., 2020). In contrast, an observational study based on administrative health care data collected in the United States from 2012 to 2018 found female youth, ages 4–17, were 3.3–5.7 times more likely to be diagnosed with bipolar disorder than male counterparts. The study was based on individuals with commercial health insurance, which may contribute to the skew in study findings. Similar to previous research, the prevalence of bipolar disorder remained 0.3% throughout the study (Tkacz & Brady, 2021).

When examining the age of onset, Lewinsohn et al. (2000) previously noted the peak first incidence of bipolar-spectrum disorders was at age 14, with a decline in incidence throughout adolescence. Based on a recent meta-analysis of 192 studies examining the global age of onset of mental health disorders, the earliest peak age of onset of bipolar-spectrum disorders was 19.5 years old, with 5.1% having onset by age 14 and 13.7% having onset by age 18. The median age of onset was age 33 (Solmi et al., 2022).

Cirone et al. (2021) further explored long-term outcomes of early-onset bipolar disorder through a systematic literature review. Most individuals retained their bipolar diagnosis when followed up to 10 years. The most common comorbid disorders were ADHD, anxiety, and substance use. Additionally, bipolar disorder was associated with high rates of suicidality. In a study by Goldstein et al. (2012) looking at suicidality in youth with bipolar disorder, 18% of youth in the study attempted suicide at least once over a 5-year period, and 8% of youth had multiple attempts. Girls were found to have higher rates of suicide attempts. Additional factors associated with increased risk of suicide attempts included the severity of depression, family history of depression, mixed mood symptoms, and substance use (Goldstein et al., 2012).

Anxiety Disorders

Anxiety disorders are characterized by excessive fears and persistent worry that interferes with daily functioning. In children and adolescents, anxiety often presents as somatic symptoms, such as fatigue, headaches, or stomach aches. It is important to note the anxiety must be inappropriate for the child's developmental stage to meet the criteria for an anxiety disorder (APA, 2022).

Anxiety disorders are one of the most common psychiatric disorders seen in children and adolescents. The lifetime prevalence of anxiety in U. S. adolescents (13–17 years old) was 26.8% in males and 38.3% in females (Kessler et al., 2012), and the global prevalence of any anxiety disorder was 6.5% in children and adolescents (Polanczyk et al., 2015). The 2016–2019 NSCH survey results showed that 9.4% (approximately 5.8 million) of children and adolescents aged 3–17 had a diagnosis of anxiety. The prevalence of anxiety disorders increased with age (2.0% in 3–5 year-olds, 8.6% in 6–11 year-olds, and 13.7% in 12–17 year-olds). In contrast to other studies, there were no significant differences in the prevalence of anxiety disorders between genders (Bitsko et al., 2022).

In a trend analysis of the prevalence of anxiety in 37,000 high school students based on student-completed anxiety screening during 2012–2018, the prevalence of anxiety increased with time from 34.1% in 2012 to 37.7% in 2015 and 44% in 2018 (Parodi et al., 2022). When comparing gender differences, the prevalence of anxiety in females was significantly higher than in male counterparts. Anxiety increased from 41.9% in females in 2012 (26% in males) to 50.7% in 2015 (24.1% in males) to 56.2% in 2018 (31.3% in males). The study also identified disparities in youth, who identified across the lesbian, gay, bisexual, transgender, gender diverse, inter-sex, and queer (LGBTIQ+) communities, with these groups having higher rates of anxiety (Parodi et al., 2022).

The prevalence of specific anxiety disorders varies by age. The median age of onset for any anxiety disorder is 11 years (Kessler et al., 2005). When looking at specific disorders, the median age of onset is the following: specific phobias and separation anxiety (7 years old); social anxiety disorder (13 years old); agoraphobia (20 years old); panic disorder (24 years old); and generalized anxiety disorder (30 years old) (Bandelow & Michaelis, 2015). The WHO's 2022 *World Mental Health Report* states anxiety disorders are the most prevalent mental health disorders in older adolescents, occurring in 5.5% of adolescent girls.

Given the high prevalence of anxiety disorders, the 2022 USPSTF recommends screening for anxiety in children and adolescents aged 8–18 years (USPTSF et al., 2022b). Diagnosis and treatment for early onset is especially important as anxiety disorders are associated with an increased likelihood of comorbid psychiatric disorders, including other anxiety disorders later in life.

Post-Traumatic Stress Disorder (PTSD)

PTSD is defined by exposure to a traumatic experience with subsequent re-experiencing of the trauma, avoidance of trauma reminders, and changes in mood and cognition. In children, themes of trauma may appear in play and nightmares may be non-specific (APA, 2022).

Research has shown more than 60% of children are exposed to traumatic events (Garza & Jovanovic, 2017). On a national level, approximately 8.1 in 1000 children in the United States experienced child abuse or neglect in 2021. Seventy-six percent of children experience neglect, 16% physical abuse, 10.1% sexual abuse, and 0.2% sexual trafficking. Rates of maltreatment were similar between genders, except for sexual trafficking, in which 87.3% of the victims were female (Children's Bureau, 2023). In addition to directly experiencing maltreatment, other common forms of trauma in childhood include witnessing domestic or community violence, losing a family member or friend to homicide, and exposure to a natural or man-made disaster (Saunders & Adams, 2014).

When specifically examining violence on a global level, exposure is high. The 2014 UNICEF report, *Ending Violence Against Children*, noted approximately 60% of children between ages 2 and 14 regularly experience physical punishment by their caregivers. It was also estimated approximately 25% of girls between ages 15 and 19 report histories of physical violence since age 15 and around 10% of girls under the age of 20 endorse histories of forced sexual acts (UNICEF, 2014b, September). Of note, in 2012, violence was the second leading cause of death among girls aged 10–19 globally. The risk of death by violence increases with age with the global percentage of female deaths due to violence trending from 0.4% in girls aged 0–9, 4% in girls aged 10–14, and 13% in girls aged 15–19 (UNICEF, 2014a, October 10).

Another significant factor contributing to trauma-related disorders worldwide is bullying; one in three adolescent girls (ages 13–15) experience bullying. Studies show equal rates of bullying between genders; however, girls are more likely to experience psychological bullying, such as rumors and being left out (UNICEF, 2014b, September). Due to the increased use of the internet and social media, cyber-bullying has significantly increased, with 46% of teens reporting they have experienced cyberbullying. The highest rates of cyberbullying occurred in girls aged 15–17 (54%) in comparison to 44% of boys of the same age, and they are most likely to experience multiple forms of cyberbullying (Vogels, 2022).

A meta-analysis of 192 epidemiological studies found the peak age of onset of trauma-related disorders was 15.5 years old with 16.9% presenting by age 14, 27.6% by age 18, and 43.1% by age 25 (Solmi et al., 2022). Despite significant trauma exposure in all children, lifetime prevalence of PTSD is higher in adolescent girls ages 13–17 in comparison to male counterparts (6.9% vs 2.3%, respectively) (Kessler et al., 2012). Similarly, a longitudinal cohort study in the UK found rates of post-traumatic stress symptoms were similar between genders at ages 8 and 10; however, girls were more likely to report symptoms at ages 13 and 15 (Haag et al., 2020). Several factors are suspected in contributing to gender differences; these include type of trauma exposure (with girls being more likely to experience sexual trauma), exposure to higher cumulative trauma (Haag et al., 2020), higher rates of internalizing symptoms in females, higher levels of fear-potentiated startle in girls during puberty, and the influence of hormones, particularly estrogen (Garza & Jovanovic, 2017).

In regards to symptom presentation, previous research has noted that girls have higher levels of avoidance symptoms than boys, who are more likely to experience intrusive symptoms (Garza & Jovanovic, 2017). Additionally, a study of 167 children ages 3–18 who experienced complex trauma (defined as exposure to multiple, severe traumatic events) found, based on caregiver report, that girls were more likely to experience depression, dissociation, hyperarousal, and total PTSD symptoms. Additionally, girls were more likely to self-report higher sexual concerns as well as slightly higher levels of re-experiencing and total PTSD symptoms (Wamser-Nanney & Cherry, 2018). In a cohort study of 159,500 adolescents aged 12–18 who were hospitalized, the majority of participants who had a primary diagnosis of PTSD were female (75.7%), and the most common comorbidities were anxiety disorders (100%), mood disorders (89.4%), and ADHD/conduct/behavioral disorders (36.5%). The PTSD cohort had higher rates of suicidal behavior (Eskander et al., 2020).

Schizophrenia-Spectrum Disorders

Schizophrenia and the spectrum of psychotic disorders are characterized by hallucinations, delusions, disorganized thought process, and negative symptoms (APA, 2022). Globally, schizophrenia-spectrum disorders are uncommon prior to adolescence (Dalsgaard et al., 2020; WHO, 2022). The worldwide prevalence of schizophrenia is approximately 0.1% in 15–19 year-olds (WHO, 2022), and the peak age of onset is approximately 20.5 years (Solmi et al., 2022).

Although presentations meeting criteria for schizophrenia-spectrum disorders are rare in childhood, subclinical psychotic-like experiences are common in adolescents. A study of 302 adolescents aged 14–18 in the UK found that 74.3% of females self-reported at least one psychotic-like symptom occurring "often or almost always" (in comparison to 58.3% of males in the study). Additionally, females self-reported higher rates of bizarre experiences and persecutory ideation as well as higher levels of distress than male peers. Although only a small percentage of individuals who have psychotic-like experiences go on to develop a psychotic disorder, these experiences can be precursors to schizophrenia-spectrum disorders later in life (Stainton et al., 2021).

Further exploring gender differences, a cohort study in Denmark found the cumulative incidence of schizophrenia by age 18 was higher in females (0.76%) than in males (0.48%;) (Dalsgaard et al., 2020). In contrast, other research has associated the male gender with higher rates of schizophrenia. An umbrella review found that males aged 15–35 are at higher risk of psychosis (Radua et al., 2018). An observational study based on 2012–2018 administrative health care data in the United States found male youth ages 4–17 are 1.2–1.5 times more likely to be diagnosed with schizophrenia than female counterparts (Tkacz and Brady, 2021). Additionally, a meta-analysis of 192 epidemiological studies discovered the median age of onset of schizophrenia-spectrum and primary psychotic disorders was 1 year later for females (26 years of age in females vs 25 years of age in males) (Solmi et al., 2022).

Exposure to several environmental factors in childhood and adolescence has been associated with the development of psychosis. Urban living environments (such as proximity to roads, living environments with lead paint risk, family poverty, and income disparity) have been associated with increased risk of psychotic-like experiences in pre-adolescents (Saxena & Dodell-Feder, 2022). Childhood adversity, such as abuse, neglect, bullying, and parental loss or parental separation, has also been associated with the development of psychosis in late adolescence (Brasso et al., 2021). A cohort study of 4433 youth in the UK discovered exposure to any form of trauma (between birth and age 17) was associated with increased risk of psychotic experiences at age 18. Repeated traumatic exposures, including exposure to multiple trauma types and exposure at different ages, were associated with higher risk of psychotic experiences. Further, exposure to trauma during adolescence was the age group most strongly associated with development of psychotic experiences at age 18 (Croft et al., 2019). Additionally, cannabis, psychostimulant, and tobacco use in adolescence also has been associated with increased risk of psychosis (Brasso et al., 2021). Cannabis use has been strongly associated with increased risk of primary psychotic disorders, particularly if cannabis use starts before age 15 or is used heavily, and the cannabis is high potency (Brasso et al., 2021; Murray et al., 2020).

Eating Disorders

Eating disorders are characterized by distorted thoughts about food and body image and persistent, irregular eating patterns. Disordered eating patterns include restricting caloric intake, binge eating, or purging via various methods, such as vomiting, compulsive exercise, or misuse of medications, such as laxatives. The most common eating disorders in female youth are anorexia nervosa, bulimia nervosa, and binge eating disorder (APA, 2022).

A meta-analysis of 192 epidemiological studies found the peak age of onset of disordered eating occurred at 15.5 years, with a median age of onset at 18 years (Solmi et al., 2022). When comparing specific disorders, anorexia nervosa and bulimia nervosa had the same peak age of onset (15.5) and similar median ages of onset (17 and 18 respectively). In contrast, binge eating disorder had a later peak age of onset (19.5) and median age of onset (20) (Solmi et al., 2022). A meta-analysis of 14 studies involving 11 high-income countries found the global prevalence of eating disorders to be 0.2% in adolescents aged 12–18 (Barican et al., 2022). Similarly, per WHO's 2022 World Mental Health Report, the global prevalence of eating disorders (including anorexia nervosa and bulimia nervosa) was 0.1% in 10–14 year-olds, 0.3% in 15–19 year-olds, and 0.4% in 20–24 year-olds.

Examining trends in eating disorder rates over time, a study based on the Norwegian National Patient Register data found that the incidence of anorexia nervosa was overall stable from 2010 to 2016; however, there was a significant increase in the annual incidence of anorexia nervosa in 10–14 year-old girls. Additionally, there was an increase in the annual incidence of broadly defined anorexia nervosa in 15–19-year-old girls between 2010 and 2012, but incidence rates subsequently leveled off for the remainder of the study. In comparison, incidence rates of bulimia nervosa overall decreased in females as the study progressed. In contrast, incidence rates of anorexia nervosa and bulimia nervosa in males remained stable and were lower than female counterparts throughout the study (Reas & Rø, 2018). During a similar time period, an observational study based on administrative health care data collected from commercially insured American youth ages 4–17 documented a 96%

increase in the prevalence of eating disorders from 2012 to 2018 (0.1–0.2%) (Tkacz & Brady, 2021).

Research has consistently shown female youth are at higher risk for eating disorders. Per the WHO's 2022 World Mental Health Report, eating disorders primarily occur in young women (0.6% of females aged 20–24 vs 0.3% of males). A recent cohort study of Danish youth also found girls are at high risk of eating disorders (1.80% of females vs 0.28% of males) (Dalsgaard et al., 2020). The point prevalence of anorexia in young women is around 0.3–0.4% (vs 0.1% in young men) and is around 1.0% for bulimia in young women (vs 0.1% in young men). Although binge eating disorder typically presents in early adulthood, approximately 1.6% of adolescent females meet criteria for subthreshold binge eating disorder (National Eating Disorders Association, 2021).

Additionally, an 8-year longitudinal study of 496 American adolescent girls examined the prevalence of both threshold and subthreshold eating disorders. Prevalence of threshold eating disorders by age 20 was 0.8% for anorexia nervosa, 2.6% for bulimia nervosa, 3.0% for binge eating disorder, 2.8% for atypical anorexia nervosa, 4.4% for subthreshold bulimia nervosa, and 3.6% for subthreshold binge eating disorder. Of note, the 1-year recovery rate was 71–100%, which may be related to the high number of participants with subthreshold symptoms (Stice et al., 2013). This study highlights the large number of female youth who are struggling with disordered eating patterns, which is important to consider when screening for psychiatric symptoms in patients.

Several environmental factors may contribute to higher eating disorder rates in girls. Primarily, societal pressure and social media influence to be thin is a significant contributor to disordered eating patterns. This influence may occur as early as elementary school (National Eating Disorders Association, 2021) and may persist into adulthood. A cross-sectional survey of American young adults aged 19–32 found higher social media use is associated with worsening eating concerns (Sidani et al., 2016). Pressure to be thin may also be precipitated by spending more time with peers and dating partners in adolescence (Stice et al., 2009). Additionally, girls who often pursue sports that encourage having a lean physique, such as dancing, cheerleading, figure skating, and gymnastics, are at increased risk (National Eating Disorders Association, 2021).

Autism Spectrum Disorder (ASD)

ASD is characterized by deficits in social communication and interaction, fixed interests, and repetitive behaviors (APA, 2022). The global prevalence of ASD ranges from 0.4% to 0.5% between birth and age 19 (WHO, 2022). On a national level, the prevalence of having a current ASD diagnosis among youth (age 3–17) ranges from 2.0% to 2.9% based on the NSCH and the NHIS (Bitsko et al., 2022). Furthermore, a recent study of American 8 year olds found the prevalence of ASD to be around 1 in 36 children (Maenner et al., 2023). The prevalence of ASD has significantly increased with time. Per the NHIS, parent-reported ASD diagnosis increased 122% between 2009 and 2017 (Zablotsky et al., 2019). Several factors are thought to have contributed to the increasing prevalence, including implementation of universal screenings by pediatricians (Zablotsky et al., 2019), increase in autism awareness in the general public, changes in the diagnostic criteria with each DSM edition, and potential inaccurate diagnoses based on the clinician's training and skill level (Matson & Kozlowski, 2011).

When comparing gender differences, the Centers for Disease Control and Prevention (CDC) Mental Health Surveillance Among Children project, which compiled studies from 2013 to 2019, found there was a higher prevalence of ASD in boys than girls in all studies included, which is consistent with previous research (Bitsko et al., 2022). A systematic review of 71 studies calculated the median ratio of male-to-female individuals with ASD was around 4.2:1 (Zeidan et al., 2022). Similarly, a study of 8-year-olds across 11 Autism and Developmental Disabilities Monitoring sites in the United States found the male-to-female ratio to be approximately 3.8:1 (Maenner et al., 2023). Researchers have speculated about a possible "female protective factor" in which females need to inherit a higher burden of genetic factors in order to exhibit the same level of ASD symptomatology as males; however, the exact mechanism is unknown (Elsabbagh, 2020).

On a national level, Maenner et al. (2023) found the median age of the first known ASD diagnosis was 49 months based on a study of 8-year-olds across the country. Of note, youth with comorbid intellectual disability had a younger median age of first diagnosis of 43 months (about 3.5 years) vs 53 months (about 4.5 years), respectively. Globally, the peak age of onset, defined as age of first diagnosis, was around 5.5 years per a meta-analysis of 192 epidemiological studies (Solmi et al., 2022).

Despite having a similar age of symptom onset between genders, girls often go undiagnosed or are misdiagnosed. A Danish cohort study found most girls were diagnosed with neurodevelopmental disorders, such as ASD, in late adolescence despite the disorder having an early age of onset (Dalsgaard et al., 2020). Lockwood Estrin et al. (2021) conducted a mixed-methods systematic review to further explore factors contributing to delayed diagnosis. Factors identified included girls having improved ability to mask their symptoms in social situations as well as girls exhibiting less restricted and repetitive behaviors and interests. Additionally, parents of girls with ASD often voiced fewer concerns about ASD or different concerns than parents of boys, which may in part be due to parents reporting they had a lack of information available about females with ASD, limiting their awareness of symptoms. Clinician bias was identified as another factor, with physicians being more hesitant to diagnose ASD in girls, even if there were documented symptoms, due to the perception that ASD is a "male disorder".

Although ASD is less common in girls, females often have a more severe presentation than male counterparts when diagnosed. A study comparing gender differences in individuals diagnosed with ASD found that females had greater social communication deficits, lower cognitive and adaptive abilities, and more externalizing behaviors in comparison to male counterparts; however, girls also had lower levels of restrictive interests (Frazier et al., 2014). Furthermore, a national study of 8-year-olds with ASD found that girls are more likely to be diagnosed with comorbid intellectual disability than boys (42.1% vs 36.9%, respectively) (Maenner et al., 2023). A mixed-method systematic review of 22 articles noted that since ASD may be overlooked in females, girls generally need more significant symptoms, such as verbal or behavioral difficulties, in order to be diagnosed (Lockwood Estrin et al., 2021).

Attention-Deficit/Hyperactivity Disorder (ADHD)

ADHD is one of the most common neurodevelopmental disorders characterized by a persistent pattern of inattention, impulsivity, and hyperactivity alone or in combination that interferes with everyday functioning in multiple settings (APA, 2022).

The prevalence of ADHD in the United States from parent-reported data of their child having been diagnosed by a health care professional was 9.6–9.8%. Prevalence increases with age in children and adolescents ages 3–17 as published by the 2017–2018 National Health Interview Survey (NHIS) and 2016–2019 National Survey of Children's Health (NSCH), respectively. The national surveys observed that the prevalence of ADHD was higher in children and adolescents with public insurance, the lowest household income, and living in rural areas (Bitsko et al., 2022). Teacher report in addition to the parent report in a community-based study of four U. S. school districts provided complementary data regarding ADHD prevalence with 5.1–9.4% of children and adolescents meeting diagnostic criteria (Danielson et al., 2021). Consistent with prior literature, the prevalence of ADHD in male children and adolescents was approximately double (13.3% vs 6.2%) that of females (Bitsko et al., 2022; Willcutt, 2012).

Globally, ADHD prevalence was informed by systematic reviews and meta-analyses. In one such review, an analysis of 171,756 children and adolescents globally calculated a prevalence of 5.3% of ADHD with no significant difference between youth in North America and Europe (Polanczyk et al., 2007). More recently, a systematic review of over 175 community- and school-based global studies revealed an overall pooled estimated prevalence of 7.2% for children and adolescents (Thomas et al., 2015).

Symptomatic presentation has been noted to differ between females and males. Girls with ADHD are more likely to manifest internalizing problems and have a predominance of inattention, whereas boys exhibit higher levels of hyperactivity, impulsivity, and externalizing behaviors (Hinshaw et al., 2022). Similarly, a meta-analysis of sex differences in ADHD also found girls to be less hyperactive and have fewer difficulties with motor response inhibition and cognitive flexibility compared to boys. As a result, girls are often less disruptive, so their symptoms may be overlooked, which likely contributes to delayed diagnosis as well as underdiagnosis (Loyer Carbonneau et al., 2021). As mentioned previously, a Danish cohort study found that girls had a delayed peak incidence of ADHD in comparison to boys (age

17 in females vs. age 8 in males), even though the disorder has an onset in early childhood, suggesting the diagnosis was delayed (Dalsgaard et al., 2020). Despite ADHD being a common disorder, research in the past decade has largely focused on males, leaving a knowledge gap for female children and adolescents with ADHD. Thankfully, national and global efforts from organizations, such as the National Institute of Mental Health and World Federation of ADHD International Consensus, have worked toward reducing misconceptions about ADHD and bringing awareness to underrepresented populations, including females and ethnic minorities, who have not previously been studied.

Suicide

Suicide continues to be a public health emergency in the United States and across the world, especially for the youth population. It is estimated that globally there are 1.3 billion adolescents, who account for more than 15% of the world population (UNICEF, 2022, April). In the United States, suicide was found to be the second leading cause of death (21.3%) for 10–17 year-olds from 2008 to 2020, having increased from the fourth leading cause (10.7%) in 2007 (CDC, 2023). In 2019, suicide was found to be the fourth leading cause of death for adolescents ages 15–19; however, for female adolescents, it was estimated to be the third leading cause of death (WHO, 2021).

The 2019 Youth Risk Behavior Survey (YRBS) reported linear trends on suicidal ideation and behaviors in U. S. adolescents from 2009 to 2019. The YRBS is a cross-sectional, school-based survey conducted every 2 years since 1991 from a nationally representative sample of public and private students in grades 9–12. Trends over time revealed an increase in adolescent reports of having seriously considered attempting suicide (18.8% in 2019 vs 13.8% in 2009), having planned how they would attempt suicide (15.7% in 2019 vs 10.9% in 2009), having attempted suicide (8.9% in 2019 vs 6.3% in 2009), and having been injured from a suicide attempt (2.5% in 2019 vs 1.9% in 2009). The YRBS study showed a higher prevalence of female high school student suicidal thoughts and behaviors compared to male peers. In the most recent survey of 2019, 24.1% of females (compared to 13.3% of males) reported having seriously considered attempting suicide during the 12 months prior to the survey, 19.9% of females (vs 11.3% males) reported having planned how they would attempt suicide, and 11% of females (vs 6.6% males) reported having attempted suicide. In 2019, female students expressed persistent feelings of sadness or hopelessness 46.6% and were nearly twice as likely to make a suicide plan compared to male students (CDC, 2022). The summary of results shows minimal progress has been made in mental health and suicide-related behaviors and perhaps worsened by the COVID-19 pandemic.

Although historically studies found that males had higher rates of completed suicide while females had higher rates of suicidal ideation and attempts, recent data shows that this gender gap is closing. Analysis of two decades (2000–2019) of suicide mortality data from the U. S. National Vital Statistics System found that females ages 10–14 had the steepest increase in suicide rates, more than doubling, from 0.9 to 2 per 100,000. The CDC reported that suicide attempt by firearm and suffocation in females had significantly increased compared to suicide attempts by poisoning (Hedegaard et al., 2021).

There is a disproportionate decline in mental health among female adolescents. Following analysis of data from 275,000 adolescents from regions of varying income among 82 countries, Biswas et al. (2020) found the prevalence of suicidal ideation (13.0%) and anxiety (9.2%) was higher for female youth compared to males, whose prevalence was 10.1% and 7.4%, respectively. Multiple logistic regression analysis identified the following risk factors to be associated with adolescent suicidal ideation and anxiety: being female; older age; low socioeconomic status; and absence of close friends. Specific risk factors for suicide attempts in adolescent females include having an eating disorder, PTSD, bipolar disorder, symptoms of depression, being victim to dating violence, interpersonal problems, and history of abortion (Miranda-Mendizabal et al., 2019).

Global Pandemic Impact on Adolescent Mental Health

COVID-19 was declared a global pandemic in March 2020. The announcement disrupted and altered life irreversibly and redefined the picture of home, school, and community. While research on mental health of individuals exposed to disasters has shown the majority of those exposed are able to cope well, research of past disasters shows a substantial number of individuals suffer psychological distress and a proportion of those develop mental health disorders. Risk factors for developing a post-disaster mental health condition include female gender, younger age, pre-existing mental health disorders, ethnic minorities, low socioeconomic status, and poor social support (Goldmann & Galea, 2014). Death in the family impacted child psychological distress as 140,000 children lost a caregiver to COVID-19 in the United States as of June 2021 (Hillis et al., 2021).

The preexisting youth mental health crisis was exacerbated by the pandemic. Children and adolescents with intellectual and developmental disabilities, including ASD, were negatively impacted by the inability to access services typically offered in school settings, such as occupational and speech therapies, counseling, and special education, and they struggled to cope with disruption to routines and school. Masi et al. (2021) surveyed caregivers of children ages 2–7 with neurodevelopmental disorders, including ADHD and ASD, and found that 64.7% of the children had worsened symptoms of the disorder or a comorbid psychiatric disorder and 76.9% had worsened well-being by the COVID-19 pandemic from caregiver reports (Masi et al., 2021). Mental health conditions also impacted physical illness, as it was found the risk of severe COVID-19 illness increased in children with schizophrenia-spectrum disorders or mood disorders (Office of the Surgeon General, 2021).

For some children and adolescents, being made to stay at home is likely to have increased the risk of family stress or abuse, which are known risk factors for mental health problems (WHO, 2022). During the pandemic, there was an increase in emergency calls of child victims of violence in France. Additionally, there was an increase in the risk of sexual exploitation of children online in Europe (Thibaut & van Wijngaarden-Cremers, 2020). Signs of abuse and mental health conditions may have been more difficult to identify in children and adolescents with reduced in-person contact outside the home due to quarantine measures. The 2021 U. S. Surgeon General's advisory, *Protecting Youth Mental Health,* called for a rapid and coordinated response to the unprecedented impacts from the pandemic on mental health.

A meta-analysis of 29 studies involving about 81,000 youths found the global prevalence in anxiety and depression doubled during the pandemic and significantly worsened with time in girls and older adolescents (Racine et al., 2021). *The Mental Health of Children and Young People in England* wave 2 survey examined the mental health of children and adolescents in 2021 compared to 2017. The survey's findings for adolescent girls were alarming, with approximately one in four girls between the ages of 17 and 19 (24.8%) likely having a mental health disorder in 2021, almost twice the rate of one in seven girls (13.4%) in 2017 (Newlove-Delgado et al., 2021). A study that analyzed the pandemic's impact on mental well-being across the lifespan in the United States found adolescents had an increased rate of clinically significant symptoms of PTSD, anxiety, depression, and suicidal ideation compared to adults (Murata et al., 2021). Females disproportionately had a greater increase in depression and anxiety than males following the COVID-19 pandemic, likely related to school closures and limited peer interaction for both sexes.

Emergency department (ED) visits related to adolescent mental health increased by 31% in 2020 compared to 2019. Analyzing data from the National Syndromic Surveillance Program, the CDC examined ED visits for suspected suicide attempts in ages 12–25 during three distinct phases of the COVID-19 pandemic during January 1st, 2019 to May 15th, 2021 and compared it to the 2019 data to analyze trends. In May 2020, adolescent ED visits for suspected suicide attempts began to increase, with up to 50.6% higher mean weekly visits during February 21st to March 20th, 2021 among female adolescents aged 12–17 compared to 4% increase in males in the same period of 2019 (Yard et al., 2021).

The COVID-19 pandemic has additionally contributed to worsening disordered eating over the last few years. Per a systematic review, there was an 83% increase in hospital admissions for pediatric patients with eating disorders during the pandemic (Devoe et al., 2023). A retrospective review of medical records of pediatric patients on an eating disorder unit during the 8-week COVID-19 lockdown in Spain found that 41.9% of patients experienced resurfacing of disordered eating as well as emotional distress during the lockdown. In addition, 93.3% of patients were admitted during that time due to self-injury and suicide risk as well as reactivation of eating disorder symptoms (Graell et al., 2020).

Although there were many negatives from the pandemic, some teens reported improved mental health during the pandemic due to reported reduction in perceived academic stress, decreased bullying, more schedule flexibility, improved amount of sleep, and increased quality time with their family (Office of the Surgeon General, 2021). Despite some unexpected positives, the negative impact of the COVID-19 pandemic on mental health, social life, school disruption, and loss of loved ones disproportionately affected vulnerable children and adolescents and widened disparities (Jones, 2021).

Implications for Women's Behavioral Health

On a global level, female adolescents across 73 countries were found to have poorer mental health than male counterparts based on 4 measures (psychological distress, life satisfaction, eudaemonia, hedonia). The most significant differences were found on the measures for psychological distress and life satisfaction. Interestingly, countries with higher GDP per capita and more gender equality had greater gender gaps on the mental health measures (Campbell et al., 2021).

As highlighted throughout this chapter, girls are often diagnosed with certain disorders later than male counterparts. In a Danish cohort study, girls had a later peak incidence of ASD, ADHD, oppositional defiant disorder, conduct disorder, other developmental disorders, and attachment disorders than boys. As most of these disorders typically present at an early age, the findings suggest delayed diagnosis in female study participants (Dalsgaard et al., 2020). Delays in the treatment of mental health disorders have been associated with poorer long-term outcomes, including worse mental and physical health (Cheung et al., 2017; McLaughlin, 2004). Additionally, mental illness has been associated with having a lower income, educational level, and level of employment, which again highlights the importance of early detection and treatment of mental health disorders (McLaughlin, 2004).

Initiatives from the U. S. Surgeon General, WHO, UNICEF, and other organizations and task forces highlight the need for mental health and well-being to be a priority for all, yet it is underfunded and underinvested particularly for adolescents. Global mental health research investments between 2015 and 2019 of $3.7 billion annually translates to about 50 cents per person per year while only one-third of that investment is allocated to youth mental health research, despite knowledge of peak onset in this age group and importance of early intervention to minimize suffering (Hayes et al., 2023). Improvements in mental health surveillance would assist in identifying protective and risk factors in children for mental health disorders, recognizing most indicated prevention measures and treatments, and guide public health initiatives to promote and support mental health in children of all ages. Furthermore, surveillance provides identification of structural and systemic differences to help toward the promotion of health equity (Bitsko et al., 2022).

One of the first steps to better understand child and adolescent mental health is access to data, which makes efforts like the "Measurement of Mental Health Among Adolescents at the Population Level" from a global collaboration so important (Carvajal-Velez et al., 2023). Epidemiological studies allow us to identify and assess the impact of mental health disorders, recognize gaps and inequities, and guide early interventions from both a clinical and public health perspective.

Although the focus of this chapter was on female biological sex, the term female gender was used interchangeably due to referenced studies not clearly differentiating between sex and gender; a current evidence gap exists for individuals who identify as gender nonconforming or nonbinary (Keyes & Platt, 2023). Future research studies should be aimed at investigating vulnerable children and adolescents belonging to gender minority, ethnic minority, and low- and middle-income countries.

In summary, it is imperative to thoroughly assess female youth to avoid overlooking important etiology and symptoms. Understanding gender differences in mental health disorders can aid clinicians in appropriately diagnosing mental health conditions and improve global and national health care delivery systems. Ultimately, all should be striving to reduce gender gaps, which will in turn improve long-term functioning of females and decrease the global mental health burden.

References

American Psychiatric Association. (2022). *Diagnostic and statistical manual of mental disorders, Fifth edition, Text revision (DSM-5-TR)* [Book]. Author.

Bandelow, B., & Michaelis, S. (2015). Epidemiology of anxiety disorders in the 21st century. *Dialogues in Clinical Neuroscience, 17*(3), 327–335. https://doi.org/10.31887/DCNS.2015.17.3/bbandelow

Barican, J. L., Yung, D., Schwartz, C., Zheng, Y., Georgiades, K., & Waddell, C. (2022). Prevalence of childhood mental disorders in high-income countries: A systematic review and meta-analysis to inform policymaking. *Evidence-Based Mental Health, 25*(1), 36–44. https://doi.org/10.1136/ebmental-2021-300277

Biswas, T., Scott, J. G., Munir, K., Renzaho, A. M. N., Rawal, L. B., Baxter, J., & Mamun, A. A. (2020). Global variation in the prevalence of suicidal ideation, anxiety and their correlates among adolescents: A population based study of 82 countries. *EClinicalMedicine, 24*, 100395. https://doi.org/10.1016/j.eclinm.2020.100395

Bitsko, R. H., Claussen, A. H., Lichstein, J., Black, L. I., Jones, S. E., Danielson, M. L., Hoenig, J. M., Davis Jack, S. P., Brody, D. J., Gyawali, S., Maenner, M. J., Warner, M., Holland, K. M., Perou, R., Crosby, A. E., Blumberg, S. J., Avenevoli, S., Kaminski, J. W., & Ghandour, R. M. (2022). Mental health surveillance among children—United States, 2013-2019. *MMWR Supplements, 71*(2), 1–42. https://doi.org/10.15585/mmwr.su7102a1

Bor, W., Dean, A. J., Najman, J., & Hayatbakhsh, R. (2014). Are child and adolescent mental health problems increasing in the 21st century? A systematic review. *Australian and New Zealand Journal of Psychiatry, 48*(7), 606–616. https://doi.org/10.1177/0004867414533834

Brasso, C., Giordano, B., Badino, C., Bellino, S., Bozzatello, P., Montemagni, C., & Rocca, P. (2021). Primary psychosis: Risk and protective factors and early detection of the onset. *Diagnostics (Basel), 11*(11). https://doi.org/10.3390/diagnostics11112146

Campbell, O. L. K., Bann, D., & Patalay, P. (2021). The gender gap in adolescent mental health: A cross-national investigation of 566,829 adolescents across 73 countries. *SSM Population Health, 13*, 100742. https://doi.org/10.1016/j.ssmph.2021.100742

Cantwell, D. P., Lewinsohn, P. M., Rohde, P., & Seeley, J. R. (1997). Correspondence between adolescent report and parent report of psychiatric diagnostic data. *Journal of the American Academy of Child and Adolescent Psychiatry, 36*(5), 610–619. https://doi.org/10.1097/00004583-199705000-00011

Carvajal-Velez, L., Harris Requejo, J., Ahs, J. W., Idele, P., Adewuya, A., Cappa, C., Guthold, R., Kapungu, C., Kieling, C., Patel, V., Patton, G., Scott, J. G., Servili, C., Wasserman, D., & Kohrt, B. A. (2023). Increasing data and understanding of adolescent mental health worldwide: UNICEF's measurement of mental health among adolescents at the population level initiative. *Journal of Adolescent Health, 72*(1s), S12–s14. https://doi.org/10.1016/j.jadohealth.2021.03.019

Centers for Disease Control and Prevention. (2022). *1991–2021 high school youth risk behavior survey data* [Report]. https://www.cdc.gov/healthyyouth/data/yrbs/pdf/YRBSDataSummaryTrendsReport2019-508.pdf

Centers for Disease Control and Prevention, & National Center for Injury Prevention and Control. (2023). *Leading causes of death and years of potential life lost data visualization 2001–2020* [Web-based Injury Statistics Query and Reporting System (WISQARS) Dataset: Elements selected: Years 2007–2020 & custom age range 10–17]. U. S. Department of Health & Human Services. https://wisqars.cdc.gov/data/icd/home

Cheung, R., O'Donnell, S., Madi, N., & Goldner, E. (2017). Factors associated with delayed diagnosis of mood and/or anxiety disorders. *Health Promotion and Chronic Disease Prevention in Canada: Research, Policy and Practice, 37*(5), 137–148. https://doi.org/10.24095/hpcdp.37.5.02

Children's Bureau. (2023). *Child maltreatment 2021* [Report]. U. S. Department of Health & Human Services & Administration on Children, Youth & Families. https://www.acf.hhs.gov/sites/default/files/documents/cb/cm2021.pdf

Cirone, C., Secci, I., Favole, I., Ricci, F., Amianto, F., Davico, C., & Vitiello, B. (2021). What do we know about the long-term course of early onset bipolar disorder? A review of the current evidence. *Brain Sciences, 11*(3). https://doi.org/10.3390/brainsci11030341

Copeland, W. E., Angold, A., Costello, E. J., & Egger, H. (2013). Prevalence, comorbidity, and correlates of DSM-5 proposed disruptive mood dysregulation disorder. *American Journal of Psychiatry, 170*(2), 173–179. https://doi.org/10.1176/appi.ajp.2012.12010132

Croft, J., Heron, J., Teufel, C., Cannon, M., Wolke, D., Thompson, A., Houtepen, L., & Zammit, S. (2019). Association of trauma type, age of exposure, and frequency in childhood and adolescence with psychotic experiences in early adulthood. *JAMA Psychiatry, 76*(1), 79–86. https://doi.org/10.1001/jamapsychiatry.2018.3155

Dalsgaard, S., Thorsteinsson, E., Trabjerg, B. B., Schullehner, J., Plana-Ripoll, O., Brikell, I., Wimberley, T., Thygesen, M., Madsen, K. B., Timmerman, A., Schendel, D., McGrath, J. J., Mortensen, P. B., & Pedersen, C. B. (2020). Incidence rates and cumulative incidences of the full spectrum of diagnosed mental disorders in childhood and adolescence. *JAMA Psychiatry, 77*(2), 155–164. https://doi.org/10.1001/jamapsychiatry.2019.3523

Danielson, M. L., Bitsko, R. H., Holbrook, J. R., Charania, S. N., Claussen, A. H., McKeown, R. E., Cuffe, S. P., Owens, J. S., Evans, S. W., Kubicek, L., & Flory, K. (2021). Community-based prevalence of externalizing and internalizing disorders among school-aged children and adolescents in four geographically dispersed school districts in the United States. *Child Psychiatry and Human Development, 52*(3), 500–514. https://doi.org/10.1007/s10578-020-01027-z

Devoe, J., Han, A., Anderson, A., Katzman, D. K., Patten, S. B., Soumbasis, A., Flanagan, J., Paslakis, G., Vyver, E., Marcoux, G., & Dimitropoulos, G. (2023). The impact of the COVID-19 pandemic on eating disorders: A systematic review. *International Journal of Eating Disorders, 56*(1), 5–25. https://doi.org/10.1002/eat.23704

Elsabbagh, M. (2020). Linking risk factors and outcomes in autism spectrum disorder: Is there evidence for resilience? *BMJ, 368*, l6880. https://doi.org/10.1136/bmj.l6880

Eskander, N., Vadukapuram, R., Zahid, S., Ashraf, S., & Patel, R. S. (2020). Post-traumatic stress disorder and suicidal behaviors in American adolescents: Analysis of 159,500 psychiatric hospitalizations. *Cureus, 12*(5), e8017. https://doi.org/10.7759/cureus.8017

Figas, K., Giannouchos, T. V., & Crouch, E. (2023). Child and adolescent anxiety and depression prior to and during the COVID-19 pandemic in the United States. *Child Psychiatry and Human Development*, 1–11. https://doi.org/10.1007/s10578-023-01536-7

Frazier, T. W., Georgiades, S., Bishop, S. L., & Hardan, A. Y. (2014). Behavioral and cognitive characteristics of females and males with autism in the Simons Simplex Collection. *Journal of the American Academy of Child and Adolescent Psychiatry, 53*(3), 329-340.e321-323. https://doi.org/10.1016/j.jaac.2013.12.004

Garza, K., & Jovanovic, T. (2017). Impact of gender on child and adolescent PTSD. *Current Psychiatry Reports, 19*(11), 87. https://doi.org/10.1007/s11920-017-0830-6

Ghandour, R. M., Sherman, L. J., Vladutiu, C. J., Ali, M. M., Lynch, S. E., Bitsko, R. H., & Blumberg, S. J. (2019). Prevalence and treatment of depression, anxiety, and conduct problems in US children. *Journal of Pediatrics, 206*, 256–267.e253. https://doi.org/10.1016/j.jpeds.2018.09.021

Goldmann, E., & Galea, S. (2014). Mental health consequences of disasters. *Annual Review of Public Health, 35*, 169–183. https://doi.org/10.1146/annurev-publhealth-032013-182435

Goldstein, T. R., Ha, W., Axelson, D. A., Goldstein, B. I., Liao, F., Gill, M. K., Ryan, N. D., Yen, S., Hunt, J., Hower, H., Keller, M., Strober, M., & Birmaher, B. (2012). Predictors of prospectively examined suicide attempts among youth with bipolar disorder. *Archives of General Psychiatry, 69*(11), 1113–1122. https://doi.org/10.1001/archgenpsychiatry.2012.650

Graell, M., Morón-Nozaleda, M. G., Camarneiro, R., Villaseñor, Á., Yáñez, S., Muñoz, R., Martínez-Núñez, B., Miguélez-Fernández, C., Muñoz, M., & Faya, M. (2020). Children and adolescents with eating disorders during COVID-19 confinement: Difficulties and future challenges. *European Eating Disorders Review: The Journal of the Eating Disorders Association, 28*(6), 864–870. https://doi.org/10.1002/erv.2763

Haag, K., Fraser, A., Hiller, R., Seedat, S., Zimmerman, A., & Halligan, S. L. (2020). The emergence of sex differences in PTSD symptoms across development: Evidence from the ALSPAC cohort. *Psychological Medicine, 50*(10), 1755–1760. https://doi.org/10.1017/s0033291719001971

Hayes, J., Carvajal-Velez, L., Hijazi, Z., Ahs, J. W., Doraiswamy, P. M., El Azzouzi, F. A., Fox, C., Herrman, H., Gornitzka, C. P., Staglin, B., & Wolpert, M. (2023). You can't manage what you do not measure: Why adolescent mental health monitoring matters. *Journal of Adolescent Health, 72*(1s), S7–s8. https://doi.org/10.1016/j.jadohealth.2021.04.024

Hedegaard, H., Curtin, S. C., & Warner, M. (2021). Suicide mortality in the United States, 1999-2019. *NCHS Data Brief, 398*, 1–8. https://www.cdc.gov/nchs/data/databriefs/db398-H.pdf

Hillis, S. D., Blenkinsop, A., Villaveces, A., Annor, F. B., Liburd, L., Massetti, G. M., Demissie, Z., Mercy, J. A., Nelson Iii, C. A., Cluver, L., Flaxman, S., Sherr, L., Donnelly, C. A., Ratmann, O., & Unwin, H. J. T. (2021). COVID-19-associated orphanhood and caregiver death in the United States. *Pediatrics, 148*(6). https://doi.org/10.1542/peds.2021-053760

Hinshaw, S. P., Nguyen, P. T., O'Grady, S. M., & Rosenthal, E. A. (2022). Annual research review: Attention-deficit/hyperactivity disorder in girls and women: Underrepresentation, longitudinal processes, and key directions. *Journal of Child Psychology and Psychiatry, and Allied Disciplines, 63*(4), 484–496. https://doi.org/10.1111/jcpp.13480

Jones, K. (2021, August). *The initial impact of COVID-19 on children and youth (birth to 24 years): Literature review in brief* [Report]. U. S. Department of Health and Human Services & Office of the Assistant Secretary for Planning and Evaluation. https://aspe.hhs.gov/reports/impact-covid-19-children-youth

Kessler, R. C., Berglund, P., Demler, O., Jin, R., Merikangas, K. R., & Walters, E. E. (2005). Lifetime prevalence and age-of-onset distributions of DSM-IV disorders in the National Comorbidity Survey Replication. *Archives of General Psychiatry, 62*(6), 593–602. https://doi.org/10.1001/archpsyc.62.6.593

Kessler, R. C., Petukhova, M., Sampson, N. A., Zaslavsky, A. M., & Wittchen, H. U. (2012). Twelve-month and lifetime prevalence and lifetime morbid risk of anxiety and mood disorders in the United States. *International Journal of Methods in Psychiatric Research, 21*(3), 169–184. https://doi.org/10.1002/mpr.1359

Keyes, K. M., & Platt, J. M. (2023). Annual research review: Sex, gender, and internalizing conditions among adolescents in the 21st century—Trends, causes, consequences. *Journal of Child Psychology and Psychiatry, and Allied Disciplines*. https://doi.org/10.1111/jcpp.13864

Lewinsohn, P. M., Klein, D. N., & Seeley, J. R. (2000). Bipolar disorder during adolescence and young adulthood in a community sample. *Bipolar Disorders, 2*(3 Pt 2), 281–293. https://doi.org/10.1034/j.1399-5618.2000.20309.x

Lockwood Estrin, G., Milner, V., Spain, D., Happé, F., & Colvert, E. (2021). Barriers to autism spectrum disorder diagnosis for young women and girls: A systematic review. *Review Journal of Autism and Developmental Disorders, 8*(4), 454–470. https://doi.org/10.1007/s40489-020-00225-8

Loyer Carbonneau, M., Demers, M., Bigras, M., & Guay, M. C. (2021). Meta-analysis of sex differences in ADHD symptoms and associated cognitive deficits. *Journal of Attention Disorders, 25*(12), 1640–1656. https://doi.org/10.1177/1087054720923736

Maenner, M. J., Warren, Z., Williams, A. R., Amoakohene, E., Bakian, A. V., Bilder, D. A., Durkin, M. S., Fitzgerald, R. T., Furnier, S. M., Hughes, M. M., Ladd-Acosta, C. M., McArthur, D., Pas, E. T., Salinas, A., Vehorn, A., Williams, S., Esler, A., Grzybowski, A., Hall-Lande, J., Nguyen, R. H. N., Pierce, K., Zahorodny, W., Hudson, A., Hallas, L., Mancilla, K. C., Patrick, M., Shenouda, J., Sidwell, K., DiRienzo, M., Gutierrez, J., Spivey, M. H., Lopez, M., Pettygrove, S., Schwenk, Y. D., Washington, A., & Shaw, K. A. (2023). Prevalence and characteristics of autism spectrum disorder among children aged 8 years—Autism and developmental disabilities monitoring network, 11 sites, United States, 2020. *MMWR Surveillance Summaries, 72*(2), 1–14. https://doi.org/10.15585/mmwr.ss7202a1

Masi, A., Mendoza Diaz, A., Tully, L., Azim, S. I., Woolfenden, S., Efron, D., & Eapen, V. (2021). Impact of the COVID-19 pandemic on the well-being of children with neurodevelopmental disabilities and their parents. *Journal of Paediatrics and Child Health, 57*(5), 631–636. https://doi.org/10.1111/jpc.15285

Matson, J. L., & Kozlowski, A. M. (2011). The increasing prevalence of autism spectrum disorders. *Research in Autism Spectrum Disorders, 5*(1), 418–425. https://doi.org/10.1016/j.rasd.2010.06.004

McLaughlin, C. G. (2004). Delays in treatment for mental disorders and health insurance coverage. *Health Services Research, 39*(2), 221–224. https://doi.org/10.1111/j.1475-6773.2004.00224.x

Melton, T. H., Croarkin, P. E., Strawn, J. R., & McClintock, S. M. (2016). Comorbid anxiety and depressive symptoms in children and adolescents: A systematic review and analysis. *Journal of Psychiatric Practice, 22*(2), 84–98. https://doi.org/10.1097/pra.0000000000000132

Merikangas, K. R., Nakamura, E. F., & Kessler, R. C. (2009). Epidemiology of mental disorders in children and adolescents. *Dialogues in Clinical Neuroscience, 11*(1), 7–20. https://doi.org/10.31887/DCNS.2009.11.1/krmerikangas

Miranda-Mendizabal, A., Castellví, P., Parés-Badell, O., Alayo, I., Almenara, J., Alonso, I., Blasco, M. J., Cebrià, A., Gabilondo, A., Gili, M., Lagares, C., Piqueras, J. A., Rodríguez-Jiménez, T., Rodríguez-Marín, J., Roca, M., Soto-Sanz, V., Vilagut, G., & Alonso, J. (2019). Gender differences in suicidal behavior in adolescents and young adults: Systematic review and meta-analysis of longitudinal studies. *International Journal of Public Health, 64*(2), 265–283. https://doi.org/10.1007/s00038-018-1196-1

Murata, S., Rezeppa, T., Thoma, B., Marengo, L., Krancevich, K., Chiyka, E., Hayes, B., Goodfriend, E., Deal, M., Zhong, Y., Brummit, B., Coury, T., Riston, S., Brent, D. A., & Melhem, N. M. (2021). The psychiatric sequelae of the COVID-19 pandemic in adolescents, adults, and health care workers. *Depression and Anxiety, 38*(2), 233–246. https://doi.org/10.1002/da.23120

Murray, R. M., Mondelli, V., Stilo, S. A., Trotta, A., Sideli, L., Ajnakina, O., Ferraro, L., Vassos, E., Iyegbe, C., Schoeler, T., Bhattacharyya, S., Marques, T. R., Dazzan, P., Lopez-Morinigo, J., Colizzi, M., O'Connor, J., Falcone, M. A., Quattrone, D., Rodriguez, V., Tripoli, G., La Barbera, D., La Cascia, C., Alameda, L., Trotta, G., Morgan, C., Gaughran, F., David, A., & Di Forti, M. (2020). The influence of risk factors on the onset and outcome of psychosis: What we learned from the GAP study. *Schizophrenia Research, 225*, 63–68. https://doi.org/10.1016/j.schres.2020.01.011

National Eating Disorders Association. (2021). *Statistics & research on eating disorders* [Web page]. Author [NEDA]. https://www.nationaleatingdisorders.org/statistics-research-eating-disorders

Newlove-Delgado, T., Williams, T., Robertson, K., McManus, S., Sadler, K., Vizard, T., Cartwright, C., Mathews, F., Norman, S., Marcheselli, F., & Ford, T. (2021). *Mental health of children and young people in England, 2021: Wave 2 follow up to the 2017 survey* [Report]. NHS Digital. https://digital.nhs.uk/data-and-information/publications/statistical/mental-health-of-children-and-young-people-in-england/2021-follow-up-to-the-2017-survey#

Office of the Surgeon General. (2021). *Protecting youth mental health: The U.S. Surgeon General's advisory* [Report]. U. S. Department of Health and Human Services. https://www.ncbi.nlm.nih.gov/books/NBK575985/

Parodi, K. B., Holt, M. K., Green, J. G., Porche, M. V., Koenig, B., & Xuan, Z. (2022). Time trends and disparities in anxiety among adolescents, 2012-2018. *Social Psychiatry and Psychiatric Epidemiology, 57*(1), 127–137. https://doi.org/10.1007/s00127-021-02122-9

Piao, J., Huang, Y., Han, C., Li, Y., Xu, Y., Liu, Y., & He, X. (2022). Alarming changes in the global burden of mental disorders in children and adolescents from 1990 to 2019: A systematic analysis for the Global Burden of Disease study. *European Child and Adolescent Psychiatry, 31*(11), 1827–1845. https://doi.org/10.1007/s00787-022-02040-4

Polanczyk, G., de Lima, M. S., Horta, B. L., Biederman, J., & Rohde, L. A. (2007). The worldwide prevalence of ADHD: A systematic review and metaregression analysis. *American Journal of Psychiatry, 164*(6), 942–948. https://doi.org/10.1176/ajp.2007.164.6.942

Polanczyk, G. V., Salum, G. A., Sugaya, L. S., Caye, A., & Rohde, L. A. (2015). Annual research review: A meta-analysis of the worldwide prevalence of mental disorders in children and adolescents. *Journal of Child Psychology and Psychiatry, and Allied Disciplines, 56*(3), 345–365. https://doi.org/10.1111/jcpp.12381

Racine, N., McArthur, B. A., Cooke, J. E., Eirich, R., Zhu, J., & Madigan, S. (2021). Global prevalence of depressive and anxiety symptoms in children and adolescents during COVID-19: A meta-analysis. *JAMA Pediatrics, 175*(11), 1142–1150. https://doi.org/10.1001/jamapediatrics.2021.2482

Radua, J., Ramella-Cravaro, V., Ioannidis, J. P. A., Reichenberg, A., Phiphopthatsanee, N., Amir, T., Yenn Thoo, H., Oliver, D., Davies, C., Morgan, C., McGuire, P., Murray, R. M., & Fusar-Poli, P. (2018). What causes psychosis? An umbrella review of risk and protective factors. *World Psychiatry, 17*(1), 49–66. https://doi.org/10.1002/wps.20490

Reas, D. L., & Rø, Ø. (2018). Time trends in healthcare-detected incidence of anorexia nervosa and bulimia nervosa in the Norwegian National Patient Register (2010-2016). *International Journal of Eating Disorders, 51*(10), 1144–1152. https://doi.org/10.1002/eat.22949

Roberson-Nay, R., Leibenluft, E., Brotman, M. A., Myers, J., Larsson, H., Lichtenstein, P., & Kendler, K. S. (2015). Longitudinal stability of genetic and environmental influences on irritability: From childhood to young adulthood. *American Journal of Psychiatry, 172*(7), 657–664. https://doi.org/10.1176/appi.ajp.2015.14040509

Saunders, B. E., & Adams, Z. W. (2014). Epidemiology of traumatic experiences in childhood. *Child and Adolescent Psychiatric Clinics of North America, 23*(2), 167–184., vii. https://doi.org/10.1016/j.chc.2013.12.003

Saxena, A., & Dodell-Feder, D. (2022). Explaining the association between urbanicity and psychotic-like experiences in pre-adolescence: The indirect effect of urban exposures. *Frontiers in Psychiatry, 13*(March), 831089. https://doi.org/10.3389/fpsyt.2022.831089

Sidani, J. E., Shensa, A., Hoffman, B., Hanmer, J., & Primack, B. A. (2016). The association between social media use and eating concerns among US young adults. *Journal of the Academy of Nutrition and Dietetics, 116*(9), 1465–1472. https://doi.org/10.1016/j.jand.2016.03.021

Solmi, M., Radua, J., Olivola, M., Croce, E., Soardo, L., Salazar de Pablo, G., Il Shin, J., Kirkbride, J. B., Jones, P., Kim, J. H., Kim, J. Y., Carvalho, A. F., Seeman, M. V., Correll, C. U., & Fusar-Poli, P. (2022). Age at onset of mental disorders worldwide: Large-scale meta-analysis of 192 epidemiological studies. *Molecular Psychiatry, 27*(1), 281–295. https://doi.org/10.1038/s41380-021-01161-7

Spoelma, M. J., Sicouri, G. L., Francis, D. A., Songco, A. D., Daniel, E. K., & Hudson, J. L. (2023). Estimated prevalence of depressive disorders in children from 2004 to 2019: A systematic review and meta-analysis. *JAMA Pediatrics*. https://doi.org/10.1001/jamapediatrics.2023.3221

Stainton, A., Chisholm, K., Woodall, T., Hallett, D., Reniers, R., Lin, A., & Wood, S. J. (2021). Gender differences in the experience of psychotic-like experiences and their associated factors: A study of adolescents from the general population. *Schizophrenia Research, 228*, 410–416. https://doi.org/10.1016/j.schres.2021.01.008

Stice, E., Marti, C. N., Shaw, H., & Jaconis, M. (2009). An 8-year longitudinal study of the natural history of threshold, subthreshold, and partial eating disorders from a community sample of adolescents. *Journal of Abnormal Psychology, 118*(3), 587–597. https://doi.org/10.1037/a0016481

Stice, E., Marti, C. N., & Rohde, P. (2013). Prevalence, incidence, impairment, and course of the proposed DSM-5 eating disorder diagnoses in an 8-year prospective community study of young women. *Journal of Abnormal Psychology, 122*(2), 445–457. https://doi.org/10.1037/a0030679

Thapar, A., Collishaw, S., Pine, D. S., & Thapar, A. K. (2012). Depression in adolescence. *Lancet, 379*(9820), 1056–1067. https://doi.org/10.1016/s0140-6736(11)60871-4

Thibaut, F., & van Wijngaarden-Cremers, P. J. M. (2020). Women's mental health in the time of Covid-19 pandemic. *Frontiers in Global Women's Health, 1*, 588372. https://doi.org/10.3389/fgwh.2020.588372

Thomas, R., Sanders, S., Doust, J., Beller, E., & Glasziou, P. (2015). Prevalence of attention-deficit/hyperactivity disorder: A systematic review and meta-analysis. *Pediatrics, 135*(4), e994–e1001. https://doi.org/10.1542/peds.2014-3482

Tkacz, J., & Brady, B. L. (2021). Increasing rate of diagnosed childhood mental illness in the United States: Incidence, prevalence and costs. *Public Health in Practice, 2*, 100204. https://doi.org/10.1016/j.puhip.2021.100204

U. S. Preventive Services Task Force, Mangione, C. M., Barry, M. J., Nicholson, W. K., Cabana, M., Chelmow, D., Coker, T. R., Davidson, K. W., Davis, E. M., Donahue, K. E., Jaén, C. R., Kubik, M., Li, L., Ogedegbe, G., Pbert, L., Ruiz, J. M., Silverstein, M., Stevermer, J., & Wong, J. B. (2022a). Screening for depression and suicide risk in children and adolescents: US Preventive Services Task Force recommendation statement. *JAMA, 328*(15), 1534–1542. https://doi.org/10.1001/jama.2022.16946

U. S. Preventive Services Task Force, Mangione, C. M., Barry, M. J., Nicholson, W. K., Cabana, M., Coker, T. R., Davidson, K. W., Davis, E. M., Donahue, K. E., Jaén, C. R., Kubik, M., Li, L., Ogedegbe, G., Pbert, L., Ruiz, J. M., Silverstein, M., Stevermer, J., & Wong, J. B. (2022b). Screening for anxiety in children and adolescents: US Preventive Services Task Force recommendation statement. *JAMA, 328*(14), 1438–1444. https://doi.org/10.1001/jama.2022.16936

UNICEF. (2014a, October). *A statistical snapshot of violence against adolescent girls* [Report; Download link]. United Nations Children's Fund. https://data.unicef.org/resources/statistical-snapshot-violence-adolescent-girls/

UNICEF. (2014b, September). *Ending violence against children: Six strategies for action* [Report]. United Nations Children's Fund. https://www.unicef.org/media/66906/file/Ending-Violence-Against-Children-Six-strategies-For-Action.pdf

UNICEF. (2021, October). *The state of the world's children 2021: On my mind: Promoting, protecting and caring for children's mental health* [Report]. United Nations Children's Fund. https://www.unicef.org/media/114636/file/SOWC-2021-full-report-English.pdf

UNICEF. (2022, April). *Adolescents* [Web page]. United Nations Children's Fund. https://data.unicef.org/topic/adolescents/overview/

Vasileva, M., Graf, R. K., Reinelt, T., Petermann, U., & Petermann, F. (2021). Research review: A meta-analysis of the international prevalence and comorbidity of mental disorders in children between 1 and 7 years. *Journal of Child Psychology and Psychiatry, 62*(4), 372–381. https://doi.org/10.1111/jcpp.13261

Vogels, E. A. (2022). *Teens and cyberbullying 2022* [Web Report]. Pew Research Center. https://www.pewresearch.org/internet/2022/12/15/teens-and-cyberbullying-2022/

Wamser-Nanney, R., & Cherry, K. E. (2018). Children's trauma-related symptoms following complex trauma exposure: Evidence of gender differences. *Child Abuse and Neglect, 77*, 188–197. https://doi.org/10.1016/j.chiabu.2018.01.009

Whitney, D. G., & Peterson, M. D. (2019). US national and state-level prevalence of mental health disorders and disparities of mental health care use in children. *JAMA Pediatrics, 173*(4), 389–391. https://doi.org/10.1001/jamapediatrics.2018.5399

Willcutt, E. G. (2012). The prevalence of DSM-IV attention-deficit/hyperactivity disorder: A meta-analytic review. *Neurotherapeutics, 9*(3), 490–499. https://doi.org/10.1007/s13311-012-0135-8

World Health Organization. (2021). *Suicide worldwide in 2019: Global health estimates* [Report]. Author [WHO]. https://apps.who.int/iris/bitstream/handle/10665/341728/9789240026643-eng.pdf?sequence=1&isAllowed=y

World Health Organization. (2022, June 16). *World mental health report: Transforming mental health for all* [Report]. Author [WHO]. https://apps.who.int/iris/rest/bitstreams/1433523/retrieve

Yard, E., Radhakrishnan, L., Ballesteros, M. F., Sheppard, M., Gates, A., Stein, Z., Hartnett, K., Kite-Powell, A., Rodgers, L., Adjemian, J., Ehlman, D. C., Holland, K., Idaikkadar, N., Ivey-Stephenson, A., Martinez, P., Law, R., & Stone, D. M. (2021). Emergency department visits for suspected suicide attempts among persons aged 12-25 years before and during the COVID-19 pandemic—United States, January 2019-May 2021. *MMWR. Morbidity and Mortality Weekly Report, 70*(24), 888–894. https://doi.org/10.15585/mmwr.mm7024e1

Zablotsky, B., Black, L. I., Maenner, M. J., Schieve, L. A., Danielson, M. L., Bitsko, R. H., Blumberg, S. J., Kogan, M. D., & Boyle, C. A. (2019). Prevalence and trends of developmental disabilities among children in the United States: 2009-2017. *Pediatrics, 144*(4). https://doi.org/10.1542/peds.2019-0811

Zeidan, J., Fombonne, E., Scorah, J., Ibrahim, A., Durkin, M. S., Saxena, S., Yusuf, A., Shih, A., & Elsabbagh, M. (2022). Global prevalence of autism: A systematic review update. *Autism Research, 15*(5), 778–790. https://doi.org/10.1002/aur.2696

Chapter 3
Epidemiology of Mental Disorders in Adult Women

Rachel Carpenter, Michael Carpenter, and Steven Cuffe

Introduction

Despite its unfortunate beginnings rooted in female "hysteria" and questionable demonological etiologies, women's mental health has maintained a ubiquitous interest throughout time (Tasca et al., 2012). One of the most extensively demonstrated findings in psychiatric epidemiology has been gender differences, even when considering age and cultural variation (Blehar, 2006). This difference was solely once attributed to the uterus as an explanation of female's vulnerable physiology and psychology (Tasca et al., 2012). We now understand that women have a unique biopsychosocial experience that may play a role in the development of mental health disorders (Tasca et al., 2012).

This understanding continues to evolve in the context of the COVID-19 pandemic. The Global Burden of Disease analyses report depression and anxiety alone are among the top causes of poor health globally. Women reported 52 million more cases of anxiety disorders and more than 35 million major depressive disorder cases in 2020 compared to 2019. This is in contrast to their male counterparts who increased by 24 million and 18 million cases in anxiety and depressive disorders, respectively (COVID-19 Mental Disorders Collaborators, 2021). These alarming numbers call for further exploration and understanding of the epidemiology of

R. Carpenter (✉) · S. Cuffe
Department of Psychiatry, University of Florida, College of Medicine—Jacksonville, Jacksonville, FL, USA
e-mail: Rachel.carpenter@jax.ufl.edu; Steven.cuffe@jax.ufl.edu

M. Carpenter
Department of Emergency Medicine, University of Florida, College of Medicine—Jacksonville, Jacksonville, FL, USA
e-mail: Michael.carpenter@jax.ufl.edu

49

A. Hanson, B. L. Levin (eds.), *Women's Behavioral Health*,
https://doi.org/10.1007/978-3-031-58293-6_3

women's mental disorders, specifically through the lens of distinct lifespan milestones.

It is additionally important to note that our definition of "woman" has expanded over time as well and that most of the current data are based on traditional binary gender. While we understand that rigid gender norms negatively affect individuals with diverse gender identities, we also acknowledge this chapter cannot adequately explore the mental health complexities of both women and the transgender and nonbinary populations. Thus, we will primarily explore the epidemiology of individuals assigned female at birth.

This chapter provides an overview of major mental health diagnoses among adult women in, primarily, the United States but also underscores noteworthy global statistics. Conditions are organized per their *Diagnostic and Statistical Manual of Mental Disorders, Fifth Edition (DSM-V)* classifications, discussing the most prevalent mood disorders, anxiety disorders, trauma-related disorders, obsessive-compulsive and related disorders, and psychotic disorders. Hopefully, by better understanding the unique challenges women face, specifically during the reproductive period, we can target public mental health services along with policy changes that empower women and allow them to feel in control of their lives during an extremely critical life cycle stage.

Reproductive Age

At its physiologic roots, this period of a woman's life is characterized by their period or menstruation. Menarche through menopause defines reproductive age, and this stage in the life cycle presents noteworthy biological and psychological transformations. In the United States (U.S.), there are currently over 77,000,000 women of reproductive age (World Health Organization (WHO), 2023). Worldwide, it is expected this population of women will grow to almost two billion by 2025 (Elflein, 2019).

Menstruation, pregnancy, childbirth, lactation, and the post-partum period present varying hormonal and biological shifts for women, all of which can affect mental health. Regrettably, most of the exact physiologic mechanisms of mental health disorders are still poorly understood. However, there are many well-regarded theories attempting to explain possible biological aberrations that result in mental illness including (but not limited to) genetics, epigenetics, hormonal impacts, prenatal exposures, brain injury, and infections. Ultimately, the role of sex steroids in the etiology, expression, and trajectory of mental illness is a major component of "women's mental health." While it is not in the scope of this chapter to explain these biological theories, the notable organic changes a female goes through during her reproductive years must be considered in the distribution of disease in this population.

Other considerations of both the biological and psychosocial impacts of this stage of the female experience are emphasized in menarche itself. The global average age of menarche has been 12 years old but that age has been steadily decreasing in recent years. There are many theories as to why this decrease has taken place, including environmental causes and social causes. However, one clear correlation that has been noted is between early menarche and an elevated risk for depression (Canelón & Boland, 2020).

Added impacts during this life stage stem from psychosocial contributions. Per Eriksons' stages of psychosocial development, individuals in their reproductive reign are solidifying their identity, forming relationships and families, and begin nurturing a future generation that will outlast them (Orenstein & Lewis, 2023). This period of interpersonal growth continues to change with women's morphing role in modern society. Ultimately, specific consideration of how policy, law, custom, research, and practice play a part in the female capacity for resilience is necessary to understand women's mental health as a whole. This is of particular concern and interest in the context of changing abortion laws in the United States. The COVID-19 pandemic has also emphasized clear inequalities that exist between the modern role of women and men (for more on the COVID-19 pandemic, see Chap. 4 in this volume). While detailed policy discussions and implications are beyond the scope of the chapter, understanding the epidemiological data provides insight into patterns of disease and allows us to identify crucial points in practice about the mental health needs of women. In addition, these findings can form the basis of public health decisions to improve the mental health of women and strengthen women's role in society.

Mood Disorders

We begin our discussion with mood disorders as they are the most prevalent and are associated with significant impairment for adult women. Based on the last data from the National Comorbidity Survey Replication (NCS-R) completed from 2001 to 2003, about 21.4% of U. S. adults experience a mood disorder during their lifetime (Alegria et al., 2016). In the sample of 9282 individuals included in the survey, roughly 25% of these adults were women and 17.5% were men (Alegria et al., 2016). However, during the COVID-19 pandemic, numerous surveys demonstrate a trend of increased prevalence of mental health disorders, specifically depression. In a systematic literature review of studies between Jan 1, 2020 and Jan 29, 2021, it was found that females were affected more by the pandemic than males (COVID-19 Mental Disorders Collaborators, 2021). There were an estimated 35.5 million additional cases of major depressive disorder among women compared to 17.7 million additional cases in males. Additionally, younger age groups were affected more than older age groups (COVID-19 Mental Disorders Collaborators, 2021).

Unipolar Depressive Disorders

The diagnosis of major depressive disorder (MDD) requires at least 2 weeks of sadness or anhedonia as well as four additional symptoms that can include concentration impairment, deviations in sleep patterns, feelings of worthlessness or disproportionate feelings of guilt, loss of energy, psychomotor agitation or slowing, suicidal thoughts, or weight or appetite changes (American Psychiatric Association, 2022). Based on the 2019 Global Burden of Disease (GBD) study, 280 million people are struggling with depression worldwide with 101 million being women ages 15–49 (Institute of Health Metrics and Evaluation, 2019). The incidence of depression has been increasing over the past half-century with the number of U. S. adults with MDD increasing by 12.9% between 2010 and 2018 (Greenberg et al., 2021). With this rising trend, depression is now the second leading cause of disability globally (Yoch, 2021).

The National Survey on Drug Use and Health (NSDUH) is an annual survey that examines data on the use of tobacco, alcohol, illicit drugs, and mental health in the United States. It is one of the primary sources of data for population-based prevalence estimates of mental health indicators in the United States (Hedden et al., 2012). The most recent statistics reported by the Substance Abuse and Mental Health Services Administration (SAMHSA) are sobering and continue to demonstrate the growing mental health problem in the U. S. (Twenge et al., 2019). Utilizing the NSDUH from 2005 to 2017, a cohort study assessed age, period and trends in mood disorders, and suicide-related outcomes. It found that compared to the comparable male cohorts, women aged 18–25 had the highest percentage of major depressive episodes (MDE) followed by women aged 26–49. When considering severe impairment due to their MDE, women aged 18–25 were twice as likely to experience severe impairment when compared to women aged 26 or older (Twenge et al., 2019). These differences involving both age and sex beg the question of what unique biopsychosocial factors of women result in the markedly increased rate of depression during their reproductive years. Of note, more than 10% of pregnant women and post-partum women experience depression with prevalence being higher in women from low- and middle-income countries (Woody et al., 2017).

This cohort study also considered those experiencing serious psychological distress (as defined by the Kessler-6 Distress Scale (Kessler et al., 2002)) who are impaired but not meeting the diagnostic criteria for a psychiatric disorder. When considering race and ethnicity, Hispanic Americans had the largest increase in serious psychological distress between 2008 and 2017 while Black Americans had the smallest change. White Americans had the largest increase in adult MDE, suicidal ideations, making a suicidal plan, and in suicide attempts. Finally, when considering socioeconomic status, with the exception of MDE and suicide attempts, increases were consistently largest among Americans with higher incomes. The increase in suicide attempts was largest in the second-lowest income group and the increase in adult MDE was largest in the lowest income group (Center for Behavioral Health Statistics and Quality, 2018; Twenge et al., 2019).

There are meaningful consequences that result from depressive disorders. While not the only diagnosis associated with suicide, an obvious impact of depression is on mortality rates and increasing deaths by suicide. Again, drawing from the NSDUH, rates of suicide deaths increased between 2008 and 2017. Similar to the increasing rate for 25 year olds and younger, suicide rates have also increased at the same rate among those in their late 20s and early 30s. Additionally, suicide-related outcomes (including suicidal thoughts, suicidal plans, and suicide attempts) were consistently more significant among women when compared to men. Specifically for suicide attempts, women demonstrated a 38% increase in prevalence from 2008 to 2017. Men, in contrast, had a 20% increase in prevalence (Twenge et al., 2019).

Mortality rates alone do not capture the overwhelming impact of the burden of disease associated with unipolar depression. Disability-adjusted life years (DALYs), the years of life lost due to premature mortality (YLLs), and the years lived with a disability (YLDs) also account for the prevalence of disease or health condition in a population. One DALY represents the loss of the equivalent of 1 year of full health (Global Health Observatory, 2023). The most recent GBD study demonstrated women with depression aged 15–49 account for 4.69% DALYs and 7.77% YLDs globally. In the U. S. alone, in the same cohort, depression accounts for 6.91% DALYs and 9.28% YLDs. For reference, in the U. S. for all ages and genders, the top cause of death is ischemic heart disease. It accounts for 7.9% DALYs but only 0.56% YLDs (Institute of Health Metrics and Evaluation, 2019).

Translating this to actual dollars, the incremental economic burden of adults with MDD rose from approximately $US 236 billion in 2010 to $US 326 billion in 2018 (Greenberg et al., 2021). This represents an increase of nearly 38% over this 8-year period. Adults with MDD, aged 18–34 years, had the largest increases in total incremental direct costs (i.e., 73.7% and 40.6%, respectively). In contrast, costs associated with adults aged ≥35 years decreased by 16.5% during this same 8-year time period (Greenberg et al., 2021).

It is clear that depression impacts women and men differently. While there have been studies attempting to explore why that may be, including hormonal considerations, there are limitations in pinpointing an exact etiology. Women are more likely to develop depressive symptoms after a major life stressor and are more likely to report recent stressful life events overall (Burt & Stein, 2002). Men are more likely to report symptoms of anger/aggression, irritability, substance use, and risk-taking behaviors over other symptoms, such as isolating behaviors, sleep problems, and expressing dissatisfaction (Martin et al., 2013). Potential psychosocial contributors to the gender discrepancies in the prevalence and experience of disease are explored later in this chapter.

We cannot discuss depression in reproductive women without exploring the rates of post-partum depression. It has been challenging to study post-partum depression globally due to the cultural barriers of how mothers conceptualize or explain symptoms of depression. Many mothers also feel immense guilt and adhere to expectations to fulfill this social role as "mother" without complaint (Dennis & Chung-Lee, 2006). In a landmark study of 10,000 mothers at an urban academic women's hospital, 21.9% experienced depression up to 1 year after birth. Of those women, 26.5%

had episodes prior to pregnancy, 33.4% had onset during pregnancy, and 40.1% had symptoms beginning post-partum (Wisner et al., 2013). These numbers are alarming and made worse by the finding that only 8.6% of women with antenatal depression and 6.3% of women with post-partum depression received adequate treatment (Cox et al., 2016).

Exacerbating psychosocial risk factors related to post-partum mood disorders include barriers to care/institutional racism, childcare stressors, climate stressors, complications in pregnancy/birth/breastfeeding, financial stress, health challenges in baby or parents, inadequate partner/social support, interpersonal violence (IPV), recent loss or move, relationship stress, returning to work, temperament of baby, or unresolved grief (American Psychological Association, 2022; Yim et al., 2015). Some of these issues disproportionately affect Black and other minority mothers in the United States, which is represented in data showing that Black and Latina women have a prevalence of post-partum depression of 35–67%. This is drastically higher than the 10–15% in the general population (Pao et al., 2019). Updated post-partum depression prevalence data during and post COVID-19 pandemic would be very enlightening as we imagine these numbers have only increased with isolation/ quarantines, as well as forced separation of SARS-CoV-2-positive mothers and infants, increased cesarean sections among infected mothers, and visitor restrictions during labor (Connor et al., 2020).

Bipolar Disorder

Based on 2019 WHO data, bipolar disorder internationally affects one in 50 adults, with 14 million being females 15–49 years of age. It accounts for 4% of mental health disorder diagnoses globally and roughly 2.8% in the United States (Dell'Osso et al., 2021; Institute of Health Metrics and Evaluation, 2019). Bipolar disorders differ from unipolar depression with the added component of mania or hypomania. Bipolar disorder is classified in the *DSM-V-TR*, as Bipolar I Disorder (BP-I) and Bipolar II Disorder (BP-II) with BP-I accounting for more severe impairment (American Psychiatric Association, 2022). BP-I does not require a depressive episode for diagnosis; however, most will experience debilitating depression (Merikangas et al., 2011). A diagnosis of Bipolar I disorder only requires one episode of mania. Mania is characterized by at least 1 week (or any duration if hospitalization occurs) of persistent elevated or irritable mood with at least three additional symptoms of grandiosity, increased energy despite limited sleep, increased talkativeness, distractibility, increased goal-directed activity, impulsive or high-risk behaviors, such as unrestrained spending, hypersexuality, or racing thoughts. If mood is irritable instead of elevated, then 4 of the aforementioned criteria are required. Distinct from mania is hypomania which involves 4 consecutive days of less severe symptoms as mentioned above. Hypomania does not require hospitalization and there tends to be no marked social or occupational impairment. There is also no evidence of psychotic symptoms. Bipolar type 2 requires a hypomanic episode and at least one MDE for diagnosis.

Bipolar I disorder has previously been thought to equally affect males and females while Bipolar II disorder has been more frequently associated with females. The NCS-R estimated prevalence to be 2.9% for males and 2.8% for females (Alegria et al., 2016). However, an international study in 2021 examined large clinical sample studies completed after 2010 to get a better understanding of the gender distribution of this disorder. They concluded, at least in the last 10+ years, there has been a predominance of the female gender in samples of bipolar patients (Dell'Osso et al., 2021). The systematic review concluded this could be due to females being more likely to seek treatment and/or better awareness of symptomology and improved diagnosis (Dell'Osso et al., 2021). Regardless, the trend is important to note and requires further research.

In contrast to MDD, bipolar disorders have a far stronger genetic risk (Smoller & Finn, 2003). First-degree relatives of affected individuals have roughly a ten-fold increased risk of the disorder compared to relatives of unaffected controls (Smoller & Finn, 2003). Twin studies have additionally confirmed strong familial transmission of the disease (Smoller & Finn, 2003). Substance use is another notable risk factor. A systematic review determined that 66.7% of the studies assessing overall substance use confirmed that substance use was a risk factor with cannabis use, nonmedical use of prescription medications, nicotine, and alcohol being the main culprits (Lalli et al., 2021). Finally, stress is suspected to be a leading risk factor. A meta-analysis completed in 2017 supported that patients with bipolar affective disorder experienced an increased number of stressful life events before an acute mood episode when compared to when they were stable (Lex et al., 2017). The COVID-19 pandemic (social implications along with disease process itself) has certainly presented the opportunity for more stressful life events which requires further investigation on a population level evaluating mania incidence.

When considering the sensitivity of this illness to stressful life events, the percentage of the first onset of illness in childbirth was noted to be associated more with bipolar disorder than unipolar depression. It is hypothesized this may be due to bipolar disorder being more sensitive to disruptions in social and circadian rhythms which childbirth obviously offers (Lex et al., 2017). Other potential explanations include the overlap between peak reproductive years and age of onset of disease as well as the hormonal/physiologic changes that transpire in pregnancy. Despite these associations, there has been a paucity of good data on the prevalence of bipolar disorders in the perinatal period. A meta-analysis done by Masters et al. (2022) attempted to explore this and found the perinatal period has an even higher risk of bipolar-spectrum mood episodes than previous estimates proposed. This is true of both those individuals with a history of psychiatric illness and those individuals never diagnosed (Masters et al., 2022). The prevalence of BD outside the perinatal period is 2–3%, but the study estimated that 20.1% of women had manic/hypomanic, mixed, or depressive episodes associated with bipolar disorder in the perinatal period. The paper describes the phenomena to potentially be due to women only having these episodes in the perinatal period with no diagnosis or lifelong illness, thus, the discrepancy in numbers (Masters et al., 2022). Additionally, BD symptoms (as opposed to a formal BD diagnosis) may occur as part of other psychiatric diagnoses such as borderline personality disorder or attention-deficit/hyperactivity disorder which would skew data as well (Masters et al., 2022).

Beyond the age of onset of bipolar-spectrum disorders which occur at such a crucial time in a woman's life cycle, the diagnosis can also be more fatal than unipolar depression. The rates of suicide attempts (30–50%) and deaths (15–20%) are twice as high as those with MDD and ultimately the highest of any mental health disorder except schizophrenia (Monson et al., 2021). Additionally, the relative likelihood of dying by suicide among women with BD was significantly higher than in men with BD (Yeh et al., 2019). Again, looking at the most recent GBD study, women with bipolar disorder aged 15–49 account for 0.8% DALYs and 1.37% YLDs globally. In the United States, it accounts for 0.88% DALYs and 1.10% YLDs. Bipolar I disorder has been associated with higher likelihood of unemployment, missing work, reducing work hours, and being fired than those with no mood disorder (Bessonova et al., 2020). Additionally, in an analysis of the national burden of bipolar I disorder in the United States, projections indicated caregivers' productivity loss and direct health care costs accounted for more than 30% of the total annual indirect costs of the disorder (Cloutier et al., 2018). Direct costs are also very high with this diagnosis. Patients are 70% more likely to use inpatient, mental health ER services, or crisis residential visits 3+ times in a year relative to those with depression (Bessonova et al., 2020). In summary, it is estimated the total U. S. costs of bipolar I disorder in 2015 alone was $202.1 billion when considering direct as well as indirect costs (Cloutier et al., 2018).

Anxiety Disorders

There are several distinct types of anxiety disorders including, but not limited to, generalized anxiety disorder (GAD), panic disorder, social anxiety disorder, and separation anxiety disorder. Although we will discuss anxiety disorders as a whole, we will focus on GAD and specific phobias due to their high prevalence. Globally, anxiety disorders affect 114 million women aged 15–49 (Institute of Health Metrics and Evaluation, 2019). With data from the GBD 2019 and a systematic review, it was estimated, during the COVID-19 pandemic, anxiety disorders increased by 25% globally, with female cases increasing by 51.8 million, compared to a 24 million case increase among men (36) (COVID-19 Mental Disorders Collaborators, 2021). When looking at a series of four national surveys to analyze predictors of 12-month anxiety prevalence, it was found that 12.7% met the criteria.

Considering race/ethnicity, white Americans had the highest 12-month prevalence at 13.4% while Asians had the lowest prevalence at 7.7%. Interestingly, when analyzing the relationship between race/ethnicity and prevalence of anxiety, when controlling for educational achievement/income, there was no significant difference in prevalence between groups (this was in contrast to mood and substance use disorders) (Vilsaint et al., 2019).

GAD is defined in the *DSM* as 6 months or more of persistent and excessive worry about different things that may cause irritability, restlessness, sleep impairment, muscle tension, and other somatic complaints. Women have a greater lifetime prevalence of GAD (~6%) when compared to men (~3%) (Kessler et al., 2005). A systematic review noted perinatal GAD prevalence ranges from 0% to 10% (Goodman et al., 2014); however, there is a paucity of studies examining anxiety incidence during the peri- and post-partum periods. Nine studies reported prevalence rates of GAD during pregnancy ranging from 0.9% to 22.7% (Viswasam et al., 2019). This enormous range beckons for further research on perinatal anxiety and how the changes occurring in women during their reproductive years contribute to the risk of developing clinically significant anxiety.

Specific phobias are some of the most common anxiety disorders, with a lifetime prevalence roughly twice the rate for women (12–27%) when compared to men (6–12%) (Hantsoo & Epperson, 2017). Women additionally tend to have more environmental and animal phobias than men (Hantsoo & Epperson, 2017). Of note, a study done in Korea on women with premenstrual dysphoric disorder found significant overlap with specific phobia diagnoses (Hong et al., 2012). Also considering the reproductive era, it is estimated that the prevalence of phobia in pregnancy is 3.2–19.9% (Goodman et al., 2014). While post-partum depression has become a more highlighted disorder, only 20% of obstetricians report screening for anxiety in pregnancy (Coleman et al., 2008). Anxiety during this life stage requires significant attention as there are potential impacts on offspring which include low birth weight, impaired cognitive development, mental health disorders, individual differences in reaction to stressful life events, and even medical disorders such as asthma, coronary artery disease, and endocrine abnormalities (Shahhosseini et al., 2015).

OCD Spectrum Disorders

Obsessive-compulsive disorder (OCD) was historically conceptualized as an anxiety disorder, however, in the *DSM-V*, it was moved into its own distinct category. While OCD has a component of anxiety, it has been proposed there is also a uniqueness to the repetitive thoughts and behaviors that exist in this spectrum of disorders that anxiety disorder pathology cannot quite capture. Additionally, OCD is associated with dysregulation of serotonergic and dopaminergic systems and frontal-striatal abnormalities, while anxiety disorders are associated with the amygdala, hippocampus, and pre-frontal cortical structures (Bartz & Hollander, 2006). Anxiety seems to rely on serotonin alone, with dopamine only implicated in social anxiety disorder (Bartz & Hollander, 2006). Per the *DSM-V,* the disease is characterized by obsessions (defined as recurrent and persistent thoughts/urges/impulses that are unwanted and distressing) and/or compulsions (defined as repetitive behaviors or mental acts individuals are driven to perform secondary to their obsessions or to reduce anxiety/distress revolving around their obsessions) (American Psychiatric Association, 2022).

Remarkably, despite causing significant disability, OCD is not included as a standalone diagnosis in the GBD data. However, the WHO does note it is one of the ten most debilitating disorders when considering loss of income and decreased quality of life (Veale & Roberts, 2014). According to the National Comorbidity Survey, 50% of adults with OCD had serious impairment (Harvard Medical School, 2007). Lifetime prevalence in the U. S. is estimated to be 2.3%, with slightly higher prevalence among women. Notable gender differences include females tending to have later onset of symptoms and continuing in an episodic versus chronic illness course characterized by cycling of symptomatology (Sharma & Mazmanian, 2021). Women also tend to have compulsive washing while men tend to have more sexual obsessions, preoccupation with magical numbers, or obsessional slowness (Veale & Roberts, 2014).

The reproductive cycle plays a noteworthy role in OCD. One study determined that 10% of women with OCD had onset of symptoms during pregnancy or the post-partum period (Fairbrother et al., 2022). It has also been estimated that 80% of women with OCD pre-gravid had exacerbation of symptoms during and after pregnancy (Fairbrother et al., 2022). A meta-analysis completed in 2013 surmised prevalence rates in the general population were 1.08%, but were 2.07% and 2.43% in pregnancy and post-partum, respectively (Russell et al., 2013). This demonstrated an almost two times greater risk for OCD in pregnancy vis-à-vis the general population (Russell et al., 2013).

Psychosis Spectrum Disorders

Psychotic spectrum disorders include schizophrenia, schizoaffective disorder, and delusional disorder. For simplicity, we will focus on schizophrenia and touch on post-partum psychosis. While most people conceive of schizophrenia encompassing positive symptoms, such as hallucinations and delusions, it is important to note that marked decline in cognitive functioning is also a crucial aspect of the disease, and this ultimately is the main source of disability for individuals (Barch, 2023). *DSM-5* criteria require greater than 6 months of two or more of the following symptoms (with one being one of the first three): hallucinations; delusions; disorganized speech; disorganized behavior; or negative symptoms (avolition, affective flattening) (American Psychiatric Association, 2022). These criteria do not account for the dramatic cognitive deficits that result from the illness, including poor episodic memory, poor working memory, and diminished processing speed (Barch, 2023).

Globally, prevalence rose from 13.1 million cases in 1990 to 20.9 million cases in 2016 per GBD 2016. Overall, schizophrenia has a relatively low prevalence estimated at 0.28% and has been found to have no gender differences in its prevalence (Charlson et al., 2018). Despite this, schizophrenia has significant morbidity and mortality, contributing to 13.4 million years of life lived with disability to burden of disease. It is ranked the 12th most disabling disorder worldwide as of 2016 data (Charlson et al., 2018). It is also the costliest mental disorder per person (Christensen et al., 2020). The average age of death in individuals with schizophrenia is 15–20 years younger than the general population (Vancampfort et al., 2017), and the diagnosis comes with one of the highest mortality risks of all psychiatric disorders (Vermeulen et al., 2017). When compared to the general population, a meta-analysis estimated the all-cause mortality of schizophrenia to have a relative risk of 2.94. When specifically looking at increased mortality by suicide in comparison with the general population, the relative risk was 9.76, signifying suicide is the greatest relative risk factor for mortality in patients with schizophrenia (Correll et al., 2022).

Although prevalence was found to be equal between males and females, there are definitive gender differences that exist in the disease course. One area of heterogeneity is the age of onset. Men tend to develop the illness between ages 18 and 25, while women do not generally exhibit symptoms until 25–35. Additionally, women have a bimodal onset distribution curve with onset at younger ages as well as late onset at ages greater than 40 (coinciding with menopause, according to the estrogenic hypothesis of schizophrenia (Riecher-Rössler et al., 1994)). In regard to symptoms, men tend to have more severe negative symptoms than women. Finally, one study suggested that women had improved premorbid social functioning compared to their male counterparts. This is an important point as it tends to align with improved outcomes and prognosis (Li et al., 2016; Ochoa et al., 2012).

While different than schizophrenia, post-partum psychosis demands mention in this section, as it is a unique experience of women and is related to significant mortality as well. Global prevalence of post-partum psychosis is roughly 0.089–2.6 per 1000 births (VanderKruik et al., 2017). Unfortunately, these numbers may be underreported since there are no standard screening procedures in place during the perinatal period (Rai et al., 2015). Despite its presumed low incidence, it has critical consequences, with an estimated 5% of women with post-partum psychosis dying by suicide and 4.5% committing infanticide (Brockington, 2017). As previously mentioned, a history of bipolar disorder is a significant risk factor; however, it is projected that about half of women who present with post-partum psychosis actually had no psychiatric history at all. The largest study assessing risk factors for this illness was done in Sweden from 1983 to 2000 utilizing the Swedish Medical Birth Registry. This study found that mothers >35 years old are 2.4 times more likely to experience post-partum psychosis when compared to mothers under 19 years of age. Low birth weight, first pregnancy, obstetric complications, and perinatal or neonatal loss were also noted as potential risk factors. Finally, most episodes tend to occur in the first month after delivery (Valdimarsdóttir et al., 2009).

While post-partum psychosis has dire consequences, it is also very responsive to treatment. Only one-third of women will have a subsequent episode in other pregnancies (Wesseloo et al., 2016). In fact, a meta-analysis estimated that about 40% of women experiencing post-partum psychosis did not have additional episodes outside the perinatal period during a mean follow-up period of 16 years (Gilden et al., 2020). Due to this favorable prognosis, finding ways to intervene as soon as possible is essential in improving maternal and infant outcomes.

Post-traumatic Stress Disorder

A traumatic event is defined as exposure to threatened death, serious injury, or sexual violence which can occur directly or indirectly. Being exposed to a traumatic event is the first of the diagnostic criteria of post-traumatic stress disorder (PTSD) per the DSM-5. Additionally, one must experience symptoms of intrusion, avoidance, negativity in cognition/mood, and arousal disturbance for more than 1 month after the inciting event. A large study done across six continents and sampling almost 69,000 adults found that 70% of respondents experienced a traumatic event and roughly one-third were exposed to four or more traumatic events (Benjet et al., 2016). Despite these alarming numbers, the reported prevalence of PTSD is lower than the aforementioned study suggests. Data analyzed from WHO World Mental Health Surveys suggest the lifetime prevalence of PTSD in those experiencing a traumatic event is roughly 5.6% globally. It was also found that high-income countries had twice the proportion of PTSD cases as lower- and middle-income countries. In addition, the age of onset was earlier on average in high-income countries, with half of these respondents reporting PTSD onset before age 30. This is in comparison with an average age of 43 for lower-income countries (Koenen et al., 2017).

When considering gender differences among PTSD diagnoses, the lifetime prevalence is double in women (10–12%) when compared to men (5–6%) (Ditlevsen & Elklit, 2010). Women also tend to experience PTSD from sexual assault or abuse events, whereas men tend to suffer from symptoms after accidents, natural disasters, and military combat (Tolin & Foa, 2006). There are several theories as to why these differences manifest including differences in genes, including physiological response to fear, hormones, evolutional factors, higher prevalence of experiencing a traumatic event, and socialized gender roles (Benjet et al., 2016; Hu et al., 2017).

In line with the other diagnoses discussed, there is also a specific phenomenon of perinatal PTSD. This includes both having a difficult or traumatic birth where the baby and mother's lives are at risk or previous PTSD that is retriggered by events of pregnancy or birth. One meta-analysis determined the mean prevalence of PTSD during pregnancy was 4.6% in community samples but was as high as 18.95% in high-risk populations (defined as current maternal depression, history of psychiatric illness, and/or infant complications). Mean prevalence of PTSD during the first post-partum year was 5.44%. PTSD specifically attributed to the birth was 5.9% (Yildiz et al., 2017). Given the association of PTSD with poor maternal and child outcomes, there are clearly noteworthy implications for health services and clinical practice (Cook et al., 2018).

Social Determinants of Health, Cultural, and Political Considerations

Beyond the biological differences and theories attempting to explain the gender differences in the prevalence of psychiatric disorders, the social determinants of health, cultural components, and political environment potentially drive these disorders that explicitly and disproportionately impact women.

Caretaker Role

In Western societies, women continue to enter the "productive world" at increasing rates without men entering the "reproductive world" at an equivalent rate (Toosi, 2002). Women still find themselves overwhelmingly in the caregiver role and this inequitable relationship between men and women must be acknowledged as a potential element in the difference of their mental health experiences (Blehar, 2006). This inequality worsened during the COVID-19 pandemic, particularly early on with school closures. After a study in Italy found the amount of household labor remained greater for women during the early period of the COVID-19 pandemic, a cross-sectional study in the U. S. investigated the association between childcare facilities and employment status among women versus men in the first year of the COVID-19 pandemic. It found that state-level childcare facility closures were associated with greater reductions in female employment than male employment (Feyman et al., 2021). Despite this, there is still significant resistance to U. S. policies that support universal childcare. These policies would inevitably provide improved support to families and to women, in particular, who take on these caregiver burdens at a disproportionate rate.

Equity in Health Care/Reproductive Health

An additional stress in this age group that may increase the risk of mental illness includes the limited access to health care exacerbated during the pandemic and specifically to reproductive health care and comprehensive family planning. While one-third of U. S. women reported delays or cancellations in sexual and reproductive health care, higher percentage of reports came from Black, Latino, LGBTQ+, and low-income women (Connor et al., 2020). With abortion utilized by one million women annually in the U. S., the current changes in legislation and political atmosphere will also undoubtedly alter women's lives, including their health and economic status as well as their sense of control and autonomy over their bodies. Gendered social roles and power differentials also contribute to loss of agency and increased risk of chronic stress (Connor et al., 2020). Another COVID influence on the potential for developing mood disorders has been increasing rates of intimate partner- (IPV) and gender-based violence. Sixteen percent of women reported an IPV experience in 2020, with one-third of those reporting challenges accessing resources after these incidents due to the pandemic (Lindberg et al., 2020).

Maternal health has also worsened throughout the pandemic according to the most recent United States Government Accountability Office report (GAO, 2022). In 2018, the maternal death rate in the U. S. was more than two times greater than in Canada and the United Kingdom. However, since 2018, these numbers have only grown in the wake of the pandemic: 658 maternal deaths in 2018; 754 in 2019; 861 in 2020; and 1178 in 2021. The rate of maternal deaths per 100,000 live births doubled from 17.4 in 2018 to 32.2 in 2021. Racial health disparities have been specifically poignant during this time as well with rates of deaths among Black women increasing more than for White women (Twenge et al., 2019: GAO, 2022; Hoyert, 2021). Notably, perinatal mental health conditions are now cited as one of the leading obstetric complications in the United States and are a preventable cause of maternal mortality (Davis et al., 2019; Kendig et al., 2017; Organization for Economic Co-operation and Development, 2023). This beckons for standardization of maternal mental health screening, resources, and changes in health policy to support women and families and reduce mortality.

Social Media, Age, and Technology

Other considerations as to why young women are more at risk include the increased use of electronic communication and social media. This has also undoubtedly increased during the pandemic when in-person interactions were put on pause. Those who spend more time on social media and less time with others face-to-face reported lower well-being and higher likelihood of depression. Increased internet use further exposes individuals to cyberbullying as well (Twenge et al., 2019).

Online communities geared toward misogynistic attitudes with self-proclaimed "incels" (involuntary celibates) have also been on the rise. A recent study examined this group more comprehensively and found the core of their belief system is the capacity for a woman's "inherent evil nature." This feels reminiscent to antiquated ideas of female "hysteria." They possess other misogynistic beliefs, such as the female brain being smaller or women being less evolved than men (Grunau et al., 2022; O'Malley et al., 2022). Technology allows the mobilization of these extremist ideas that can be damaging to women on both a micro and macro level. This is especially true in light of legislation that continues to undermine women's ability to make decisions about their own bodies. These patriarchal groups, whose ideology is based on oppression, are a cultural phenomenon that requires further examination regarding their impact on women's mental health.

Social Determinants of Health

In addition to acknowledging these unique, contemporary social circumstances that contribute to the mental health of women, obviously there are more generalized social determinants of health at play as well. From the Adverse Childhood Experiences study, it is clear that psychological, physical, or sexual abuse exposure greatly impacts the future well-being of children (Felitti et al., 1998). Girls are ultimately more likely to be sexually abused than boys leading to higher risk of developing mental health and substance abuse disorders (MacMillan et al., 2001).

Poverty is another clear component contributing to poor mental health outcomes among women. Seventy percent of those living in poverty are women (Buvinic & King, 2007). Clear consequences of poverty include food insecurity and housing insecurity. Beyond that, balancing home and work responsibilities, while also having lower salaries in comparison to men, has detrimental health impacts too (Onarheim et al., 2016). Additionally, the gender disparities in primary education are likely linked to this gender discrepancy in poverty and ultimately mental health as well. In 2008, 64% of the 796 million illiterate adults worldwide were women (UNESCO Institute for Statistics, 2010). However, when women have more schooling, future generations have more opportunities at their dispense. This is due to the tendency of working women allocating more resources to their children's' food, education, and health care in comparison to their male counterparts. This leads to greater wellbeing of themselves and their families (Buvinic & King, 2007).

Finally, another recognized contributor to poor health outcomes in women is the higher degree of violence they are exposed to compared to men. Human rights violations and societal violence including, but not limited to, property ownership, voting rights, and human trafficking exploit women disproportionately. Women and girls represent 99% of victims of forced labor in the commercial sex industry and 58% in other sectors (International Labour Organization, 2017). Violence in the domestic setting is also more profound with over half of female homicide victims in the U. S. being killed by a current or former male intimate partner (Jack et al., 2018). Outside the fragile physical state of pregnancy, women are even more vulnerable considering that homicide is the leading cause of death for pregnant women in the U. S. (Modest et al., 2022). Excluding homicide, interpersonal violence alone is experienced more by females. Between 2017 and 2019, 19% of adolescent females reported sexual or physical violence by a dating partner compared to only 9.4% of adolescent males (Kann et al., 2018). Thus, it is evident that particularly throughout their reproductive age, women are at extremely high risk of brutality and all the consequent physical and mental health sequela that accompanies it.

Implications for Women's Behavioral Health

Ultimately, public health initiatives can be developed once problems are identified and access to care and treatment are improved. By reducing the prevalence of mental illnesses, diminishing health inequities, and rehabilitating disabilities, women are more able to flourish. More opportunities to take part in raising safe and healthy children will be available. Opportunities to take part in their own agency and health can be cultivated.

The WHO's *Comprehensive Mental Health Action Plan 2013–2030* recognizes the critical role of mental health in achieving health for all people. This plan includes four objectives: (1) "strengthen effective leadership and governance for mental health; (2) provide comprehensive, integrated, and responsive mental health and social services in community-based settings; (3) implement strategies for promotion and prevention in mental health; and (4) strengthen information systems, evidence, and research for mental health" (WHO, 2021).

Public health endeavors should continue to focus on modifiable social conditions, such as poverty, access to health care, access to work, access to childcare, as well as expanding treatment options that nurture and empower women, while responding to the misogynist dogmas that have historically affected women's health, mental health, and well-being.

References

Alegria, M., Jackson, J. S., Kessler, R. C., & Takeuchi, D. (2016, March 23). *Collaborative Psychiatric Epidemiology Surveys (CPES), 2001–2003*. National Comorbidity Survey (NCS) Series; Inter-university Consortium for Political and Social Research [United States]. https://doi.org/10.3886/ICPSR20240.v8

American Psychiatric Association. (2022). *Diagnostic and statistical manual of mental disorders, text revision (DSM-5-TR)* (5th ed.). Author.

American Psychological Association. (2022). *Postpartum depression: Causes, symptoms, risk factors, and treatment options*. [Web page]. APA. https://www.apa.org/topics/women-girls/postpartum-depression

Barch, D. M. (2023). Schizophrenia spectrum disorders. In R. Biswas-Diener, & E. Diener (Eds.), *Noba textbook series: Psychology* (p. HTML). DEF publishers. https://nobaproject.com/modules/schizophrenia-spectrum-disorders

Bartz, J. A., & Hollander, E. (2006). Is obsessive–compulsive disorder an anxiety disorder? *Progress in Neuro-Psychopharmacology and Biological Psychiatry, 30*(3), 338–352. https://doi.org/10.1016/j.pnpbp.2005.11.003

Benjet, C., Bromet, E., Karam, E. G., Kessler, R. C., McLaughlin, K. A., Ruscio, A. M., Shahly, V., Stein, D. J., Petukhova, M., Hill, E., Alonso, J., Atwoli, L., Bunting, B., Bruffaerts, R., Caldas-de-Almeida, J. M., de Girolamo, G., Florescu, S., Gureje, O., Huang, Y., Lepine, J. P., Kawakami, N., Kovess-Masfety, V., Medina-Mora, M. E., Navarro-Mateu, F., Piazza, M., Posada-Villa, J., Scott, K. M., Shalev, A., Slade, T., ten Have, M., Torres, Y., Viana, M. C., Zarkov, Z., & Koenen, K. C. (2016). The epidemiology of traumatic event exposure worldwide: Results from the World Mental Health Survey Consortium. *Psychological Medicine, 46*(2), 327–343. https://doi.org/10.1017/s0033291715001981

Bessonova, L., Ogden, K., Doane, M. J., O'Sullivan, A. K., & Tohen, M. (2020). The economic burden of bipolar disorder in the United States: A systematic literature review. *ClinicoEconomics and Outcomes Research, 12*, 481–497. https://doi.org/10.2147/ceor.S259338

Blehar, M. C. (2006). Women's mental health research: The emergence of a biomedical field. *Annual Review of Clinical Psychology, 2*(1), 135–160. https://doi.org/10.1146/annurev.clinpsy.2.022305.095344

Brockington, I. (2017). Suicide and filicide in postpartum psychosis. *Archives of Women's Mental Health, 20*(1), 63–69. https://doi.org/10.1007/s00737-016-0675-8

Burt, V. K., & Stein, K. (2002). Epidemiology of depression throughout the female life cycle. *Journal of Clinical Psychiatry, 63*(Suppl 7), 9–15.

Buvinic, M., & King, E. M. (2007). Smart economics. *Finance and Development, 44*(2), HTML. https://www.imf.org/external/pubs/ft/fandd/2007/06/king.htm

Canelón, S. P., & Boland, M. R. (2020). A systematic literature review of factors affecting the timing of menarche: The potential for climate change to impact women's health. *International Journal of Environmental Research and Public Health, 17*(5), 1703.

Center for Behavioral Health Statistics and Quality. (2018). *National survey on drug use and health 2019* [Report; NSDUH-2019-DS0001]. U.S. Department of Health and Human Services, Substance Abuse and Mental Health Services Administration. https://www.samhsa.gov/data/release/2019-national-survey-drug-use-and-health-nsduh-releases

Charlson, F. J., Ferrari, A. J., Santomauro, D. F., Diminic, S., Stockings, E., Scott, J. G., McGrath, J. J., & Whiteford, H. A. (2018). Global epidemiology and burden of schizophrenia: Findings from the global burden of disease study 2016. *Schizophrenia Bulletin, 44*(6), 1195–1203. https://doi.org/10.1093/schbul/sby058

Christensen, M. K., Lim, C. C. W., Saha, S., Plana-Ripoll, O., Cannon, D., Presley, F., Weye, N., Momen, N. C., Whiteford, H. A., Iburg, K. M., & McGrath, J. J. (2020). The cost of mental disorders: A systematic review. *Epidemiology & Psychiatric Sciences, 29*, e161. https://doi.org/10.1017/s204579602000075x

Cloutier, M., Greene, M., Guerin, A., Touya, M., & Wu, E. (2018). The economic burden of bipolar I disorder in the United States in 2015. *Journal of Affective Disorders, 226*, 45–51. https://doi.org/10.1016/j.jad.2017.09.011

Coleman, V. H., Carter, M. M., Morgan, M. A., & Schulkin, J. (2008). Obstetrician-gynecologists' screening patterns for anxiety during pregnancy. *Depression and Anxiety, 25*(2), 114–123. https://doi.org/10.1002/da.20278

Connor, J., Madhavan, S., Mokashi, M., Amanuel, H., Johnson, N. R., Pace, L. E., & Bartz, D. (2020). Health risks and outcomes that disproportionately affect women during the Covid-19 pandemic: A review. *Social Science and Medicine, 266*, 113364. https://doi.org/10.1016/j.socscimed.2020.113364

Cook, N., Ayers, S., & Horsch, A. (2018). Maternal posttraumatic stress disorder during the perinatal period and child outcomes: A systematic review. *Journal of Affective Disorders, 225*, 18–31. https://doi.org/10.1016/j.jad.2017.07.045

Correll, C. U., Solmi, M., Croatto, G., Schneider, L. K., Rohani-Montez, S. C., Fairley, L., Smith, N., Bitter, I., Gorwood, P., Taipale, H., & Tiihonen, J. (2022). Mortality in people with schizophrenia: A systematic review and meta-analysis of relative risk and aggravating or attenuating factors. *World Psychiatry, 21*(2), 248–271. https://doi.org/10.1002/wps.20994

COVID-19 Mental Disorders Collaborators. (2021). Global prevalence and burden of depressive and anxiety disorders in 204 countries and territories in 2020 due to the COVID-19 pandemic. *Lancet, 398*(10312), 1700–1712. https://doi.org/10.1016/s0140-6736(21)02143-7

Cox, E. Q., Sowa, N. A., Meltzer-Brody, S. E., & Gaynes, B. N. (2016). The perinatal depression treatment cascade: Baby steps toward improving outcomes. *Journal of Clinical Psychiatry, 77*(9), 1189–1200. https://doi.org/10.4088/JCP.15r10174

Davis, N. L., Smoots, A. N., & Goodman, D. A. (2019). *Pregnancy-related deaths: Data from 14 U.S. Maternal Mortality Review Committees, 2008–2017* [Report; Maternal Mortality Review Information Application]. U. S. D. o. H. a. H. S. Centers for Disease Control and

Prevention. https://www.cdc.gov/reproductivehealth/maternal-mortality/erase-mm/mmr-data-brief_2019-h.pdf

Dell'Osso, B., Cafaro, R., & Ketter, T. A. (2021). Has Bipolar Disorder become a predominantly female gender related condition? Analysis of recently published large sample studies. *International Journal of Bipolar Disorders, 9*(1), 3. https://doi.org/10.1186/s40345-020-00207-z

Dennis, C.-L., & Chung-Lee, L. (2006). Postpartum depression help-seeking barriers and maternal treatment preferences: A qualitative systematic review. *Birth, 33*(4), 323–331. https://doi.org/10.1111/j.1523-536X.2006.00130.x

Ditlevsen, D. N., & Elklit, A. (2010). The combined effect of gender and age on post traumatic stress disorder: Do men and women show differences in the lifespan distribution of the disorder? *Annals of General Psychiatry, 9*, 32. https://doi.org/10.1186/1744-859x-9-32

Elflein, J. (2019, August 15). *Population of women aged 15–49 in the U.S. and worldwide in 2013 and 2025* [Web page]. Statista. https://www.statista.com/statistics/654630/female-population-aged-15-49-us-worldwide/

Fairbrother, N., Collardeau, F., Albert, A., & Stoll, K. (2022). Screening for perinatal anxiety using the Childbirth Fear Questionnaire: A new measure of fear of childbirth. *International Journal of Environmental Research and Public Health, 19*(4). https://doi.org/10.3390/ijerph19042223

Felitti, V. J., Anda, R. F., Nordenberg, D., Williamson, D. F., Spitz, A. M., Edwards, V., Koss, M. P., & Marks, J. S. (1998). Relationship of childhood abuse and household dysfunction to many of the leading causes of death in adults. The Adverse Childhood Experiences (ACE) study. *American Journal of Preventive Medicine, 14*(4), 245–258. https://doi.org/10.1016/s0749-3797(98)00017-8

Feyman, Y., Fener, N. E., & Griffith, K. N. (2021). Association of childcare facility closures with employment status of US women vs men during the COVID-19 pandemic. *JAMA Health Forum, 2*(6), e211297. https://doi.org/10.1001/jamahealthforum.2021.1297

Gilden, J., Kamperman, A. M., Munk-Olsen, T., Hoogendijk, W. J. G., Kushner, S. A., & Bergink, V. (2020). Long-term outcomes of postpartum psychosis: A systematic review and meta-analysis. *Journal of Clinical Psychiatry, 81*(2). https://doi.org/10.4088/JCP.19r12906

Global Health Observatory. (2023). *Disability-adjusted life years (DALYs)* [Web page]. World Health Organization. https://www.who.int/data/gho/indicator-metadata-registry/imr-details/158

Goodman, J. H., Chenausky, K. L., & Freeman, M. P. (2014). Anxiety disorders during pregnancy: A systematic review. *Journal of Clinical Psychiatry, 75*(10), e1153–e1184. https://doi.org/10.4088/JCP.14r09035

Greenberg, P. E., Fournier, A. A., Sisitsky, T., Simes, M., Berman, R., Koenigsberg, S. H., & Kessler, R. C. (2021). The economic burden of adults with major depressive disorder in the United States (2010 and 2018). *PharmacoEconomics, 39*(6), 653–665. https://doi.org/10.1007/s40273-021-01019-4

Grunau, K., Bieselt, H. E., Gul, P., & Kupfer, T. R. (2022). Unwanted celibacy is associated with misogynistic attitudes even after controlling for personality. *Personality and Individual Differences, 199*, 111860. https://doi.org/10.1016/j.paid.2022.111860

Hantsoo, L., & Epperson, C. N. (2017). Anxiety disorders among women: A female lifespan approach. *Focus (American Psychiatric Publishing), 15*(2), 162–172. https://doi.org/10.1176/appi.focus.20160042

Harvard Medical School. (2007). *Table 2: 12-month prevalence DSM-IV/WMH-CIDI disorders by sex and cohort* [Table]. https://www.hcp.med.harvard.edu/ncs/ftpdir/table_ncsr_12monthprevgenderxage.pdf

Hedden, S., Gfroerer, J., Barker, P., Smith, S., Pemberton, M. R., Saavedra, L. M., Forman-Hoffman, V. L., Ringeisen, H., & Novak, S. P. (2012, March). *Comparison of NSDUH mental health data and methods with other data sources* (CBHSQ Data Review). SAMHSA, Center for Behavioral Health Statistics and Quality. https://www.samhsa.gov/data/sites/default/files/CBHSQ_Data_Review_C2_MentalHealth_2012/CBHSQ_Data_Review_C2_MentalHealth_2012.pdf

Hong, J. P., Park, S., Wang, H. R., Chang, S. M., Sohn, J. H., Jeon, H. J., Lee, H. W., Cho, S. J., Kim, B. S., Bae, J. N., & Cho, M. J. (2012). Prevalence, correlates, comorbidities, and suicidal tendencies of premenstrual dysphoric disorder in a nationwide sample of Korean women. *Social Psychiatry and Psychiatric Epidemiology, 47*(12), 1937–1945. https://doi.org/10.1007/s00127-012-0509-6

Hoyert, D. L. (2021). *Maternal mortality rates in the United States, 2019* [NCHS Health E-Stats]. National Center for Health Statistics. https://www.cdc.gov/nchs/data/hestat/maternal-mortality-2021/E-Stat-Maternal-Mortality-Rates-H.pdf

Hu, J., Feng, B., Zhu, Y., Wang, W., Xie, J., & Zheng, X. (2017). Gender differences in PTSD: Susceptibility and resilience. In A. Alvinius (Ed.), *Gender differences in different contexts* (pp. 21–42). InTechOpen. https://doi.org/10.5772/65287

Institute of Health Metrics and Evaluation. (2019). *Global Health Data Exchange (GHDx)* [Online; Mental disorders]. https://vizhub.healthdata.org/gbd-results/

International Labour Organization. (2017). *Global estimates of modern slavery: Forced labour and forced marriage* [Report]. International Labour Organization & Walk Free Foundation. https://www.ilo.org/wcmsp5/groups/public/@dgreports/@dcomm/documents/publication/wcms_575479.pdf

Jack, S. P. D., Petrosky, E., Lyons, B. H., Blair, J. M., Ertl, A. M., Sheats, K. J., & Betz, C. J. (2018). Surveillance for violent deaths: National Violent Death Reporting System, 27 states, 2015. *MMWR: Surveillance Summaries, 67*(11), 1–32. https://doi.org/10.15585/mmwr.ss6711a1

Kann, L., McManus, T., Harris, W. A., Shanklin, S. L., Flint, K. H., Queen, B., Lowry, R., Chyen, D., Whittle, L., Thornton, J., Lim, C., Bradford, D., Yamakawa, Y., Leon, M., Brener, N., & Ethier, K. A. (2018). Youth risk behavior surveillance – United States, 2017. *MMWR: Surveillance Summaries, 67*(8), 1–114. https://doi.org/10.15585/mmwr.ss6708a1

Kendig, S., Keats, J. P., Hoffman, M. C., Kay, L. B., Miller, E. S., Moore Simas, T. A., Frieder, A., Hackley, B., Indman, P., Raines, C., Semenuk, K., Wisner, K. L., & Lemieux, L. A. (2017). Consensus bundle on maternal mental health: Perinatal depression and anxiety. *Obstetrics and Gynecology, 129*(3), 422–430. https://doi.org/10.1097/aog.0000000000001902

Kessler, R. C., Andrews, G., Colpe, L. J., Hiripi, E., Mroczek, D. K., Normand, S. L., Walters, E. E., & Zaslavsky, A. M. (2002). Short screening scales to monitor population prevalences and trends in non-specific psychological distress. *Psychological Medicine, 32*(6), 959–976. https://doi.org/10.1017/s0033291702006074

Kessler, R. C., Berglund, P., Demler, O., Jin, R., Merikangas, K. R., & Walters, E. E. (2005). Lifetime prevalence and age-of-onset distributions of DSM-IV disorders in the National Comorbidity Survey Replication. *Archives of General Psychiatry, 62*(6), 593–602. https://doi.org/10.1001/archpsyc.62.6.593

Koenen, K. C., Ratanatharathorn, A., Ng, L., McLaughlin, K. A., Bromet, E. J., Stein, D. J., Karam, E. G., Meron Ruscio, A., Benjet, C., Scott, K., Atwoli, L., Petukhova, M., Lim, C. C. W., Aguilar-Gaxiola, S., Al-Hamzawi, A., Alonso, J., Bunting, B., Ciutan, M., de Girolamo, G., Degenhardt, L., Gureje, O., Haro, J. M., Huang, Y., Kawakami, N., Lee, S., Navarro-Mateu, F., Pennell, B. E., Piazza, M., Sampson, N., Ten Have, M., Torres, Y., Viana, M. C., Williams, D., Xavier, M., & Kessler, R. C. (2017). Posttraumatic stress disorder in the World Mental Health Surveys. *Psychological Medicine, 47*(13), 2260–2274. https://doi.org/10.1017/s0033291717000708

Lalli, M., Brouillette, K., Kapczinski, F., & de Azevedo Cardoso, T. (2021). Substance use as a risk factor for bipolar disorder: A systematic review. *Journal of Psychiatric Research, 144,* 285–295. https://doi.org/10.1016/j.jpsychires.2021.10.012

Lex, C., Bäzner, E., & Meyer, T. D. (2017). Does stress play a significant role in bipolar disorder? A meta-analysis. *Journal of Affective Disorders, 208,* 298–308. https://doi.org/10.1016/j.jad.2016.08.057

Li, R., Ma, X., Wang, G., Yang, J., & Wang, C. (2016). Why sex differences in schizophrenia? *Journal of Translational Neurosciences (Beijing), 1*(1), 37–42.

Lindberg, L. D., VandeVusse, A., Mueller, J., & Kirstein, M. (2020, June). *Early impacts of the COVID-19 pandemic: Findings from the 2020 Guttmacher survey of reproductive health experiences.* Guttmacher Institute. https://www.guttmacher.org/report/early-impacts-covid-19-pandemic-findings-2020-guttmacher-survey-reproductive-health

MacMillan, H. L., Fleming, J. E., Streiner, D. L., Lin, E., Boyle, M. H., Jamieson, E., Duku, E. K., Walsh, C. A., Wong, M. Y., & Beardslee, W. R. (2001). Childhood abuse and lifetime psychopathology in a community sample. *American Journal of Psychiatry, 158*(11), 1878–1883. https://doi.org/10.1176/appi.ajp.158.11.1878

Martin, L. A., Neighbors, H. W., & Griffith, D. M. (2013). The experience of symptoms of depression in men vs women: Analysis of the National Comorbidity Survey Replication. *JAMA Psychiatry, 70*(10), 1100–1106. https://doi.org/10.1001/jamapsychiatry.2013.1985

Masters, G. A., Hugunin, J., Xu, L., Ulbricht, C. M., Moore Simas, T. A., Ko, J. Y., & Byatt, N. (2022). Prevalence of bipolar disorder in perinatal women: A systematic review and meta-analysis. *Journal of Clinical Psychiatry, 83*(5). https://doi.org/10.4088/JCP.21r14045

Merikangas, K. R., Jin, R., He, J. P., Kessler, R. C., Lee, S., Sampson, N. A., Viana, M. C., Andrade, L. H., Hu, C., Karam, E. G., Ladea, M., Medina-Mora, M. E., Ono, Y., Posada-Villa, J., Sagar, R., Wells, J. E., & Zarkov, Z. (2011). Prevalence and correlates of bipolar spectrum disorder in the world mental health survey initiative. *Archives of General Psychiatry, 68*(3), 241–251. https://doi.org/10.1001/archgenpsychiatry.2011.12

Modest, A. M., Prater, L. C., & Joseph, N. T. (2022). Pregnancy-associated homicide and suicide: An analysis of the national violent death reporting system, 2008–2019. *Obstetrics and Gynecology, 140*(4), 565–573. https://doi.org/10.1097/aog.0000000000004932

Monson, E. T., Shabalin, A. A., Docherty, A. R., DiBlasi, E., Bakian, A. V., Li, Q. S., Gray, D., Keeshin, B., Crowell, S. E., Mullins, N., Willour, V. L., & Coon, H. (2021). Assessment of suicide attempt and death in bipolar affective disorder: A combined clinical and genetic approach. *Translational Psychiatry, 11*(1), 379. https://doi.org/10.1038/s41398-021-01500-w

O'Malley, R. L., Holt, K., & Holt, T. J. (2022). An exploration of the involuntary celibate (incel) subculture online. *Journal of Interpersonal Violence, 37*(7–8), NP4981–NP5008. https://doi.org/10.1177/0886260520959625

Ochoa, S., Usall, J., Cobo, J., Labad, X., & Kulkarni, J. (2012). Gender differences in schizophrenia and first-episode psychosis: A comprehensive literature review. *Schizophrenia Research and Treatment, 2012*, 916198. https://doi.org/10.1155/2012/916198

Onarheim, K. H., Iversen, J. H., & Bloom, D. E. (2016). Economic benefits of investing in women's health: A systematic review. *PLoS One, 11*(3), e0150120. https://doi.org/10.1371/journal.pone.0150120

Orenstein, G. A., & Lewis, L. (2023). Erikson's stages of psychosocial development. In *StatPearls*. StatPearls Publishing. https://www.ncbi.nlm.nih.gov/books/NBK556096/

Organisation for Economic Co-operation and Development. (2023). *Maternal and infant mortality* [Dataset; Health Status: Maternal and nfant mortality; Date: 2017]. OECD. https://stats.oecd.org/index.aspx?queryid=30116

Pao, C., Guintivano, J., Santos, H., & Meltzer-Brody, S. (2019). Postpartum depression and social support in a racially and ethnically diverse population of women. *Archives of Women's Mental Health, 22*(1), 105–114. https://doi.org/10.1007/s00737-018-0882-6

Rai, S., Pathak, A., & Sharma, I. (2015). Postpartum psychiatric disorders: Early diagnosis and management. *Indian Journal of Psychiatry, 57*(Suppl 2), S216–S221. https://doi.org/10.4103/0019-5545.161481

Riecher-Rössler, A., Häfner, H., Stumbaum, M., Maurer, K., & Schmidt, R. (1994). Can estradiol modulate schizophrenic symptomatology? *Schizophrenia Bulletin, 20*(1), 203–214. https://doi.org/10.1093/schbul/20.1.203

Russell, E. J., Fawcett, J. M., & Mazmanian, D. (2013). Risk of obsessive-compulsive disorder in pregnant and postpartum women: A meta-analysis. *Journal of Clinical Psychiatry, 74*(4), 377–385. https://doi.org/10.4088/JCP.12r07917

Shahhosseini, Z., Pourasghar, M., Khalilian, A., & Salehi, F. (2015). A review of the effects of anxiety during pregnancy on children's health. *Mater Sociomed, 27*(3), 200–202. https://doi.org/10.5455/msm.2015.27.200-202

Sharma, V., & Mazmanian, D. (2021). Are we overlooking obsessive-compulsive disorder during and after pregnancy? Some arguments for a peripartum onset specifier. *Archives of Women's Mental Health, 24*(1), 165–168. https://doi.org/10.1007/s00737-020-01038-8

Smoller, J. W., & Finn, C. T. (2003). Family, twin, and adoption studies of bipolar disorder. *American Journal of Medical Genetics. Part C: Seminars in Medical Genetics, 123c*(1), 48–58. https://doi.org/10.1002/ajmg.c.20013

Tasca, C., Rapetti, M., Carta, M. G., & Fadda, B. (2012). Women and hysteria in the history of mental health. *Clinical Practice and Epidemiology in Mental Health, 8,* 110–119. https://doi.org/10.2174/1745017901208010110

Tolin, D. F., & Foa, E. B. (2006). Sex differences in trauma and posttraumatic stress disorder: A quantitative review of 25 years of research. *Psychological Bulletin, 132*(6), 959–992. https://doi.org/10.1037/0033-2909.132.6.959

Toosi, M. (2002, May). A century of change: The U.S. labor force, 1950–2050. *Monthly Labor Review,* 15–28. https://www.bls.gov/opub/mlr/2002/05/art2full.pdf

Twenge, J. M., Cooper, A. B., Joiner, T. E., Duffy, M. E., & Binau, S. G. (2019). Age, period, and cohort trends in mood disorder indicators and suicide-related outcomes in a nationally representative dataset, 2005–2017. *Journal of Abnormal Psychology, 128*(3), 185–199. https://doi.org/10.1037/abn0000410

U. S. Government Accountability Office. (2022, October). *Maternal health: Outcomes worsened and disparities persisted during the pandemic: Report to Congressional addressees* [Report; GAO-23-105871]. U. S. GAO. https://www.gao.gov/assets/730/723432.pdf

UNESCO Institute for Statistics. (2010). *Adult and youth literacy: Global trends in gender parity* [Report; UIS Fact Sheet no. 3]. U. I. f. Statistics. https://uis.unesco.org/sites/default/files/documents/fs3-adult-and-youth-literacy-global-trends-in-gender-parity-2010-en.pdf

Valdimarsdóttir, U., Hultman, C. M., Harlow, B., Cnattingius, S., & Sparén, P. (2009). Psychotic illness in first-time mothers with no previous psychiatric hospitalizations: A population-based study. *PLoS Medicine, 6*(2), e13. https://doi.org/10.1371/journal.pmed.1000013

Vancampfort, D., Rosenbaum, S., Schuch, F., Ward, P. B., Richards, J., Mugisha, J., Probst, M., & Stubbs, B. (2017). Cardiorespiratory fitness in severe mental illness: A systematic review and meta-analysis. *Sports Medicine, 47*(2), 343–352. https://doi.org/10.1007/s40279-016-0574-1

VanderKruik, R., Barreix, M., Chou, D., Allen, T., Say, L., & Cohen, L. S. (2017). The global prevalence of postpartum psychosis: A systematic review. *BMC Psychiatry, 17*(1), 272. https://doi.org/10.1186/s12888-017-1427-7

Veale, D., & Roberts, A. (2014). Obsessive-compulsive disorder. *BMJ: British Medical Journal, 348,* g2183. https://doi.org/10.1136/bmj.g2183

Vermeulen, J., van Rooijen, G., Doedens, P., Numminen, E., van Tricht, M., & de Haan, L. (2017). Antipsychotic medication and long-term mortality risk in patients with schizophrenia; a systematic review and meta-analysis. *Psychological Medicine, 47*(13), 2217–2228. https://doi.org/10.1017/s0033291717000873

Vilsaint, C. L., NeMoyer, A., Fillbrunn, M., Sadikova, E., Kessler, R. C., Sampson, N. A., Alvarez, K., Green, J. G., McLaughlin, K. A., Chen, R., Williams, D. R., Jackson, J. S., & Alegría, M. (2019). Racial/ethnic differences in 12-month prevalence and persistence of mood, anxiety, and substance use disorders: Variation by nativity and socioeconomic status. *Comprehensive Psychiatry, 89,* 52–60. https://doi.org/10.1016/j.comppsych.2018.12.008

Viswasam, K., Eslick, G. D., & Starcevic, V. (2019). Prevalence, onset and course of anxiety disorders during pregnancy: A systematic review and meta analysis. *Journal of Affective Disorders, 255,* 27–40. https://doi.org/10.1016/j.jad.2019.05.016

Wesseloo, R., Kamperman, A. M., Munk-Olsen, T., Pop, V. J., Kushner, S. A., & Bergink, V. (2016). Risk of postpartum relapse in bipolar disorder and postpartum psychosis: A systematic review and meta-analysis. *American Journal of Psychiatry, 173*(2), 117–127. https://doi.org/10.1176/appi.ajp.2015.15010124

Wisner, K. L., Sit, D. K. Y., McShea, M. C., Rizzo, D. M., Zoretich, R. A., Hughes, C. L., Eng, H. F., Luther, J. F., Wisniewski, S. R., Costantino, M. L., Confer, A. L., Moses-Kolko, E. L., Famy, C. S., & Hanusa, B. H. (2013). Onset timing, thoughts of self-harm, and diagnoses in postpartum women with screen-positive depression findings. *JAMA Psychiatry, 70*(5), 490–498. https://doi.org/10.1001/jamapsychiatry.2013.87

Woody, C. A., Ferrari, A. J., Siskind, D. J., Whiteford, H. A., & Harris, M. G. (2017). A systematic review and meta-regression of the prevalence and incidence of perinatal depression. *Journal of Affective Disorders, 219*, 86–92. https://doi.org/10.1016/j.jad.2017.05.003

World Health Organization. (2021). *Comprehensive mental health action plan 2013–2030* [Report]. WHO. https://apps.who.int/iris/handle/10665/345301

World Health Organization. (2023). *Women of reproductive age (15–49 years) population (thousands)* [Table: WHO regions: Americas; Date: 2023]. https://www.who.int/data/maternal-newborn-child-adolescent-ageing/indicator-explorer-new/mca/women-of-reproductive-age-(15-49-years)-population-(thousands)

Yeh, H. H., Westphal, J., Hu, Y., Peterson, E. L., Williams, L. K., Prabhakar, D., Frank, C., Autio, K., Elsiss, F., Simon, G. E., Beck, A., Lynch, F. L., Rossom, R. C., Lu, C. Y., Owen-Smith, A. A., Waitzfelder, B. E., & Ahmedani, B. K. (2019). Diagnosed mental health conditions and risk of suicide mortality. *Psychiatric Services, 70*(9), 750–757. https://doi.org/10.1176/appi.ps.201800346

Yildiz, P. D., Ayers, S., & Phillips, L. (2017). The prevalence of posttraumatic stress disorder in pregnancy and after birth: A systematic review and meta-analysis. *Journal of Affective Disorders, 208*, 634–645. https://doi.org/10.1016/j.jad.2016.10.009

Yim, I. S., Tanner Stapleton, L. R., Guardino, C. M., Hahn-Holbrook, J., & Dunkel Schetter, C. (2015). Biological and psychosocial predictors of postpartum depression: Systematic review and call for integration. *Annual Review of Clinical Psychology, 11*, 99–137. https://doi.org/10.1146/annurev-clinpsy-101414-020426

Yoch, M. (2021). *New Global Burden of Disease analyses show depression and anxiety among the top causes of health loss worldwide, and a significant increase due to the COVID-19 pandemic | The Institute for Health Metrics and Evaluation.* [Blog]. IHME. https://www.healthdata.org/news-events/insights-blog/acting-data/new-global-burden-disease-analyses-show-depression-and

Chapter 4
Epidemiology of Mental Health Conditions in Older Adult Women

Fern J. Webb, Phildra Swagger, and Selena Webster-Bass

Introduction

This chapter focuses on the epidemiology of mental health conditions which have a high incidence, prevalence, and mortality among women aged 65 years or older living in the United States (U. S.). The etiology of mental health conditions, including risk and protective factors, and the estimated impact of the COVID-19 pandemic (with the highest incidence and mortality from March 2020 to December 2021) are also presented throughout this chapter. The epidemiology of mental health conditions and their associative factors among older women living in the U. S. is of high relevance.

From a public health perspective consistent with the World Health Organization's (WHO) 2022 *Mental Health Report*, the term "mental health conditions" is used broadly throughout this chapter to describe mental states associated with psychological distress or psychosocial disability. Specifically, the *International Classification of Diseases 11th Revision (ICD-11)* defines mental health conditions or illness as a "syndrome or condition characterized by clinical disruptions in cognition, emotion or behavior resulting in significant impairment with personal, family, social, educational, or occupational areas of life function" (WHO, 2022, p. 8).

F. J. Webb (✉)
Department of Surgery, Center for Health Equity and Engagement Research (CHEER),
University of Florida, Jacksonville, FL, USA
e-mail: Fern.Webb@jax.ufl.edu

P. Swagger
Combined Expertise Inc., Tampa, FL, USA
e-mail: pswagger@combinedexpertise.com

S. Webster-Bass
Voices Institute LLC, Jacksonville, FL, USA
e-mail: Selena@voicesinst.org

A. Hanson, B. L. Levin (eds.), *Women's Behavioral Health*,
https://doi.org/10.1007/978-3-031-58293-6_4

Psychosocial disability is characterized as the "inability to fully and effectively function in society on an equal basis with others due to societal barriers, or lack of access to adequate health care and medical treatment" (WHO, 2022, p. 8). Throughout this chapter, the term "mental health condition" is used interchangeably with the term "mental illness" or "psychological distress".

Population Impact of Mental Health Conditions

Globally, 12.5% of the worldwide population or 970 million people (1 in 8 people) were living with a mental health condition in 2019 (Institute of Health Metrics and Evaluation, 2019). More than 580 million people globally were living with either depression or anxiety, the two most prevalent mental health conditions related to *psychological distress* (WHO, 2022). Changes in mental health conditions on a global scale have been steadily increasing over the last 20 years. Estimates of the percentage of the population having at least one mental health condition increased by 20% between 1993 and 2014 (McManus et al., 2014).

In 2021, estimates were that 23% of all adults living in the U. S., representing about 58 million people, lived with a mental condition or illness (SAMHSA, 2022). Globally, women are two times more likely to experience a mental health condition compared with men (WHO, 2022). In 2021, the *National Survey on Drug Use and Health* (*NSDUH*) results show nearly 34% of U. S. adults aged 18–25 report having any type of mental illness (AMI) compared with 28% of U. S. adults aged 26–49, and 15% of U. S. adults aged 50 years of age or older (SAMHSA, 2022). The prevalence of AMI was highest among U. S. adults of two or more races/ethnicities (almost 35%), with U. S. adults of Asian ethnicity (16%) reporting the lowest percentage of past year prevalence of AMI (SAMHSA, 2022).

On the other hand, serious mental illness (SMI), defined as "extreme psychological distress experienced on an ongoing persistent basis" (WHO, 2022), is much lower in the U. S. with similar trends observed globally (SAMHSA, 2022). In 2021, 6.5% of the U. S. adult population, or approximately 14 million people, had a SMI (SAMHSA, 2022). Similar to the prevalence of AMI in the U. S. population, adults aged 18–25 (approximately 11%) had higher SMI prevalence when compared with adults aged 26–49 (7%), or older than 50 (2.5%) (SAMHSA, 2022). Regarding race/ethnicity, American Indian/Alaskan Native (AI/AN) had the highest prevalence of SMI at approximately 9% compared with Asian adults having the lowest prevalence of SMI at nearly 3% (SAMHSA, 2022). While the prevalence of SMI has remained steady over the last two decades (Rice-Oxley, 2019), the incidence of mental health conditions is projected to increase in the U. S. and global populations given public health efforts to increase awareness, prevention, treatment, and acceptance (da Silva et al., 2020) as well as increased projections in individual and societal trauma resulting from societal injustices and discrimination (Compton & Shim, 2015; Thornicroft et al., 2016).

Disability, Comorbidity and Mortality of Mental Health Conditions

Globally, mental conditions account for ~5% of the overall disease burden with more women affected than men (SAMHSA, 2022). Reports indicate that the types of mental health conditions that burden the population change throughout the life course (Vigo et al., 2016). Mental health illness on an individual/intrapersonal level impacts one's activities of daily living (ADL) (Linden, 2017). According to the *ICF*, poor mental health or high levels of psychological distress are associated with limitations of ADLs (Linden, 2017). The *ICF* defines disability as an "umbrella term for impairments, activity limitations, or participation restrictions", and that "environment", "life situation", or "context" are essential when seeking to understand the epidemiology and impact of mental health conditions (Federici et al., 2017; Linden, 2017). The *ICF* further divides functionality and disability into "body functions and structures" to include *physiological* functions captured by "temperament and personality functions", "energy and drive functions", and "emotion functions" (Linden, 2017). These conceptual functions directly relate to psychological distress diagnosed or characterized as conditions like depression, anxiety, and other emerging conditions of "imposter" and "superwoman" syndromes (Holden et al., 2021; Rivera et al., 2021).

The *World Health Organization Disability Assessment Schedule* (WHODAS 2.0) is an assessment tool created to measure the ability to provide self-care or to interact socially with others (Federici et al., 2017). WHODAS measures the degree of disability in the population. Almazán-Isla et al. (2014) found disability scores (as measured by WHODAS) were higher among women and among persons with severe mental illness. Disability-adjusted life years (DALYs) is another measure created to describe years of life lost (YLL) due to a certain condition (WHO, 2020). DALYs are measured by summing one's estimated years of living with a disability (YLD) added to the estimated number of years of life lost due to premature death (WHO, 2020). DALYs create a standard measure to compare the impact of disability caused by various health conditions, including mental illnesses, which helps when describing morbidity (including disability and comorbidity) and premature mortality. Research shows that DALYs are higher for persons living with a mental health condition given comorbidity with other chronic or infectious diseases (Chesney et al., 2014).

Severe mental illness, or extreme psychological distress, also has a substantial impact on mortality given that populations with a high proportion of persons with mental health conditions report significantly higher mortality rates compared with other populations. Globally, people living with mental health conditions are projected to die 10–20 years earlier compared with people who do not have a reported or diagnosed mental health condition (WHO, 2022). Mortality attributed to mental health conditions will continue to increase globally (Charlson et al., 2015) since physiological conditions such as cardiovascular, respiratory, and infectious diseases are exacerbated among persons with mental health conditions (Chesney et al.,

2014). This is supported by research findings that mental health conditions are associated with cardiovascular underdiagnosis and treatment (Thornicroft, 2011), contributing to higher cardiovascular-related mortality in this population (Smith et al., 2013a, b). The theory is that persons with mental health conditions oftentimes neglect care for other life-threatening conditions, which serve as the primary cause of death (Chesney et al., 2014).

Epidemiology of Mental Health Conditions Among Older Women

Epidemiology is defined as "the study of the distribution and determinants of health-related states or events in specified populations, and the application of this study to the control of health problems" (Last, 2001, p. 61). From an epidemiological perspective, diseases are not randomly distributed in the population. Further, individuals may have certain characteristics which increase or decrease their risks for developing different diseases or maintaining health. The epidemiology of mental health conditions in older populations is complex given exposure and responses to infinite risk and protective factors throughout the life course (Lilford & Hughes, 2020). Examining the epidemiology of mental health conditions in older women is of high importance since women comprise the majority of the world's population. In fact, more than half of the approximately 56 million adults aged 65 years or older in the U. S. in 2020 are women (U. S. Administration for Community Living, 2021).

Women are also expected to live, on average, 6 years longer than men. According to the Centers for Disease Control and Prevention, the average life expectancy for women in the U. S. is 79 years compared with men's average life expectancy of 73 years old (Arias et al., 2022). While life expectancy and health outcomes for individuals with chronic diseases are improving (as compared to prior generations), the need for more information regarding mental health conditions, risks, and protective factors, as well as effective oral and behavioral treatments require more discussion and information sharing to adequately address these conditions in populations of older women. This is increasingly relevant for women; the *NSDUH* 2021 study (SAMHSA, 2022) shows approximately 27% of U. S. women had any mental illness (AMI) compared with 18% of men, with more women (7%) having a SMI compared to men (4%).

Almost 20 years ago, Kessler et al. (2005) estimated approximately 50% of all Americans could meet the criteria of having at least one mental health condition given what was known about mental conditions at that time. Since then, significant advances have been made to identify and specifically characterize mental health conditions or illnesses (SAMHSA, 2022), which has contributed to more precise screening, diagnosis, and treatments. Mental illnesses include a myriad of conditions, varying in degree of severity. These include (but are not limited to) the following: anxiety; attention deficit hyperactivity disorder (ADHD); depression; bipolar;

obsessive-compulsiveness conditions; schizophrenia; post-traumatic stress disorder; and suicide (SAMHSA, 2022) briefly described below in the context of older women.

Mental Health Conditions and Associative Factors in Older Women

From a public health perspective, examining mental health conditions in women 65 years of age or older is important given variation in outcomes and associative factors by age and gender. Over the last 20 years, we have learned a great deal about the signs and symptoms of various mental health conditions as well as pharmacological, cognitive, and social-behavioral treatment approaches. To keep pace with medical treatment, ongoing assessment of the epidemiology of mental health conditions that affect older women in the U. S. is vitally important. However, medical treatment will only be relevant and effective with increased understanding of: (a) incidence, prevalence, and mortality of mental health conditions affecting older women; and (b) risks and protective factors (for a lifespan perspective, see Chaps. 2 and 3 in this volume).

Depression Depression is characterized as a state of being that negatively affects how you feel, the way you think, and the way you act or behave; as such, depression is often referred to as a mood disorder since one's mood appears to be in a persistent and constant negative affect, having a 15% annual prevalence among all adults in the U. S. (National Institute of Mental Health [NIMH], 2023a). A more recent meta-analysis estimated a global prevalence of 35% (Cai et al., 2023). A meta-analysis of population-based studies conducted with community-dwelling older adults in the U. S. shows that more women report having depression or depressive symptomatology than men (Cheung & Mui, 2023). While the incidence of depression in the U. S. is higher among women younger than 65 years old (SAMHSA, 2022), the factors influencing the onset of depression in women 65 years old or older differ substantially from factors associated with incidence and prevalence rates of depression in younger populations.

While a myriad of factors (biochemistry, genetics, personality, and environment) influence depression (NIMH, 2023a), a meta-analysis of 85 epidemiological studies found that among older persons, women are more at risk for depression due to: widowhood or living alone; cognitive decline; financial strain; and the onset of comorbidity of chronic conditions (Girgus et al., 2017). Cheung and Mui (2023) reported similar factors associated with increased prevalence of depression among older women ($n = 1600$) to include: less social participation; less emotional spousal support; having more ADL impairment; and family conflicts or disharmony.

These associative factors to depression are of high importance since research shows that older women are less likely to be married and more likely to be a widow

(Sasson & Umberson, 2014). Regarding health, women who live to older ages have more comorbid conditions than men or younger women (Noh et al., 2016). Elderly women who experience cognitive decline report more depressive symptoms (Lee et al., 2017) which may be a manifestation of increased frustration as one faces the realization of losing cognitive function. National studies also show that elderly women are more likely to have financial hardship as they age (Fiske et al., 2009; Girgus et al., 2017).

Postpartum Depression (PPD) PDD is a depressive condition that occurs when women give birth, especially at ages 35 years or older that affects up to 15% of new mothers (Woody et al., 2017). While PPD only occurs in women of childbearing age, women diagnosed with PPD are (a) significantly more likely to have AMI or SMI in later years. In addition, children of women with untreated PPD are at increased risk for developmental impairment, low self-esteem, and subsequent behavioral problems for mother and child (Patel et al., 2012). Regarding etiology, biological deficiencies like zinc supplementation have been explored where women with PPD consuming zinc had improved mental health outcomes (Anbari-Nogyni et al., 2020). More recent findings by Liu et al. (2022) report that mentally healthy women who elect to have a cesarean are more likely to develop PPD compared to mentally healthy women who opted to have a vaginal delivery (unless a cesarean was medically required or warranted). Additional associative factors for women who develop PPD include marital conflicts, low self-confidence and health efficacy, and negative labor experiences (Ahmadpour et al., 2023) which are associative factors that are prevalent among older women.

Bipolar Disorders Bipolar disorder, formerly referred to as "manic-depressive illness," is described as a condition involving alternating behavior of extreme or high energy and activity (i.e., mania) with behavior of extreme low energy or activity (i.e., depressive mood) (NIMH, 2023b). Historically considered within the spectrum of depression, bipolar conditions are now grouped into Bipolar II, changes in affect and energy that do not severely impede daily life functions and activities, and Bipolar I, which consists of severe changes in mood and energy that severely impact daily life function (NIMH, 2023b). Bipolar I affects women and men equally yet more older women than older men tend to be diagnosed with Bipolar I (NIMH, 2023b). Moreover, women with Bipolar are more likely to have other physical and mental health conditions compared with men with Bipolar (NIMH, 2023b). While all of the causes and associative factors for Bipolar I or II remain relatively unknown, research shows that physiological factors related to biology and brain chemistry, along with social environment characteristics have been associated with Bipolar I condition in women (NIMH, 2023b).

Anxiety Anxiety is a mental condition described as a severe inability to respond to situations or life events that persist beyond temporary worry or fear (Office on Women's Health [OWH], 2021a). Approximately 40 million adults in the U. S. have anxiety with women diagnosed at double the rate of men (OWH, 2021a). Moreover, the lifetime prevalence of anxiety is two times higher in women than in men with higher risk observed for developing other mental health conditions like depression and are associated with physiological (e. g., irritable bowel syndrome, chronic pain, and cardiovascular diseases) (Kaplan et al., 2014; Lackner et al., 2013) and cognitive conditions (AgingCare, 2023). Factors associated with or possibly causal to increased anxiety in women include genetics, traumatic events, and hormonal changes that begin at the onset of menstruation (OWH, 2021c). Anxiety is more prevalent in populations of women given higher incidence of trauma related to childhood, and sexual and emotional violence (WHO, 2022).

Generalized Anxiety Disorder (GAD) GAD is categorized by excessively thinking about life experiences or everyday activities where independent life functioning is negatively affected (OWH, 2021c). GAD symptoms can be described in a myriad of ways such as increased muscle tension, headaches, or gastrointestinal issues (OWH, 2021c). Panic attacks, characterized as more abrupt and sudden episodes with extremely high levels of fear resulting in an immediate physiological body response (i.e., inability to breathe; urge to use the bathroom), are more commonly diagnosed in women than in men, and more among younger aged women than older women (OWH, 2021c).

Post-traumatic Stress Disorder (PTSD) PTSD results from the lack of psychological recovery from a traumatic life event (OWH, 2021b). Traumatic events are simply defined as "events that one perceives as dangerous or scary"; while psychological distress is expected in response to any traumatic event, PTSD is characterized by the prolonged feeling of lack of control, fear, or perceived danger beyond what is considered "normal" (i.e., days, weeks, months) (OWH, 2021b). Women are more likely to be diagnosed with PTSD with a 10% lifetime prevalence for developing this condition (OWH, 2021b). Innumerable factors can lead to PTSD where anyone who experiences trauma is at risk (OWH, 2021b) and prolonged exposure to trauma is directly associated with the severity of PTSD (National Center for PTSD, 2023).

Attention Deficit/Hyperactivity Disorder (ADHD) ADHD is a mental health condition primarily studied in younger populations of school children or working adults, which persists into adulthood (Henry & Jones, 2011). ADHD is simply characterized as the inability to remain focused on an activity or goal to completion and is usually assessed by one's ability to focus on completing immediate- or less-time-consuming tasks. ADHD is more readily observed and diagnosed in populations that have high social interaction (i.e., school children, places of employment) like children and working adults. However, girls are underdiagnosed in childhood. Missed or late diagnosis can be damaging to a woman's mental health and well-being (Attoe & Climie, 2023). Thus, the incidence and prevalence of ADHD among older adults, and in particular older women, is low due to the inability to observe and diagnose this condition, especially in older women of overall high functioning.

Obsessive-Compulsive Disorder (OCD) OCD is a condition characterized by unwanted, uncontrolled thoughts (obsessions) or behaviors (compulsions) which can result in excessive repetitive behaviors that can impede daily life function (OWH, 2021c). Approximately 2.2 million, or 1 in 100 adults in the U. S. report having OCD (OWH, 2021c), and is usually co-diagnosed or associated with other mental conditions like eating conditions, panic attacks, or depression (AgingCare, 2023). Grenier et al. (2009) found that the 1-year prevalence of OCD in ~2800 older adults aged 65 years or older was 1.5%, and unlike other mental health conditions, was higher in men than women. However, Calamari et al. (2014) suggest the incidence and prevalence of OCD might be underdiagnosed in older adults due to the lack of validated tools that can detect obsessive symptoms that would characterize uncommon behavior in older adults separate from "expected" or "natural" aging. While the causes of OCD are not completely known, research indicates that genetics, physiobiological factors as well as the environment are associated factors. For example, women who have OCD report that their symptoms seem to worsen when they are on their menstrual cycle, when pregnant, or after birth (when hormonal levels naturally change) (OWH, 2021c).

Schizophrenia Approximately 2.8 million adults in the U. S. live with schizophrenia (WHO, 2022) which is defined as having unreal or distorted views of reality (WHO, 2022). The incidence and prevalence of late-onset schizophrenia (L-OS) among older persons is low compared to the incidence and prevalence of other major mood conditions (WHO, 2022). Although the incidence and prevalence of L-OS is low, representing about .3% of all mental health conditions, it is arguably the most impairing (Barbui et al., 2021). In fact, the WHO (2022) reports that schizophrenia is the most costly mental health condition worldwide. The causes and associative factors for schizophrenia are unknown although more delineation is now given to *positive* (i.e., delusions, hallucinations, lapses in coherent thinking), or *negative* (i.e., lack of emotion, loss of interest, or incoherent thinking or interaction with others) symptoms observed in persons diagnosed with schizophrenia. Regardless of sociodemographic characteristics including race/ethnicity, gender, or age at onset, persons diagnosed with schizophrenia are more likely to report adverse childhood experiences and persistent life-long trauma (Kline et al., 2016).

Suicide and Suicidal Ideations Globally, suicide accounts for one out of every 100 deaths with estimates that only 5% of suicide attempts are successful (WHO, 2022). Suicide accounts for 1% of deaths, or 1 out of every 100 deaths globally (SAMHSA, 2022) with estimates that at least 20 attempts are made for every 1 successful suicide death (WHO, 2022). Regarding gender, women are more likely to attempt suicide than men although men are two times more likely to be successful at committing suicide than women (WHO, 2022). This gender disparity becomes even more apparent in high-resourced/high-income countries where men are 3 times more likely to die by suicide compared to women (WHO, 2022). Regardless of gender, persons of younger ages are significantly more likely to die by suicide compared to older persons. For example, in 2019, death by suicide was the 3rd leading cause of death among women/girls aged 15–29 years old with approximately 58% of suicide occurring in people younger than 50 years old (SAMHSA, 2022). Suicide rates for women ≥65 years old are 5.6 persons per 10^6 population than 8.2 persons per 10^6 in 2021 (WHO, 2022).

Estimating accurate mortality, especially due to suicide, is complex since the number of suicide attempts before a successful suicide occurs is poorly measured. The incidence of suicide and suicidal ideation among older women remains substantially low compared to other segments of the population at higher risk. Although the incidence of suicide and suicide ideation is relatively low among older women, women of older ages who commit suicide or have suicidal ideations have specific associative factors and experiences related to severe comorbidities resulting in high impairment and poor life quality (WHO, 2022).

Public Health Ecological Framework for Associative Factors

As women age, the manifestation of mental health conditions is influenced by a myriad of factors, such as genetic predisposition as well as behavioral, socio-cultural, and environmental exposures unique to each woman. However, current evidence shows that the most common mental health conditions among older women in the U. S. are depression, anxiety, and bipolar II. What remains to be determined is whether increases in diagnosis/incidence among older women are due to increased societal acceptance rather than solely advances in screening and clinical diagnosis. From a public health perspective, examining mental health conditions in women 65 years of age or older is important given the variation in outcomes and associative factors by age and gender and the subsequent opportunity to provide tailored treatment.

In past editions of the *Women's Mental Health* textbooks (Kenna et al., 2010; Padgett et al., 1998), mental health conditions were referred to as "chronic conditions of the young" since the first incidence of a mental health condition typically occurs during adolescence and young adulthood. Older adults have a lower lifetime prevalence of mental health conditions. Fifteen percent of older adults have a lower lifetime prevalence of AMI compared to younger persons with AMI (SAMHSA, 2022). The initial age of onset has remained steady in 2022 when compared with findings from the National Comorbidity Survey (NCS-R) conducted 20 years ago (2001–2003). The NCS-R found one-half of the population had a mental health condition as early as age 14 while three-quarters of the population who met the criteria for a mental health diagnosis had a mental health condition by age 24 (Kessler et al., 2005).

The etiology and manifestation of mental health conditions in adolescents and younger adults are associated with major life events, such as (but not limited to) obtaining college degrees and education beyond high school, starting professional careers, forming intimate and committed relationships, and deciding to start families of their own. Women with severe mental health conditions are significantly more likely to have experienced violence during their lifetime (Khalifeh et al., 2015) compared with women who do not have a mental health condition. Specifically, experiences of intimate partner violence or sexual violence are strong risk factors for mental health conditions of depression, anxiety, stress conditions including PTSD and suicidal ideation (Oram et al., 2017).

The risk of having a mental health condition or an "episode" increases substantially when any of these life experiences are disturbed or result in a negative, unexpected, or unwanted outcome. Ongoing incidents or occurrences of mental conditions, especially manifesting at ages 24 years old or younger, are key factors that limit levels of functioning and health. Recognizing mental health conditions experienced at younger ages can provide insight to women in later years. A direct dose-response relationship is also observed between severity and impairment where women who experience three or more mental health conditions were severely more impaired compared to women with fewer reported mental health conditions (SAMHSA, 2022).

Over the last 20 years, we have learned a great deal about signs and symptoms of various mental health conditions and pharmacological, cognitive, and social-behavioral treatment approaches. Historical stigma and hesitancy to seek treatment when experiencing a mental health episode has been tracked to prior institutionalization of mental illness or fear of family or community response to diagnosis and treatment may also result in older women not seeking treatment. To keep pace with medical treatment, ongoing assessment of the epidemiology of mental health conditions affecting older women in the U. S. is vitally important. Epidemiology can describe the incidence, prevalence, and mortality of mental health conditions disproportionately affecting older women; and identify risks and protective factors for insights to inform effective prevention and treatment strategies.

During the last 10 years, the national conversation has changed from a focus on "mental illness" to supporting "mental wellness". Using a socioecological framework of "mental wellness" provides theoretical support for public health, social policy, and health practitioners to address mental health and mental health conditions. The framework offers a comprehensive model which includes factors representing the sociological levels of health influence. As a multidimensional framework, the socioecological model provides a deeper understanding of the specific areas and life events which are associated with her mental health. Acknowledgment of mental health conditions using this model for women of all ages and of varying cultures is creating a national discussion for an increased acceptance and value of one's mental health.

Although the prevalence of mental health conditions appears to be steadily increasing, why it is increasing is unclear. Possible factors include more accurate diagnoses and reporting of these diagnoses, exacerbated individual or societal trauma, the global COVID pandemic, social and institutional injustices, natural or man-made disasters, and other social determinants of health (SDOH), more recently referred to as social *drivers* of health. Each of these factors (Table 4.1) directly affects mental health and should be adequately addressed to (1) ensure prevention

Table 4.1 Associative factors of common mental health conditions

Factors	Depression	Anxiety	Bipolar	PTSD
Family history/genetics	X	X	X	
Brain changes	X		X	
Biological causes	X	X	X	X
Stress	X			X
Comorbid conditions	X	X		
Societal injustices	X	X		X

and intervention initiatives, and (2) address the creation, amendment, and implementation of public health policy.

Individual Biological Factors Genetics, hormonal changes, and societal injustices are strongly associated with the most common or prevalent mental health conditions in older women. At least four genes affecting depression (Deng et al., 2022) and anxiety have been identified (Domschke et al., 2012). In addition to genetic factors, (childhood) trauma, stress, and the onset and morbidity of chronic conditions are significantly associated with observed and diagnosed mental health conditions of depression and anxiety (WHO, 2022).

The Structural and Political Determinants of Health The SDOH, more recently coined social *drivers* of health, are defined as "social and environmental conditions experienced across the lifespan" (Centers for Disease Control and Prevention [CDC], 2018). The political determinants of health (PDOH) are defined as governing policies and practices that affect the population's health (Dawes, 2020). Structural racism is conceptualized as the implementation of policies or practices that inherently and disproportionately favor persons socially classified as "White" or those having the ability to influence or govern others (Guess, 2006; Harrell, 2000).

Structural racism is a major contributor to psychological distress in the U. S. Studies conducted in other developed countries show higher incidence and prevalence of mental health conditions among persons with African and Caribbean ancestry. Cohen and Marino (2013) determined lifetime prevalence of psychotic symptoms was higher among U. S. Blacks (15%) compared with U. S. Whites (10%). Compton and Shim (2020) conclude that mental health conditions or illnesses may be increasing in various populations given increased exposure to societal injustices, discrimination, and public policy. The perpetual systemic inequity in community-wide access to fundamental healthy life resources of healthy food, safe and clean environments and housing, affordable education, health, and childcare, along with employment opportunities have all been shown to increase cumulative stress (Assari, 2018). Neighborhood factors, such as economic and residential factors and community unrest (i.e., vandalism, and other indicators of societal loss of control like violence), are also directly associated with increased incidence and prevalence of mental health conditions in populations (Bjørndal et al., 2023).

To address structural racism, health services research is increasingly informed by the SDOH and PDOH conceptual frameworks (CDC, 2018; Dawes, 2020). Harrell's (2000) multidimensional model of social and political factors illustrates the multiple mechanisms by which structural racism increases psychological distress in persons of color over time. Compton and Shim (2015) describe how social policies that impede access to education, health care, healthy food, and safe housing directly affect overall mental health. Research by Walker et al. (2011) shows how governing policies and practices increase the risk for severe mental illness among persons who experience negative SDOH factors in early childhood.

Increasing Access to Mental Health Services

Several reasons have been cited as to why older women do not seek treatment for mental health conditions, or for mental wellness. These include (1) a lack of confidence in the health care system's ability to effectively treat patients' mental health conditions devoid of stigma and institutional discrimination; (2) low levels of understanding of the biology and importance of mental wellness, and in particular, the need to treat to increase well-being and function; and (3) lack of access to and navigation of health care systems which result in improved mental health outcomes for patients (WHO, 2022). Hence, large segments of the population may choose to live with their mental health condition, never seeking treatment or care.

Interestingly, mental health conditions are more prevalent in high-resourced, high-income countries (15%) compared to the prevalence in low-resourced/low-income countries (12%) (GBD 2019 Human Resources for Health Collaborators, 2022). Reasons for underreporting mental health conditions in low-resourced/low-income countries may include national emphasis on communicable and chronic diseases; continued stigma and discrimination of persons with mental illnesses; and poor epidemiological reporting infrastructure for behavioral health. The need for ongoing epidemiological evaluation is critical. Such evaluation will lead to better characterization of disease changes, identification of potential/new risks or protective factors that affect access to care, and more accurate diagnoses, and more specific/tailored treatment for mental health disorders.

COVID-19 Pandemic and Mental Conditions

Mental health conditions have significantly increased among the population due to the COVID-19 pandemic. The number of persons per 100,000 (10^6) living with a mental health condition significantly increased during and after the pandemic. For example, 193 million people (or 2471 persons/10^6) had a mental health condition before the pandemic while 246 million people ($3153/10^6$) reported having a mental condition during the pandemic, approximately a 28% increase (WHO, 2022). Webb and Chen (2022) reported that gender, age, social isolation, socioeconomic status, and chronic physical and psychiatric comorbidities (the same factors influencing mental among older adult women) had an even greater impact during the pandemic. Approximately 28 million people (3825 persons/10^6) had anxiety before the pandemic compared to 374 million (4802 persons/10^6) with anxiety after 2020, representing a 26% increase after the pandemic (WHO, 2022).

Older women, even before the pandemic, were at increased risk for anxiety, in particular anxiety related to fear of death, experiencing comorbid chronic conditions, and increasing need for additional assistance from others (Khademi et al., 2020). Older women (28%) compared to older men (20%), with 26% of those aged 65–74 and 19% of those 80 or older, self-reported experiencing anxiety or depression during the pandemic (Koma et al., 2020). These numbers are similar to observed percentages before the pandemic (Girgus et al., 2017). Khubchandani et al. (2021) reported that men were more likely to report depression while women were more likely to report anxiety. It is important to note that while self-reported anxiety and depression among older adults increased during the pandemic, the prevalence of these two conditions was still higher among adults younger than 65 years old (Koma et al., 2020).

Need for Community-Focused Mental Health Services for Older Adult Women

Approximately 13% of persons globally are estimated to be currently living with a mental health condition (WHO, 2022). The thrust to create mental health systems that provide preventive care and effective medical treatments to improve mental health requires a better understanding of the etiology and experiences at an individual and societal level. There has been more intentionality to create integrated, patient-centered, and evidence-based mental health systems/services. However, mental health systems embedded within large, multi-faceted health care systems are often fragmented and lack adequate resources, research, and evidence-based programs/interventions tailored to meet the need of at-risk populations.

According to WHO (2022), mental health programs must *"address the individual, social and structural determinants of mental health, and then intervening to reduce risks, build resilience and establish supportive environments for [optimal] mental health"* (pg. XVIII). However, building such programs remains a significant challenge to empirically measure each protective factor in integrated, multi-faceted, and dynamically designed systems. Moreover, mental health programs and systems have not traditionally been designed to include stakeholders' perspectives (i.e., older women) for what services will be provided, hence reducing the likelihood of relevance or effectiveness for the broader community.

Several suggestions have been offered regarding what should be incorporated into any health program designed to improve mental health among older women.

For example, individual-level strategies, in light of the reduced impact of COVID-19, include providing help/support lines for persons in crisis to call, assisting with food provision, and reducing the amount of time spent on social media (Webb & Chen, 2022). Social-level interventions should promote ongoing interaction/engagement with trusted family and friends (Webb & Chen, 2022). Community-level interventions should address ongoing interaction through virtual chats, safe in-person meetings, and discussions with trusted sources (i.e., family and friends).

Seibert et al. (2022) recommend that community-level interventions address loneliness and social isolation among older adults who are at increased risk due to retirement, decreased income, loss of significant family members and friends, and overall declining health. Another recommendation is to ensure persons at risk and their caregivers are connected to groups that provide support (Webb & Chen, 2022). Recommendations for environmental/structural interventions include creating more "green space" or open living areas (Engemann et al., 2018) and actively working to reduce exposure to environmental toxins (Attademo et al., 2017). Health care system interventions should focus on improving specificity of screening tools and providing treatment that promotes mental wellness as tailored to older women's health needs and conditions.

Programs that are designed to specifically address the mental health needs of older adult women must be developed and offered to increase opportunities for interested persons to attend (and benefit). These programs should provide a "safe space" for persons to share their past experiences that affect their mental health. In addition, older adult women living with a mental health condition should be able to seek and receive culturally sensitive, individually tailored treatment to obtain mental wellness. The WHO (2022) encourages public health practitioners, researchers, and policy experts to improve mental health (wellness) using a health equity approach, which requires providers, services, and systems to be intentional, thoughtful, and non-judgmental in the provision of care. Global and national efforts should discuss mental health issues as "conditions" or "diseases" rather than "disorders". If the psychology of "dis" implies dysfunction and promotes stigma, changes in language seek to increase awareness of mental health conditions and reduce the stigma associated with mental health conditions. However, one of the first steps to improve mental health conditions is to better address it in at-risk populations, specifically in older women.

Case Studies of Community-Engaged Mental Health Model Programs

Programs seeking to engage youth and women (of younger ages) are essential when seeking to address mental health conditions among women. However, such programs are critically important to share coping strategies like resilience, mindfulness, peer-to-peer connections, and self-efficacy and validation. The *EmpowerHER* program and *Hope and Healing Circles* are two programs designed to specifically approach mental health from a wellness perspective. The following are brief descriptions of two programs for modeling and community-wide upscaling.

EmpowerHER EmpowerHER is a transformational group coaching program for African American women created by Combined Expertise Inc. (Swagger, 2023) seeking to overcome personal obstacles and achieve professional growth. In particular, EmpowerHER is an exclusive group coaching program designed specifically for high potential African American women of all ages seeking to expand their personal leadership capacity. In recognition of the unique challenges faced by this specific demographic, this program focuses on building a supportive community and equipping women with the necessary tools and strategies to embrace personal growth, alleviate mental health symptoms, and pursue meaningful professional goals.

The 12-week program includes: Orientation and Connection (Week 1); Understanding Mindfulness and Self-Care (Week 2–4); Strengthening Personal Growth (Week 5–10); and Building a Supportive Network (Week 11–12). Working with older African American women in group coaching programs to address limiting beliefs and professional growth can yield numerous benefits. First, these women bring a wealth of wisdom, life experiences, and unique perspectives, enriching the group dynamic and fostering a supportive environment. Their resilience and ability to navigate complex societal challenges can serve as a source of inspiration and motivation for other group members.

Moreover, older African American women often possess deep cultural and community ties, which can enhance the group's cultural competence and facilitate a more inclusive approach to addressing depression and professional growth. By acknowledging and valuing their cultural heritage, the group coaching program can create a safe space that promotes healing, self-discovery, and personal growth. Furthermore, working with older African American women can address the issue of underrepresentation in wellness and professional development services. This targeted approach ensures the unique challenges faced by older African American women are recognized and addressed effectively. The intergenerational aspect of group coaching can also be advantageous, as it allows for the exchange of ideas and knowledge between younger and older participants. This intergenerational collaboration can foster mentorship opportunities and facilitate the transmission of cultural heritage, values, and lessons learned.

The *EmpowerHER* coaching program for African American women encompasses a comprehensive approach to personal wellness while simultaneously supporting professional growth. By providing a nurturing environment, essential mindfulness tools, guidance on personal development, and a robust network, participants can confidently navigate their journey toward personal and professional transformation. *EmpowerHER* empowers women to overcome adversity, enhance psychological well-being, and excel in their chosen profession with newfound resilience and confidence. The benefit may also serve the African American community by enhancing cultural understanding and, in turn, empowering women underrepresented in the community.

Hope and Healing Circles The Hope and Healing Circles program is an intergenerational aggregate of mothers and grandmothers raising children, populations known to be at increased risk for mental health conditions created by Voice Institute LLC (Webster-Bass, 2023). The purpose of the sessions is to cultivate hope, resilience, and positive transformation in families. Peer support sessions focus on mental, emotional, physical, and spiritual well-being while also addressing personal self-development and parenting skills. *Hope and Healing Circles* also provide a safe space for mothers to talk about intergenerational trauma, racial stress and trauma, adversity, and triumphs in a supportive and non-judgmental environment, promoting healing *from the inside out.*

Hope and Healing Circles began in 2021 with funding from local and regional organizations committed to community betterment—the Family Support Services of North Florida, Kids Hope Alliance, the Center for Children's Rights, and the Voices Institute. Developed with residents in the designated areas in which the program, seven prioritized community needs were determined which were: (1) activities for children/teens; (2) community togetherness, love, and unity; (3) safety and security; (4) jobs; (5) healthy living; (6) financial support and education; and (7) neighborhood beautification. These community needs were correlated with five protective factors for strengthening families: (1) parental resilience; (2) social connections; (3) knowledge of parenting and child development; (4) concrete supports in times of support; and (5) social and emotional competence of children. Hope and Healing Circles address the domains of social connection, parental resilience, community togetherness, love, and unity.

Implications for Women's Behavioral Health

Over the last 20 years, our knowledge and understanding of the epidemiology of mental disorders and effective ways to treat women having mental disorders has significantly increased. Findings further support theories that the epidemiology of mental health conditions experienced by women changes over time; for example, the incidence of mental health conditions of virtually every mental health condition decreases as women age, indicating either diagnosis inaccuracies or improved coping skills or mindsets of older women. Understanding that mental health (or any wellness or illness state) does not follow the same exact trajectory in each woman is critical and such understanding must be considered vis-à-vis a population approach to addressing mental health conditions on a global scale.

Our knowledge and understanding of the epidemiology and associative factors of mental health conditions among older women have significantly improved. While all epidemiologic measures of incidence and mortality of mental health conditions are lower for older women, the increasing population size of women aged 65 years and older warrants more attention to improve specificity for screening, diagnosis, and treatment, along with understanding coping strategies older women already employed when living with a mental health condition.

References

AgingCare. (2023). *Obsessive-compulsive disorders in elders*. [Web Article]. https://www.agingcare.com/articles/obsessive-compulsive-disorder-in-elderly-parents-138686.htm

Ahmadpour, P., Faroughi, F., & Mirghafourvand, M. (2023). The relationship of childbirth experience with postpartum depression and anxiety: A cross-sectional study. *BMC Psychology, 11*(1), 58. https://doi.org/10.1186/s40359-023-01105-6

Almazán-Isla, J., Comín-Comín, M., Damián, J., Alcalde-Cabero, E., Ruiz, C., Franco, E., Martín, G., Larrosa-Montañés, L. A., & de Pedro-Cuesta, J. (2014). Analysis of disability using WHODAS 2.0 among the middle-aged and elderly in Cinco Villas, Spain. *Disability & Health Journal, 7*(1), 78–87. https://doi.org/10.1016/j.dhjo.2013.08.004

Anbari-Nogyni, Z., Bidaki, R., Madadizadeh, F., et al. (2020). Relationship of zinc status with depression and anxeity among elderly population. *Clinical Nutrition ESPEN, 37*, 233–239. https://doi.org/10.1016/j.clnesp.2020.02.008

Arias, E., Tejada-Vera, B., Kochanek, K. D., & Ahmad, F. (2022, August). Provisional life expectancy estimates for 2021 [Report]. *NVSS Vital Statistics Rapid Release, No. 23*. https://www.cdc.gov/nchs/data/vsrr/vsrr023.pdf

Assari, S. (2018). Unequal gain of equal resources across racial groups. *International Journal of Health Policy and Management, 7*(1), 1–9. https://doi.org/10.15171/ijhpm.2017.90

Attademo, L., Bernardini, F., Garinella, R., & Compton, M. T. (2017). Environmental pollution and risk of psychotic disorders: A review of the science to date. *Schizophrenia Research, 181*, 55–59. https://doi.org/10.1016/j.schres.2016.10.003

Attoe, D. E., & Climie, E. A. (2023). Miss. Diagnosis: A systematic review of ADHD in adult women. *Journal of Attention Disorders, 27*(7), 645–657. https://doi.org/10.1177/10870547231161533

Barbui, C., Purgato, M., Abdulmalik, J., Caldas-de-Almeida, J. M., Eaton, J., Gureje, O., Hanlon, C., Nosè, M., Ostuzzi, G., Saraceno, B., Saxena, S., Tedeschi, F., & Thornicroft, G. (2021). Efficacy of interventions to reduce coercive treatment in mental health services: Umbrella review of randomised evidence. *British Journal of Psychiatry, 218*(4), 185–195. https://doi.org/10.1192/bjp.2020.144

Bjørndal, L. D., Ebrahimi, O. V., Lan, X., Nes, R. B., & Røysamb, E. (2023). Mental health and environmental factors in adults: A population-based network analysis. *American Psychologist*, Online ahead of print, https://doi.org/10.1037/amp0001208

Cai, H., Jin, Y., Liu, R., Zhang, Q., Su, Z., Ungvari, G. S., Tang, Y. L., Ng, C. H., Li, X. H., & Xiang, Y. T. (2023). Global prevalence of depression in older adults: A systematic review and meta-analysis of epidemiological surveys. *Asian Journal of Psychiatry, 80*, 103417. https://doi.org/10.1016/j.ajp.2022.103417

Calamari, J. E., Woodard, J. L., Armstrong, K. M., Molino, A., Pontarelli, N. K., Socha, J., & Longley, S. L. (2014). Assessing older adults' obsessive-compulsive disorder symptoms: Psychometric characteristics of the Obsessive Compulsive Inventory-Revised. *Journal of Obsessive Compulsion & Related Disorders, 3*(2), 124–131. https://doi.org/10.1016/j.jocrd.2014.03.002

Centers for Disease Control and Prevention. (2018). *Social determinants of health*. [Web page]. https://health.gov/healthypeople/objectives-and-data/social-determinants-health

Charlson, F. J., Baxter, A. J., Dua, T., Degenhardt, L., Whiteford, H. A., & Vos, T. (2015). Excess mortality from mental, neurological and substance use disorders in the Global Burden of Disease Study 2010. *Epidemiology & Psychiatric Sciences, 24*(2), 121–140. https://doi.org/10.1017/s2045796014000687

Chesney, E., Goodwin, G. M., & Fazel, S. (2014). Risks of all-cause and suicide mortality in mental disorders: A meta-review. *World Psychiatry, 13*(2), 153–160. https://doi.org/10.1002/wps.20128

Cheung, E. S. L., & Mui, A. C. (2023). Gender variation and late-life depression: Findings from a national survey in the USA. *Ageing Interntaional, 48*(1), 263–280. https://doi.org/10.1007/s12126-021-09471-5

Cohen, C. I., & Marino, L. (2013). Racial and ethnic differences in the prevalence of psychotic symptoms in the general population. *Psychiatric Services, 64*(11), 1103–1109. https://doi.org/10.1176/appi.ps.201200348

Compton, M. T., & Shim, R. S. (2015). The social determinants of mental health. *FOCUS: The Journal of Lifelong Learning in Psychiatry, 13*(4), 419–425. https://doi.org/10.1176/appi.focus.20150017

Compton, M. T., & Shim, R. S. (2020). Mental illness prevention and mental health promotion: When, who, and how. *Psychiatric Services, 71*(9), 981–983. https://doi.org/10.1176/appi.ps.201900374

da Silva, A. G., Baldaçara, L., Cavalcante, D. A., Fasanella, N. A., & Palha, A. P. (2020). The impact of mental illness stigma on psychiatric emergencies. *Frontiers in Psychiatry, 11*, 573. https://doi.org/10.3389/fpsyt.2020.00573

Dawes, D. E. (2020). *Political determinants of health.* [Web page]. Satcher Health Leadership Institute, Morehouse College of Medicnie. https://satcherinstitute.org/priorities/political-determinants-of-health

Deng, Y. T., Ou, Y. N., Wu, B. S., Yang, Y. X., Jiang, Y., Huang, Y. Y., Liu, Y., Tan, L., Dong, Q., Suckling, J., Li, F., & Yu, J. T. (2022). Identifying causal genes for depression via integration of the proteome and transcriptome from brain and blood. *Molecular Psychiatry, 27*(6), 2849–2857. https://doi.org/10.1038/s41380-022-01507-9

Domschke, K., Gajewska, A., Winter, B., Herrmann, M. J., Warrings, B., Mühlberger, A., Wosnitza, K., Glotzbach, E., Conzelmann, A., Dlugos, A., Fobker, M., Jacob, C., Arolt, V., Reif, A., Pauli, P., Zwanzger, P., & Deckert, J. (2012). ADORA2A Gene variation, caffeine, and emotional processing: A multi-level interaction on startle reflex. *Neuropsychopharmacology, 37*(3), 759–769. https://doi.org/10.1038/npp.2011.253

Engemann, K., Pedersen, C. B., Arge, L., Tsirogiannis, C., Mortensen, P. B., & Svenning, J. C. (2018). Childhood exposure to green space: A novel risk-decreasing mechanism for schizophrenia? *Schizophrenia Research, 199*, 142–148. https://doi.org/10.1016/j.schres.2018.03.026

Federici, S., Bracalenti, M., Meloni, F., & Luciano, J. V. (2017). World Health Organization disability assessment schedule 2.0: An international systematic review. *Disability and Rehabilitation, 39*(23), 2347–2380. https://doi.org/10.1080/09638288.2016.1223177

Fiske, A., Wetherell, J. L., & Gatz, M. (2009). Depression in older adults. *Annual Review of Clinical Psychology, 5*, 363–389. https://doi.org/10.1146/annurev.clinpsy.032408.153621

GBD 2019 Human Resources for Health Collaborators. (2022). Measuring the availability of human resources for health and its relationship to universal health coverage for 204 countries and territories from 1990 to 2019: a systematic analysis for the Global Burden of Disease Study 2019. *The Lancet, 399(10341), 2129–2154.* https://doi.org/10.1016/S0140-6736(22)00532-3

Girgus, J. S., Yang, K., & Ferri, C. V. (2017). The gender difference in depression: Are elderly women at greater risk for depression than elderly men? *Geriatrics (Basel), 2*(4), 35. https://doi.org/10.3390/geriatrics2040035

Grenier, S., Préville, M., Boyer, R., & O'Connor, K. (2009). Prevalence and correlates of obsessive-compulsive disorder among older adults living in the community. *Journal of Anxiety Disorders, 23*(7), 858–865. https://doi.org/10.1016/j.janxdis.2009.04.005

Guess, T. J. (2006). The social construction of whiteness: Racism by intent, racism by consequence. *Critical Sociology, 32*(4), 649–673. https://doi.org/10.1163/156916306779155199

Harrell, S. P. (2000). A multidimensional conceptualization of racism-related stress: Implications for the well-being of people of color. *American Journal of Orthopsychiatry, 70*(1), 42–57. https://doi.org/10.1037/h0087722

Henry, E., & Jones, S. H. (2011). Experiences of older adult women diagnosed with attention deficit hyperactivity disorder. *Journal of Women & Aging, 23*(3), 246–262. https://doi.org/10.1080/08952841.2011.589285

Holden, C. L., Wright, L. E., Herring, A. M., & Sims, P. L. (2021). Imposter syndrome among first- and continuing-generation college students: The roles of perfectionism and stress. *Journal of College Student Retention: Research, Theory & Practice, 0*(0). https://doi.org/10.1177/15210251211019379

Institute of Health Metrics and Evaluation. (2019). *Global Health Data Exchange (GHDx)* [Online databank; Mental disorders]. https://vizhub.healthdata.org/gbd-results/

Kaplan, A., Franzen, M. D., Nickell, P. V., Ransom, D., & Lebovitz, P. J. (2014). An open-label trial of duloxetine in patients with irritable bowel syndrome and comorbid generalized anxiety disorder. *International Journal of Psychiatry in Clinical Practice, 18*(1), 11–15. https://doi.org/10.3109/13651501.2013.838632

Kenna, H. A., Ghezel, T., & Rasgon, N. L. (2010). Epidemiology of mental disorders in older women. In B. L. Levin & M. Becker (Eds.), *A public health perspective of women's mental health* (pp. 65–80). Springer. https://doi.org/10.1007/978-1-4419-1526-9

Kessler, R. C., Berglund, P., Demler, O., Jin, R., Merikangas, K. R., & Walters, E. E. (2005). Lifetime prevalence and age-of-onset distributions of DSM-IV disorders in the National Comorbidity Survey Replication. *Archives of General Psychiatry, 62*(6), 593–602. https://doi.org/10.1001/archpsyc.62.6.593

Khademi, F., Moayedi, S., Golitaleb, M., & Karbalaie, N. (2020). The COVID-19 pandemic and death anxiety in the elderly. *International Journal of Mental Health Nursing, 30*(1), 346–349. https://doi.org/10.1111/inm.12824

Khalifeh, H., Moran, P., Borschmann, R., Dean, K., Hart, C., Hogg, J., Osborn, D., Johnson, S., & Howard, L. M. (2015). Domestic and sexual violence against patients with severe mental illness. *Psychological Medicine, 45*(4), 875–886. https://doi.org/10.1017/s0033291714001962

Khubchandani, J., Sharma, S., Webb, F. J., Wiblishauser, M. J., & Bowman, S. L. (2021). Post-lockdown depression and anxiety in the USA during the COVID-19 pandemic. *Joournal of Public Health, 43*(2), 246–253. https://doi.org/10.1093/pubmed/fdaa250

Kline, E., Millman, Z. B., Denenny, D., Wilson, C., Thompson, E., Demro, C., Connors, K., Bussell, K., Reeves, G., & Schiffman, J. (2016). Trauma and psychosis symptoms in a sample of help-seeking youth. *Schizophrenia Research, 175*(1–3), 174–179. https://doi.org/10.1016/j.schres.2016.04.006

Koma, W., True, S., Fuglesten Biniek, J., Cubanski, J., Orgera, K., & Garfield, R. (2020, October 9). *One in four older adults report anxiety or depression amid the COVID-19 pandemic* [Web page]. KFF. https://www.kff.org/medicare/issue-brief/one-in-four-older-adults-report-anxiety-or-depression-amid-the-covid-19-pandemic/

Lackner, J. M., Ma, C. X., Keefer, L., Brenner, D. M., Gudleski, G. D., Satchidanand, N., Firth, R., Sitrin, M. D., Katz, L., Krasner, S. S., Ballou, S. K., Naliboff, B. D., & Mayer, E. A. (2013). Type, rather than number, of mental and physical comorbidities increases the severity of symptoms in patients with irritable bowel syndrome. *Clinical Gastroenterology and Hepatology, 11*(9), 1147–1157. https://doi.org/10.1016/j.cgh.2013.03.011

Last, J. M. (2001). *Dictionary of epidemiology* (4th ed.). Oxford University Press.

Lee, J., Lee, K. J., & Kim, H. (2017). Gender differences in behavioral and psychological symptoms of patients with Alzheimer's disease. *Asian Journal of Psychiatry, 26*, 124–128. https://doi.org/10.1016/j.ajp.2017.01.027

Lilford, P., & Hughes, J. C. (2020). Epidemiology and mental illness in old age. *BJPsych Advances, 26*(2), 92–103. https://doi.org/10.1192/bja.2019.56

Linden, M. (2017). Definition and assessment of disability in mental disorders under the perspective of the International Classification of Functioning Disability and Health (ICF). *Behavioral Sciences & the Law, 35*(2), 124–134. https://doi.org/10.1002/bsl.2283

Liu, T. C., Peng, H. C., Chen, C., & Chen, C. S. (2022). Mode of delivery is associated with postpartum depression: Do women with and without depression history exhibit a difference? *Healthcare, 10*(7), 1308. https://doi.org/10.3390/healthcare10071308

McManus, S., Bebbington, P., Jenkins, R., & Brugha, T. (2014). *Mental health and wellbeing in England: Adult psychiatric morbidity survey.* [Report]. NHS Digital. https://webarchive.nationalarchives.gov.uk/ukgwa/20180328140249/http:/digital.nhs.uk/catalogue/PUB21748

National Center for PTSD. (2023, August 8). *Prolonged exposure for PTSD.* [Web page]. Department of Veterans Affairs. https://www.ptsd.va.gov/professional/treat/txessentials/prolonged_exposure_pro.asp

National Institute of Mental Health. (2023a, April). *Transforming the understanding and treatment of mental illnesses. What is depression?* [Web page]. Author. https://www.nimh.nih.gov/health/topics/depression

National Institute of Mental Health. (2023b, February). *Bipolar disorder.* [Fact sheet]. Author. https://www.nimh.nih.gov/health/topics/bipolar-disorder

Noh, J. W., Kwon, Y. D., Park, J., Oh, I. H., & Kim, J. (2016). Relationship between physical disability and depression by gender: A panel regression model. *PLoS One, 11*(11), e0166238. https://doi.org/10.1371/journal.pone.0166238

Office of Women's Health. (2021a, February 17). *Obsessive-compulsive disorder.* [Fact sheet]. U. S. Department of Health and Human Services. https://www.womenshealth.gov/mental-health/mental-health-conditions/obsessive-compulsive-disorder

Office of Women's Health. (2021b, June 3). *Post-traumatic stress disorder.* [Fact sheet]. U. S. Department of Health and Human Services. https://www.womenshealth.gov/mental-health/mental-health-conditions/post-traumatic-stress-disorder

Office of Women's Health. (2021c, February). *Anxiety disorders.* [Fact sheet]. U. S. Department of Health & Human Services. https://www.womenshealth.gov/mental-health/mental-health-conditions/anxiety-disorders

Oram, S., Khalifeh, H., & Howard, L. M. (2017). Violence against women and mental health. *Lancet Psychiatry, 4*(2), 159–170. https://doi.org/10.1016/s2215-0366(16)30261-9

Padgett, D. K., Burns, B. J., & Grau, L. A. (1998). Risk factors and resilience: Mental health needs and services use of older women. In B. L. Levin, A. K. Blanch, & A. Jennings (Eds.), *Women's mental health services: A public health perspective* (pp. 390–413). Sage.

Patel, M., Bailey, R. K., Jabeen, S., Ali, S., Barker, N. C., & Osiezagha, K. (2012). Postpartum depression: A review. *Journal of Health Care for the Poor & Underserved, 23*(2), 534–542. https://doi.org/10.1353/hpu.2012.0037

Rice-Oxley, M. (2019, June 3). Mental illness: Is there really a global epidemic? *The Guardian,* Online. https://www.theguardian.com/society/2019/jun/03/mental-illness-is-there-really-a-global-epidemic

Rivera, N., Feldman, E. A., Augustin, D. A., Caceres, W., Gans, H. A., & Blankenburg, R. (2021). Do I belong here? Confronting imposter syndrome at an individual, peer, and institutional level in health professionals. *MedEdPORTAL, 17,* 11166. https://doi.org/10.15766/mep_2374-8265.11166

Sasson, I., & Umberson, D. J. (2014). Widowhood and depression: New light on gender differences, selection, and psychological adjustment. *Journals of Gerontology. Series B: Psychological Sciences and Social Sciences, 69*(1), 135–145. https://doi.org/10.1093/geronb/gbt058

Seibert, T., Schroeder, M. W., Perkins, A. J., Park, S., Batista-Malat, E., Head, K. J., Bakas, T., Boustani, M., & Fowler, N. R. (2022). The impact of the COVID-19 pandemic on the mental health of older primary care patients and their family members. *Journal of Aging Research, 2022,* 6909413. https://doi.org/10.1155/2022/6909413

Smith, D. J., Langan, J., McLean, G., Guthrie, B., & Mercer, S. W. (2013a). Schizophrenia is associated with excess multiple physical-health comorbidities but low levels of recorded cardiovascular disease in primary care: Cross-sectional study. *BMJ Open, 3*(4). https://doi.org/10.1136/bmjopen-2013-002808

Smith, D. J., Martin, D., McLean, G., Langan, J., Guthrie, B., & Mercer, S. W. (2013b). Multimorbidity in bipolar disorder and undertreatment of cardiovascular disease: A cross sectional study. *BMC Medicine, 11,* 263. https://doi.org/10.1186/1741-7015-11-263

Substance Abuse and Mental Health Services Administration. (2022). *Key substance use and mental health indicators in the United States: Results from the 2021 National Survey on Drug Use and Health* [Report; HHS Publication No. PEP22-07-01-005, NSDUH Series H-5]. Sunstance Abuse and Mental Health Services Administration, Center for Behavioral Health Statistics and Quality. https://www.samhsa.gov/data/sites/default/files/reports/rpt39443/2021NSDUHFFRRev010323.pdf

Swagger, P. (2023). *EmpowerHER*. [Web page]. Combined Expertise Inc. https://www.combine-dexpertise.com

Thornicroft, G. (2011). Physical health disparities and mental illness: The scandal of premature mortality. *British Journal of Psychiatry, 199*(6), 441–442. https://doi.org/10.1192/bjp.bp.111.092718

Thornicroft, G., Mehta, N., Clement, S., Evans-Lacko, S., Doherty, M., Rose, D., Koschorke, M., Shidhaye, R., O'Reilly, C., & Henderson, C. (2016). Evidence for effective interventions to reduce mental-health-related stigma and discrimination. *Lancet, 387*(10023), 1123–1132. https://doi.org/10.1016/s0140-6736(15)00298-6

U. S. Administration for Community Living. (2021, May). *2020 profile of older Americans* [Report]. U. S. Department of Health & Human Services, Administration on Aging. https://acl.gov/sites/default/files/Aging%20and%20Disability%20in%20America/2020ProfileOlderAmericans.Final_.pdf

Vigo, D., Thornicroft, G., & Atun, R. (2016). Estimating the true global burden of mental illness. *Lancet Psychiatry, 3*(2), 171–178. https://doi.org/10.1016/s2215-0366(15)00505-2

Walker, S. P., Wachs, T. D., Grantham-McGregor, S., Black, M. M., Nelson, C. A., Huffman, S. L., Baker-Henningham, H., Chang, S. M., Hamadani, J. D., Lozoff, B., Gardner, J. M., Powell, C. A., Rahman, A., & Richter, L. (2011). Inequality in early childhood: Risk and protective factors for early child development. *Lancet, 378*(9799), 1325–1338. https://doi.org/10.1016/s0140-6736(11)60555-2

Webb, L. M., & Chen, C. Y. (2022). The COVID-19 pandemic's impact on older adults' mental health: Contributing factors, coping strategies, and opportunities for improvement. *International Journal of Geriatric Psychiatry, 37*(1), 1–7. https://doi.org/10.1002/gps.5647

Webster-Bass, S. (2023). *Hope and healing circles*. [Web page]. Voices Institute LLC. https://www.voicesinst.org

Woody, C. A., Ferrari, A. J., Siskind, D. J., Whiteford, H. A., & Harris, M. G. (2017). A systematic review and meta-regression of the prevalence and incidence of perinatal depression. *Journal of Affective Disorders, 219*, 86–92. https://doi.org/10.1016/j.jad.2017.05.003

World Health Organization. (2020). *WHO methods and data sources for global burden of disease estimates 2000–2019* [Report; Global Health Estimates Technical Paper WHO/DDI/DNA/GHE/2020.3]. Author. https://cdn.who.int/media/docs/default-source/gho-documents/global-health-estimates/ghe2019_daly-methods.pdf?sfvrsn=31b25009_7

World Health Organization. (2022, June 16). *World mental health report: Transforming mental health for all* [Report]. Author. https://apps.who.int/iris/rest/bitstreams/1433523/retrieve

Chapter 5
Epidemiology of Substance Use Disorders in Women

Kimberly A. Johnson

Introduction

Substance use disorders (SUD), comprised of alcohol use disorders (AUDs) and drug use disorders (DUDs), are a significant public health issue. Globally, alcohol use has increased over the past 30 years. This may be due to the global increase in living standards, as the consumption of alcohol increases with a country's average income. Globally, 8.6% of men and 1.7% of women have AUDs; however, the gender gap is much lower in the United States with only a 1%-point difference between men and women (Rehm & Shield, 2019). Mortality due to AUDs was reported to be 121,600 deaths for men and 24,000 deaths for women in 2016, the most recent global data available (Rehm & Shield, 2019). In the United States, alcohol-related deaths were increasing at a pace of about 2% per year until the start of the COVID-19 pandemic when there was a 25% increase in alcohol-related deaths from 2019 to 2020 (White et al., 2022). The rates for DUDs are much lower, with a global estimate of 0.22% for men and women combined and the rates for women are lower for all classes of drugs (Degenhardt et al., 2018; Peacock et al., 2018). Mortality due to drug use has increased dramatically over the past 20 years in the United States, with an additional 30% increase in death rate due to drug use between 2019 and 2020. The increase in drug-related deaths during the first year of the COVID-19 pandemic was 23% for women, smaller than for men, but a significant single-year increase (National Center for Health Statistics, 2021).

Adolescent girls in the United States and other high-income countries are more likely to drink alcohol than adolescent boys, and women's use of alcohol approaches that of men in old age. However, women of childbearing age are less likely to drink

K. A. Johnson (✉)
Department of Mental Health Law and Policy, College of Behavioral and Community Sciences, University of South Florida, Tampa, FL, USA
e-mail: kjohnson33@usf.edu

A. Hanson, B. L. Levin (eds.), *Women's Behavioral Health*,
https://doi.org/10.1007/978-3-031-58293-6_5

alcohol than men, and women of all ages are less likely than men to misuse other drugs. The difference is even wider in middle- and low-income countries. This difference in use accounts at least partially for the lower prevalence of SUD and related morbidity and mortality in women compared to men (White, 2020).

In the United States, women are treated in systems of care that were designed for men and that were developed separately from the rest of health care. The modern treatment systems were built on top of and in support of Alcoholics Anonymous (AA), a self-help group model that was originally developed in 1935 for professional men to support each other in maintaining abstinence (White, 1998). While new concepts, such as trauma-informed care have been incorporated into treatment, the goal of behavioral treatments remains much as it was 50 years ago, designed by and for men.

This chapter covers the history of research on SUDs in women beginning in the 1960s, what we know about biological and social determinants of SUD, and the sex and gender differences in those determinants. It covers the prevention, screening, assessment, diagnosis, and treatment of SUDs and what is known and not known regarding efficacy for girls and women. The chapter also covers adaptations that have been made for women and identifies opportunities for new research and evaluation to better prevent and treat SUD in women.

Evolution of Research on Women and SUD

During the 1960s researchers began to attempt to characterize the difference in alcohol and drug use between men and women (Ellinwood et al., 1966; Schuckit et al., 1969; Wood & Duffy, 1966), though Jellinek, a pioneer in research on alcoholism, had identified differences as early as 1947 (Jellinek, 1947, 1952). The differences identified included higher incidence of use and SUD for men (Ellinwood et al., 1966; Jellinek, 1952), higher levels of psychopathology for women who have a SUD (Ellinwood et al., 1966; Schuckit et al., 1969), and differences in drinking patterns (Wood & Duffy, 1966). These themes continue in later research.

In 1966, the National Center for Prevention and Control of Alcoholism and the Center for Studies of Narcotic and Drug Abuse were established within the National Institute of Mental Health. Research on substance use disorders accelerated in the 1970s with the passage of the Comprehensive Alcohol Abuse and Alcoholism Prevention, Treatment, and Rehabilitation Act of 1970 (Pub.L. 91–616, *aka* the Hughes Act). The Drug Abuse Office and Treatment Act (Public Law or P.L. 92–255, 1972) authorized the establishment of the National Institute on Drug Abuse ([NIDA] White, 1998). Concern over fetal alcohol syndrome and fetal drug effects led to early inclusion of the study of women in federally funded alcohol and drug research with a focus on pregnancy, and the assessment of treatment protocols for pregnant and parenting women (Kandall, 2010). This focus included a demonstration project on addiction treatment programs designed specifically for women beginning in 1973 (Beschner et al., 1981).

In the 1980s and 1990s, the focus on fetal effects of alcohol and drug use turned from alcohol and opioids to stimulants like cocaine and methamphetamine (Grella, 2008). Starting in 1984, 5% of the federal Substance Abuse Prevention and Treatment Block Grant program was required to be spent on specialized treatment for women. After a General Accounting Office report on drug-affected newborns (GAO, 1990), NIDA launched the perinatal 20 demonstration project with the aim of increasing the number of residential treatment beds for women and assessing whether housing newborns with mothers during residential treatment improved outcomes for mother or child. NIDA also conducted a one-time cross-sectional survey of postpartum women in hospital that found that in 1992 5.5% of women had used an illicit drug during pregnancy (NIDA, 1996).

At the same time, feminist perspectives on psychological development (Gilligan, 1993) and treatment for women with SUD (Covington, 1999) were emerging. The feminist perspectives focused on women's need to be treated within a context of relationships as opposed to the way men were treated as individuals (Finkelstein, 1996). This focus on context led to increasing calls for comprehensive treatment programs that addressed not just substance use, but also housing, work, childcare, and other needs (Finkelstein, 1996).

Research in the 2000s began to focus on the relationship between childhood trauma and substance use, particularly childhood sexual abuse for women. The Kaiser Adverse Childhood Experience Study (Felitti et al., 1998) established a strong correlation between the number of adverse childhood experiences (ACEs) and a variety of negative health outcomes in adulthood including substance use disorders. Research on women's substance use began to focus on addressing childhood trauma and co-occurring post-traumatic stress disorder (Covington, 2008; Hien et al., 2004). The cyclical nature of the relationship between trauma and abuse and substance use was identified as a driver of substance use problems for women with a need for treatment to interrupt the cycle (Kilpatrick et al., 1997). These women-centered themes that influenced the development of comprehensive SUD treatment programs that address multiple issues in addition to the SUD remain the focus of gender-specific treatment today.

The focus of current research is on understanding the biological (or sex) and sociological (or gender) differences in disease etiology and treatment effectiveness (McHugh et al., 2018; Guinle & Sinha, 2020). Treating pregnant and parenting women has moved from the focus on stimulants back to a focus on opioids as increases in the number of infants born with neonatal opioid withdrawal syndrome grew dramatically between 2000 and 2015 (Winkelman et al., 2018). Fortunately, while there are some differences in response to medications to treat OUDs, pregnant and postpartum women can safely be treated with the same medications, buprenorphine and methadone, used to treat women who are not pregnant (Blanco & Volkow, 2019).

Major Epidemiological Studies

Global Studies In 1996, the World Health Organization (WHO) launched the Global Alcohol Database and member states began collecting standardized data on alcohol consumption, consequences, and treatment of alcohol use disorders (Poznyak et al., 2013). The first Global Status Report on Alcohol was published in 1999, with the most recent version of the report published in 2019 (WHO, 1999, 2019). The United Nations Office on Drugs and Crime (UNODC, 2020) publishes *The World Drug Report*, an annual survey of drug use, policy, and services for drug users annually since 1997. These surveys use similar protocols in that they receive data from member states who self-report using standardized tools, but not necessarily standardized data collection protocols.

United States Studies In 1972, the National Household Survey on Drug Use and the Drug Abuse Warning Network (DAWN), two important long-term epidemiological studies, were launched. The National Household Survey continues today as the National Survey on Drug Use and Health (NSDUH). The DAWN survey, which collected data from hospital emergency departments was discontinued in 2011, however, it was refunded in federal fiscal year 2019 due to strong demand for better data on overdoses. In 1975, NIDA launched the Monitoring the Future (MTF) Survey, which assessed trends in drug and alcohol use among adolescents, a growing concern at the time (Bachman et al., 2015). Conducted annually, data from all years since 1975 is available for analysis from the MTF website. These three large epidemiological surveys provide a history of alcohol and drug-using behavior in the United States, as well as consequences and treatment receipt going back nearly 50 years. They provide a rich national and selected state-level data set to assess difference in alcohol and drug use, consequences, treatment receipt, and outcomes.

NIAAA launched its first longitudinal study, the National Longitudinal Alcohol Epidemiologic Survey (NLAES) in 1991, followed by three waves of the National Epidemiologic Survey on Alcohol and Related Conditions (NESARC) study in 2001. The second wave conducted in 2005 reinterviewed 34,000 of the original 43,000 participants (Hasin & Grant, 2015). NESARC III, a follow-up cross-sectional design conducted in 2012–2013, included collection of biospecimens for analysis (Grant et al., 2015). All these national surveys have been used to assess sex and gender differences in substance use.

Diagnosing and Assessing Alcohol and Drug Use Disorders

Alcohol and drug use disorders are part of two well-known national and international classification systems—the *Diagnostic and Statistical Manual* (*DSM*, United States) and the *International Statistical Classification of Diseases and Related Health Problems* (*ICD*), developed by the American Psychiatric Association (APA) and the WHO, respectively. In the United States, at the time of this writing, the *DSM-5* (APA, 2013) and the *ICD-10* (WHO, 1993) are the versions currently in use. However, the *ICD-11* (WHO, 2020, September) has been implemented and the WHO has encouraged member states to migrate to *ICD-11* by January 1, 2022 (Seventy-Second World Health Assembly, 2019, April 11). Both the *DSM-5* and *ICD-11* have made changes that reflect a dimensional approach, focusing on symptom severity and function rather than number of symptoms present (Reed et al., 2019; Regier et al., 2013; Saunders, 2017). *ICD-11* also addresses cultural differences in disease presentation (Reed et al., 2019.

In line with the dimensional approach used throughout DSM 5, SUDs are diagnosed on a continuum of mild, moderate, and severe based on 11 criteria that include both physical symptoms and "use despite negative consequences." In previous *DSM*s, SUDs were categorized as either abuse or dependence. If a patient met the criteria for dependence and abuse, she received the diagnosis for dependence. A diagnosis of abuse was only given if the patient did not meet the criteria for dependence. Since the most commonly met criterion for the abuse diagnosis was repeated arrests for alcohol or drug-related offenses (i.e., driving under the influence arrests), there is disagreement as to whether the SUD nosology of the previous *DSM* versions (1–4) was valid for women (Hasin et al., 1997; Lynskey et al., 2005), as the number of women arrested for drunk driving and other alcohol and drug-related crime remains far lower than for men (Navas et al., 2019; Schwartz, 2008).

Screening and Assessment Tools

The primary instruments used to screen and assess SUDs do not differentiate by gender, except for assessing dangerous levels of alcohol consumption where the cut point for men is five drinks and the cut point for women is four drinks in screening tools such as the AUDIT-C (Bradley et al., 2007). The different cut point makes the screening tools slightly less sensitive in detecting problem drinking in women (Bradley et al., 2007; Dawson et al., 2005). Widely used screening tools, such as the AUDIT-C (Bradley et al., 2007), MAST (Selzer, 1971), DAST (Skinner, 1982), and CAGE (Ewing, 1984), were normed on men and are less sensitive to screening for alcohol and drug use problems in women (Babor et al., 1989; Cherpitel, 1995; Dhalla & Kopec, 2007; Grekin et al., 2010).

The WHO currently promotes use of the Alcohol, Smoking and Substance Involvement Screening Test (ASSIST) to diagnose alcohol and drug use problems (Humeniuk et al., 2010). The validation study population for the ASSIST was nearly half women (Humeniuk et al., 2008), with the same questions and scoring for men and women (except for quantity of alcohol consumed). However, Kumar et al. (2016) suggest there should be different cut points in scoring for women.

Due to concerns about efficacy of these tools with pregnant women (Chang, 2001; Grekin et al., 2010; Ondersma et al., 2019), there are new efforts to assess the effectiveness of screening tools on pregnant women (Oga et al., 2020) and to develop new screening tools for this population (Chasnoff et al., 2007; Yonkers et al., 2010). In 2020, the United States Preventative Services Task Force (USPSTF) recommended the use of drug screening in primary care for adults including pregnant women (Patnode et al., 2020). The Task Force recommends use of simple, short tools, including the NIDA Quick Screen (The MITRE Corporation, 2020, June 22), which has a single question about alcohol, drug, and tobacco use and has been shown to be an effective screening tool for pregnant women for alcohol and cannabis use but not for other drugs (Oga et al., 2020).

The two most widely used standardized assessment tools are the Addiction Severity Index (ASI, McLellan et al., 1980) and the Global Appraisal of Individual Needs (GAIN, Dennis et al., 2003). While the ASI included women in its reliability and validity testing (McLellan et al., 1985), it received early criticism for leaving out factors specifically associated with women's substance use problems which was addressed by changes in later versions (McLellan et al., 2006; Wilke, 1994). The GAIN has been normed on adolescents and adults (Dennis et al., 2003) and includes questions that are more likely to predict women's substance use. However, the ASI is more widely used.

Disease Etiology

How we study a condition affects our perceptions of the problem and its possible solutions. Conceptual models are often used to frame the approach to research on the etiology of a condition. Addiction research benefitted from early adoption of a whole-person perspective to disease etiology, treatment, and recovery that was termed the bio-psychosocial model.

Bio-psychosocial Perspective

Since the 1980s, addiction has been called a bio-psychosocial disease, a concept first put forward by Alan Marlatt and colleagues as a way of integrating popular previous conceptual models that could only partially explain the development of substance use disorders (Collins & Marlatt, 1983; Marlatt et al., 1988). This thinking predated our understanding of epigenetics, but it incorporated what was known about the biological processes involved in the development of SUDs as well as the social and psychological factors that contribute to alcohol and drug use and disease development. The bio-psychosocial model proposes that multiple interacting determinants lead to the development of SUD.

This perspective acknowledges there are individuals who are at higher risk of developing a SUD due to genetic vulnerability (Agrawal & Lynskey, 2008). Early age of first use of alcohol or drugs also increases risk (DeWit et al., 2000). The psychological impact of childhood trauma (Felitti et al., 1998) and personality traits, such as risk-taking or novelty-seeking (Wills et al., 1994), and impulsivity (Moeller et al., 2001) are correlated with development of SUDs. The bio-psychosocial model also recognizes the importance of social factors, such as parents' use and attitudes toward use (Chassin et al., 1999), and the behaviors and attitudes of social network members (Valente, 2010). It also includes the neurobiological processes of the different drugs and the variation in abuse potential between drugs (Gable, 1993). In short, the bio-psychosocial model describes a complex interaction between biological and environmental risk, the individual's psychological profile, the effects of the specific drugs themselves, the age of initiation, and the frequency and duration of specific drug use (Sloboda et al., 2012).

Genetics and Epigenetics

The heritability of addiction, particularly to alcohol and nicotine is well documented for both men and women (Enoch & Goldman, 2001); however, there are fewer studies on heritability of other DUDs (Li & Burmeister, 2009). Finding the specific genes related to addiction has proved more difficult (Agrawal et al., 2012). Early genetic research sought to identify specific genes that might increase risk for development of SUDs. Studies have identified mechanisms that may be responsible for sex-specific preference for alcohol which is related to the quantity of alcohol an individual chooses to consume (Melo et al., 1996). Sex differences in genetic risk for SUD have been difficult to research primarily due to the large quantity of data required, the limited sample size available, and the rates of substance misuse/SUDs are lower in women than men (Datta et al., 2020). However, more recent research using genome-wide association studies (GWAS) and sequencing study methods are leading to a more polygenic model of genetic risk with hundreds or thousands of gene modifications playing a small role in the etiology of substance use disorders (Edenberg et al., 2019). Studies using GWAS are beginning to identify generalized addiction and drug specific genomic loci and the metabolic pathways that link the genetic variation to development of SUD (Hatoum et al., 2023).

Gene-Environment Interaction

Stress, particularly prenatal stress not moderated by early life care and early childhood stress, affects gene expression in brain development and function (McEwen et al., 2012), potentially leaving individuals more susceptible to the effects of alcohol and drugs (Cadet, 2016). Gene expression may be related to the development of tolerance, memory formation, and regulation. These factors are thought to cause craving and relapse that can occur many years after cessation of use (Beayno et al., 2019; Wong et al., 2011). While research has observed the physical impact of the environment on gene expression, linking these impacts to specific disease conditions has proven more difficult. Epigenetics of SUDs is an emerging field of study that is beginning to identify mechanisms to explain the interaction between genetic and environmental risk for SUDs as well as how the drug itself alters gene expression (Shepard & Nugent, 2023).

Biological Mechanisms

In considering sex differences in the etiology of SUDs, it is important to identify both biological sex and gender differences (i.e., differences based on XX chromosome pairs or female sex hormones versus risk and protective factors based on gender roles) (Sanchis-Segura & Becker, 2016). While these mechanisms have been theorized, there is inadequate data to explain the specific contribution and interaction of genetic, environmental, and sex-specific factors in both genetic and environmental risk and exposure. However, there are observed differences in use behavior, metabolism of alcohol and drugs, stress response and its relationship to use and misuse, the impact of sex hormones on stress and use, and the progression from use to SUD. While the mechanisms of why there are sex differences in alcohol and drug use and progression to SUD remain poorly defined, there are clear gender differences in the development and trajectory of SUD (Sanchis-Segura & Becker, 2016).

Gender Differences

The process of developing a substance use disorder has three stages: (1) acquisition, where a person initiates substance use; (2) escalation, where use becomes more regular and quantity and frequency of use escalate; and (3) dysregulation, where normal brain functioning becomes "hijacked" by the drug(s) leading to the inability to control use and craving for the drug (Carroll et al., 2004). Sex/gender differences occur at every step in this process. Women have higher rates of absorption than men who drink the same amount. The difference in body composition and average size between men and women leads to greater bioavailability of alcohol even at lower amounts consumed (Thomasson, 2002). Further, there are sex differences in responsivity to drugs, with females more sensitive to the rewarding effects of psychoactive substances (Fattore et al., 2008). Studies also indicate women appear to move from use to problematic use faster than men (McHugh et al., 2018). Chronic use of alcohol or drugs reduces the responsivity of the brain to dopamine and other neurochemicals and increases the tolerance to the drugs being used (Bobzean et al., 2014). Estrogen and progesterone often function as opposing forces related to cognitive functioning, impulsivity and self-control, and stress response, all of which are related to the development of SUDs (Carroll & Smethells, 2016). Differences in the balance of the two hormones in different women and at different times of the menstrual cycle may impact the probability of developing an SUD and of relapsing once an SUD has become controlled (Petersen & London, 2018).

Addiction has been described as a "spiraling dysregulation of brain reward systems" (Koob & Le Moal, 1997) characterized by an inability to control use, despite negative consequences, with a compulsion to use. Behavioral and neuroimaging studies have shown women are more likely to crave drugs when faced with stress while men are more likely to respond to drug-related cues such as images of people using or sounds or smells reminiscent of use (McHugh et al., 2018). These findings indicate differences in etiology but also potential differences in treatment targets. The NIH now requires inclusion of sex/gender as a moderator in research. Its Sex as a Biological Variable (SaBV) policy, which went into effect in January 2016, will help us to better understand how men and women progress from use to SUDs (NIH, 2015, June 9).

Environmental Factors

The primary environmental risk factor for development of a SUD is exposure to the drug. Without use, there is no SUD. Earlier exposure may increase risk of disease development regardless of other risks (DeWit et al., 2000). There is evidence that adolescent brains are particularly vulnerable to the intoxicating effects of various drugs and less capable of overcoming the desire or social pressure to use (Bava & Tapert, 2010), making adolescence a vulnerable period for initial exposure to alcohol and drugs.

People with genetic risk and other environmental risks are more likely to use early, confounding observational studies that link early exposure and development of SUD. Other environmental factors related to increased risk of SUD can be categorized as family, peer, and community-level risks (Hawkins et al., 2008; Hawkins et al., 1992). These risks might contribute to early exposure (acquisition phase), escalation or dysregulation. Within the context of the family, poor bonding in infancy and early childhood, parental use, and lax parental attitudes toward use in middle childhood and adolescents, and either poor parental controls or excessive punitiveness and abuse are all related to development of SUD. At the peer level, poor attachment to school, and friends who use alcohol and drugs create risks for SUD. At the community level, availability of alcohol and drugs as well as community attitudes permissive of use are related to early use and development of SUD (Sloboda et al., 2012). Family dysfunction appears to be more predictive of SUD development for girls than for boys (Evans et al., 2017; Skeer et al., 2011). Women with substance use sisorders are more likely to be in a relationship with a partner with a substance use disorder and to have been introduced to use by a male partner (Tuchman, 2010).

Disease Progression

Studies of treatment populations find that women progress from initiation of use to disordered use faster than men (Greenfield et al., 2010; McHugh et al., 2018). This process is called telescoping and has been found in studies of treatment populations for all drugs except cocaine (Tuchman, 2010). However, studies of the general population do not have this finding. In general population studies the time from initial use to disordered use seems to be age cohort-specific (Keyes et al., 2010). This difference in results for different populations suggests there is an unobserved difference between men and women in the treatment-seeking population. Pattern of use may affect the pace at which individuals progress from acquisition through dysregulation with binge use followed by periods of abstinence appearing to be more likely to lead to dysregulation (Lynch, 2018). A difference in use patterns may be one explanation for the difference in observed progression between men and women in studies of treatment populations.

Comorbidities

Women with SUD are more likely to have psychiatric comorbidities, particularly anxiety and depression than men with SUD (McHugh et al., 2018). PTSD has been linked to SUD in women both as cause and effect (Najavits et al., 1997). Women who have experienced violence or trauma in childhood or adolescence are more likely to develop SUD and women with SUD are more likely to experience sexual or physical violence that leads to PTSD. This circular relationship between trauma and SUD can be difficult to break and is often a focus of treatment. Similarly, depression can be both part of the cause and an effect of SUD in women. For women, the temporal relationship between anxiety, depression, and SUD is more frequently that anxiety is the precursor to both depression and SUD, while for men, SUD may be more likely a precursor to depression (Kessler, 2003). Childhood trauma is a risk factor for all three conditions (Felitti et al., 1998).

How other psychiatric diagnoses and substance use disorders are linked causally is still unknown (Castillo-Carniglia et al., 2019). Rates of substance use disorders are higher for people who have other mental illnesses than for those individuals who do not. However, the causal pathway has been demonstrated to go in both directions and there is reason to believe that common genetic and environmental risks, may play a role in the development of multiple conditions (Jang et al., 2020).

Women are more susceptible to infectious diseases related to injection drug use (e.g., HIV, HCV) (Des Jarlais et al., 2012; Iversen et al., 2015). The risk of infectious diseases may be equally related to intimate partner drug use and sex work as to IV drug use. IV drug use increases the risk of various other potentially fatal infectious disease such as thrombosis, cellulitis, and endocarditis (Strang et al., 2020). Women with AUDs are also more at risk for developing alcohol-related liver disease, cardiomyopathy, and cancers than men and have higher mortality rates (Agabio et al., 2017; Roerecke & Rehm, 2013).

Since women of childbearing age are at risk of miscarriage and other pregnancy complications related to alcohol or drug use, there has been increased focus in the United States on maternal and fetal effects of opioid use disorder (Blanco & Volkow, 2019). Rates of neonatal opioid withdrawal syndrome in the United States average 6 per 1000 births, though states have reported rates as high as 50 per 1000 births (Ko et al., 2016; Winkelman et al., 2018). Globally, fetal alcohol spectrum disorder is more prevalent with an incidence rate of nearly 8 per 1000 births (Lange et al., 2017).

Life Course Perspective

Prevalence by Age

The National Survey on Drug Use and Health (NSDUH) survey (SAMHSA, 2019) reports that AUDs have declined in the past decade for all age groups, but the rate of drug use disorders has remained relatively stable. The rate of AUDs is higher for adolescent girls (2.1%) than for boys, but at other ages it is lower for women than for men. Overall, DUDs are lower for girls and women of all ages than for boys and men, respectively (SAMHSA, 2019). The higher rate of AUDs in adolescent girls is a recent phenomenon and is thought to be related to the shift in drinking patterns over the past decade as the rate of alcohol consumption has decreased more rapidly for boys than girls.

Adolescent Brain Development

In general, SUDs are thought of as adolescent onset conditions (Volkow et al., 2016), though periods of stress and old age are also high-risk (Emiliussen et al., 2017). During periods of rapid brain development (prenatal, early childhood, and adolescence), children are at particular risk for development of mental conditions including SUDs (Bava & Tapert, 2010; Kim et al., 2015; Lupien et al., 2009; Weinstock, 2008). The adolescent brain is considered particularly vulnerable to the effects of alcohol and drugs (Casey & Jones, 2010) and use of alcohol and most drugs is commonly initiated in adolescence or early adulthood (SAMHSA, 2019). Adolescents seem particularly inclined toward risk-taking and social influences (Bava & Tapert, 2010), have a heightened reward response, and reduced experience of the negative effects of alcohol (e.g., withdrawal and sedation) (Casey & Jones, 2010). The combination of higher risk-seeking and greater response to reward makes adolescence a time that is particularly vulnerable to substance use. Childhood exposure to drugs may lead to incorporation of the response into the development of the brain and permanent structural adaptations, whereas exposure during adulthood requires an adaptive or compensating response that may be more easily overridden by behavior change or withdrawal of the exposure (Andersen, 2003). The earlier exposure occurs, the greater the impact on structural development of the brain and the greater potential for cognitive impairment as well as increased risk for development of SUD.

While the increase in gonadal hormones in adolescence affects brain development, research on the impact of these differences on substance use and substance use disorders is inconclusive. Although it appears girls are more likely to begin drinking alcohol to alleviate stress or negative affect while boys are more likely to drink for positive effects, the specific mechanisms underlying these different behaviors are still unclear (Peltier et al., 2019) (for more about girls, see Chap. 2 in this volume).

Social Factors for Adults

Women with SUDs are at particular risk for social stigma for two reasons: sexuality and their role as mother. There is a perceptual link between alcohol, drug use, and promiscuity, and women are still condemned for sexual behavior for which men are rewarded (Covington, 1997) and women are blamed (Abbey, 2002). In other words, social beliefs are that alcohol makes men less responsible for their aggression and it makes women more responsible for their victimization (Mellins et al., 2017; Jozkowski et al., 2017). Sexual assault may be a trigger for alcohol use, so the relationship between alcohol use and sexual assault is bi-directional or cyclical, with women with AUDs reporting multiple sexual assaults (Lorenz & Ullman, 2016). Drug use, prostitution, and sexual assault follow a similar pattern. Women with DUDs, who experienced sexual assault in childhood or early adulthood, use drugs at a young age, may exchange sex for drugs or money to purchase drugs, experience additional sexual trauma, and increase drug use in a spiraling decline (Potterat et al., 1998; Romero-Daza et al., 2003).

Women who have SUDs are also assumed to be bad mothers. A mother's substance use is often the primary reason for child placement in foster care (Young, 2016, February 23). As with men in the criminal justice system, minority women are over-represented in the child welfare system and their children are disproportionately placed in the foster care system (Annie E. Casey Foundation, 2020, April 13) even though national data suggest that there is a lower rate of SUDs in African American women (GAO, 2007, July 11). Social stigma and fear of losing their children are two factors that may explain the low rates of women accessing treatment for SUDs (Greenfield et al., 2007).

Women are less likely than men to be arrested for drunk driving (Schwartz, 2008) or drug crimes. The U. S. Department of Justice (2020) estimated a quarter of drunk driving arrests and a third of drug arrests in 2019 were women. While the number of men arrested for these crimes has decreased, the number of women arrested has increased (Prison Policy Initiative, 2019; Schwartz, 2008). In 1980, 26,738 women were incarcerated; in 2019, 222,455 women were incarcerated, a 700% increase in 40 years (The Sentencing Project, 2020). Women are more likely to be incarcerated for drug offenses, while men are more likely to be incarcerated for violent offenses. Since many states still bar people with felony drug convictions from public housing, certain types of employment, public welfare payments, and other support, women fall back into criminal activity, including prostitution and drug trafficking to support themselves, leading them back into the cycle of trauma and drug use (Kirk & Wakefield, 2018).

UNODC began an initiative in 2019 to target gender issues in drug policy. While no country reaches the rate of incarceration or the acceleration in the rate of incarceration of women for drug crimes in the United States, increases in Latin America and Asia have raised concern. UNODC is targeting the differential impact of drug policy on women and children, particularly as it relates to incarceration, family separation, women and children being used as "mules" or carriers of illegal drugs across country borders, and in human trafficking (UNODC, 2018). (for more about adult women, see Chap. 3 in this volume).

Older Adults

While alcohol and drug use are much lower in older populations, aging is a risk factor for the development of SUDs for those who use. Most research has been on effects of continued alcohol consumption and AUDs as use of other drugs is extremely low in older populations. Changes in physiology, particularly body composition and digestion, make old age a time of risk for development of late-onset AUD for people who continue to drink. These physiologic changes in proportion of weight that is made up of fat and the amount of alcohol dehydrogenase in the gut disproportionately affect women post menopause (Milic et al., 2018). Older people may be more sensitive to the negative effects of alcohol, such as sedation and motor impairment, which increase risks for falls or other injuries (Novier et al., 2015). In addition to the risk of late-onset AUD, alcohol consumption by older women increases blood pressure and the risk of certain cancers, including breast cancer (Milic et al., 2018). Widely disseminated research demonstrating health improvement with alcohol consumption has poor study design and biased samples (Knott et al., 2015) (for more on older adults, see Chap. 4 in this volume).

Cohort Effects

One of the difficulties in understanding SUDs in women from a life course perspective is that changing norms for women led to changing behaviors, particularly in high-income countries (Keyes et al., 2011). Assumptions made about sex/gender differences in incidence and prevalence of SUDs were based on cohorts who were born, matured, and aged under different social expectations for women. Over the past 20 years, there has been convergence in rates of use and in rates of SUDs for younger age groups (White, 2020). As this cohort ages, we may see less difference between genders in the prevalence of SUDs, or it may be that women use less during the childbearing years and cohort factors play less of a role. The baby boom generation, those born between 1945 and 1965, is a cohort with heavy lifetime use of alcohol and drugs compared to other cohorts. It appears that use is continuing into old age, with the increase in prevalence of SUDs from previous generations, particularly for women (Duncan et al., 2010; Han et al., 2017). Whether these are cohort effects or life course effects is currently unknown as the increase in use by women is a recent phenomenon.

The mandatory stay at home orders and shutdown of most business and social activity in the United States appears to have had an impact on alcohol consumption, with early reports indicating that women drank on more days and had a greater increase in the number of risky drinking days than men (Barbosa et al., 2021). This increase was greatest in women of childbearing age who were married with children (Grigsby et al., 2023) Alcohol and drug use appears to have decreased for adolescents perhaps because of lack of social pressure and access during extended school shutdowns and online teaching (Compton et al., 2023). It remains to be seen whether these changes are permanent or whether use will revert to previous trends. Easing of alcohol regulation in the United States is being made permanent in many states which may lead to higher rates of continued higher consumption.

Prevention

Two prevention models are currently in use. The first model, the chronic disease prevention model first proposed by Leavell and Clark (1958), focuses on when in the disease development process an intervention is applied. The three stages of prevention are primary, secondary, and tertiary. Primary prevention activities intervene before disease progression has begun; secondary prevention activities intervene when there has been exposure or increased risk, but no disease and tertiary prevention is disease treatment or prevention of progression of disease. The second model, an operational classification of disease prevention proposed by Gordon (1983), focuses on the population to which the intervention is delivered and is assumed to be relevant only for primary prevention. This conceptual model uses the terms universal, selective, and indicated to describe strategies used for the entire population, at-risk populations, and individuals who have exhibited risk behaviors, respectively. Gordon's model is the most widely used conceptual model for prevention of substance use and its problems (Haggerty & Mrazek, 1994). In 2020, Kahn and colleagues integrated the two models to explain the overlap and intersection so that the public health/chronic disease prevention and SUD prevention fields could interact and understand each other's language (National Academies of Sciences et al., 2020; see Fig. 5.1).

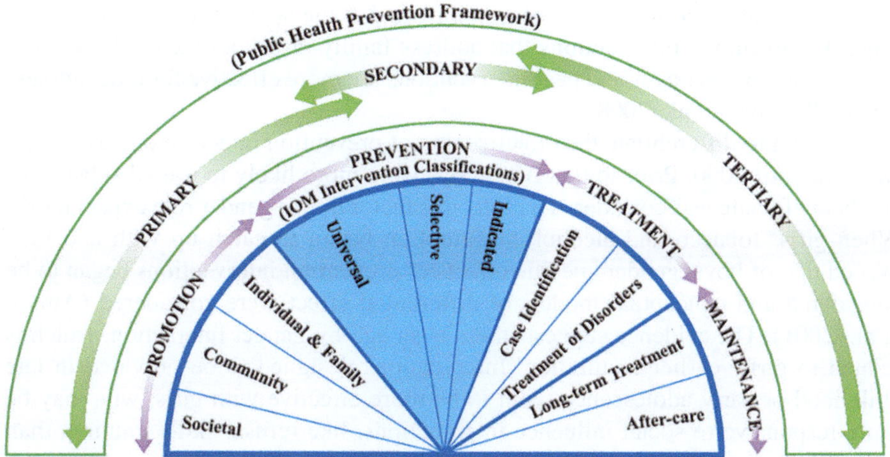

Fig. 5.1 Overlap of two prevention models: The Institute of Medicine (IOM) intervention classifications and the public health prevention framework. (National Academies of Sciences, Engineering, & Medicine, 2020, p. 19). (Used with permission of The National Academies Press, from *Promoting Positive Adolescent Health Behaviors and Outcomes: Thriving in the twenty-first Century*, The National Academies of Sciences, Engineering, & Medicine, 2020, permission conveyed through Copyright Clearance Center, Inc.)

Prevention Interventions

Most evidence-based SUD prevention interventions are primary prevention efforts targeted toward preventing or delaying initiation of alcohol and drug use by children and adolescents. While certain interventions are effective with college students, the bulk of research and practice is focused on children and adolescents up to age 18. Prevention interventions can be implemented at a policy level (e.g., restricting access through possession laws), practices (e.g., school efforts to engage children in after-school activities), or programs (e.g., LifeSkills Training Program) (Botvin & Griffin, 2004). School-based programs are the most widely used. Although randomized trials have demonstrated efficacy of U. S. school-based programs, replication studies in European samples have not demonstrated the same effect, particularly for girls (Vigna-Taglianti et al., 2009, 2014).

Prevention of early use of alcohol and drugs has focused on addressing risk and strengthening protective factors. Modifiable parental factors include attitudes and use of alcohol or drugs, parents supplying alcohol or drugs, and lack of parental supervision or support (Yap et al., 2017). Modifiable peer factors include peers who use alcohol and drugs or who have favorable attitudes toward alcohol and drugs. Where it is difficult to modify risk, such as school failure, low commitment to school, or community norms supportive of alcohol or drug use, protection can be added by strengthening other areas, such as increasing awareness of social influence and skills in resisting social pressure to use, enhancing school success or commitment to pro-social activities (Hawkins et al., 2008). As influences change over the life course, interventions should be implemented at the appropriate developmental stage. For example, interventions that address family or school factors have more influence at younger ages and peer interventions are more effective for older adolescents (Cleveland et al., 2008).

Research to differentiate the effectiveness of prevention interventions by gender was rare until 2000. Prior to that time, boys were more likely to use all substances and being female was considered a protective factor due to gender role expectations. When girls' tobacco and alcohol consumption began to catch up with and then exceed that of boys, gender-specific effects of prevention interventions began to be considered and conceptual models of differential effect were considered (Amaro et al., 2001). The evidence suggests there is an age-by-gender interaction, which is related to girls' earlier maturation. Interventions designed to be provided in late childhood or early adolescence seem to be more effective with girls, who may be more responsive to social influence interventions, like refusal skills training, than boys (Blake et al., 2001).

The UNODC (2018) *International Standards on Drug Use Prevention* summarizes the current understanding of what constitutes the evidence base for prevention of substance use and outlines the components necessary for member states to develop an effective comprehensive substance use prevention strategy. One item of interest is that while the standards note that it is important to treat childhood mental illness and behavior disorders, there is no evidence for treatment of mental illness as an effective strategy to reduce substance use. The standards document identifies few primary or secondary prevention interventions focused on adults, but there are workplace alcohol use prevention programs that appear to be effective for women but not for men. Other programs target pregnant women and mothers with information on alcohol and drug effects on the fetus and parenting training. Brief interventions for alcohol use were demonstrated to be effective with pregnant women and other populations; however, brief interventions have not been demonstrated to be effective for drug use. Training in parenting and parent-focused programming have good evidence for decreasing alcohol and drug use by adolescents (UNODC, 2018). The UNODC *Standards* were transformed into publicly available prevention and treatment curricula (International Society of Substance Use Professionals, 2020, April; see Fig. 5.2).

Treatment

Epidemiology of Treatment Receipt

Currently, there is a movement to measure the epidemiology of treatment receipt using a "cascade of care" (e.g., "continuum of care") model (CoC, Socías et al., 2016), which measures diagnosis, treatment initiation, treatment retention, and treatment outcomes compared to levels that would be desirable based on population

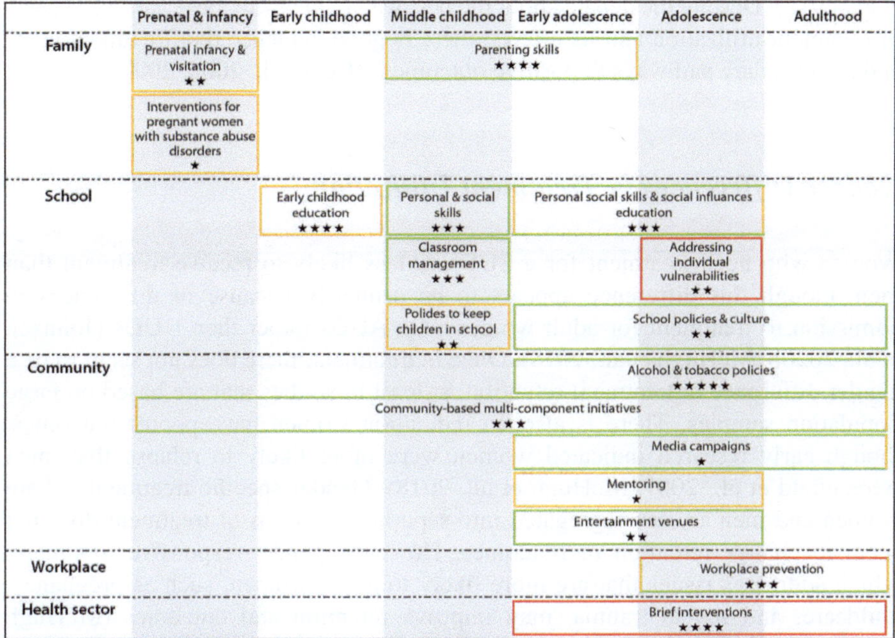

Fig. 5.2 EBP for alcohol and drug prevention. (International Society of Substance Use Professionals, 2020, April, p. 268), reprinted with permission

trends. While there is debate about whether everyone with a diagnosis of SUD requires treatment (MacKillop, 2020), currently there is no accepted tool or assessment that can differentiate those who will recover or resolve on their own. The general assumption is that everyone that receives a diagnosis would benefit from treatment, though researchers may limit the use of the model to OUD or to people who meet the criteria for severe SUD.

Because there is a lack of consensus on who needs treatment, there is lack of consensus on the rest of the cascade. Historically, in the United States, the rate of met treatment need has been calculated as the percent of people who met diagnostic criteria for SUD in the past year who received treatment for an SUD during that time. The rate of treatment receipt using those criteria has averaged 10–11% for the past 20 years, though there is wide variation by severity, specific drug, and definition of treatment (Johnson et al., 2020b). Similarly, there is lack of consensus on how long an individual should remain in treatment, but since SUD is a chronic condition, a general agreement is longer treatment is better. For OUD, most studies using a CoC model use 6 months or 1-year retention, particularly when assessing maintenance medications (Johnson et al., 2020a; Socías et al., 2018). The expected outcome for treatment is abstinence from use of alcohol or drugs; however, this outcome measure is in debate as practitioners would argue normal functioning with reduced use or return to "normal" use is a successful treatment outcome (Tiffany et al., 2012). Despite the debate about the best way to measure these various aspects of treatment utilization and its effects, there is good evidence that treatment entry and retention are pathways to positive outcomes (Hser et al., 2004, 2007).

Gender Differences in Treatment Utilization

Women who need treatment for a SUD are less likely to receive treatment than men, though this difference appears to be primarily because of differences in admission to treatment for adult women with AUDs rather than DUDs (Johnson et al., 2020b; McHugh et al., 2018). Once in treatment, there does not seem to be a gender difference in treatment retention, at least in studies that are based on large population samples. There is also no indication women have poorer outcomes, though early research indicated women were more likely to relapse than men (Greenfield et al., 2007; McHugh et al., 2018). Gender-specific treatment, where women and men are sex segregated into separate programs of treatment does not seem to change retention or outcomes. However, gender-responsive treatment, which addresses issues that are more likely to affect women, such as pregnancy, childcare, and sexual trauma, may improve retention and outcomes (McHugh et al., 2018).

Effective Treatment Strategies

Medication is currently only available to treat AUDs and OUDs. There are no medications approved for use to treat stimulant use disorder or cannabis use disorder. Medication for AUD falls into three categories: (1) opioid antagonists (naltrexone and nalmefene), (2) a glutamate receptor antagonist (acamprosate), and (3) an aldehyde dehydrogenase inhibitor (disulfiram). Other "off-label" medications include gabapentin and topiramate. However, none of these medications, FDA approved or otherwise, is widely used (Harris et al., 2012; Mason, 2022).

Use of opioid agonists, buprenorphine, and methadone, to treat OUDs has grown in the past 5 years as the U. S. federal government has significantly increased funding to cover the cost of medication and has made a concerted effort to improve use of medication, the only effective treatment for OUD (Johnson et al., 2018). During 2018/2019, only 18.1% of people who met diagnostic criteria for OUDs in the prior 12 months received medication for OUDs (MOUD) (SAMHSA, 2019). Because this figure only reflects the percent of people who met the criteria for active OUD (not in remission), it misses the population of people who are in remission from OUD who are in ongoing treatment with an opioid agonist. For people who initiate MOUD, treatment needs to be long-term, even lifelong, for successful outcomes (Hser et al., 2004). Women are less likely than men to receive MOUDs (16.2% vs.

Table 5.1 Elements of an adequate SUD system of care

Steps to treatment	SUD	Medications	Psychosocial intervention
Screening	Alcohol	Acamprosate	Behavioral Couples Therapy
Treatment		Disulfuram	Cognitive Behavioral Therapy (CBT)
Alcohol use disorder		Naltrexone	Community Reinforcement Approach (CRA)
		Topiramate	Motivation Enhancement Therapy (MET)
Opioid use disorder		Gabapentin[a]	Twelve-Step Programs
Cannabis use disorder	Opioid	Buprenorphine	Medical Management (MM)[b]
Stimulant use disorder		Methadone	Contingency Management (CM)
Promoting group mutual help		ER-Injectable	Individual Drug Counseling (IDC)[b]
Address co-occurring conditions		Naltrexone[a]	
Continuing care guided by ongoing assessment			
Stabilization and recovery	Cannabis		CBT/MET
	Stimulant		CBT/CRA/IDC ± CM

Image from Karen Drexler, personal communication, based on information from The Management of Substance Use Disorders Work Group (2015), reprinted with permission
[a]Suggested
[b]Recommended only with medication

19.7%) even though women are more likely to have Medicaid as insurance rather than have private insurance (29% vs. 16.3%) (SAMHSA, 2019).

Behavioral therapies are the treatment of choice for people with mild or moderate SUDs who may not require medication or who have SUDs that do not have available medication. Behavioral, cognitive, and contingency management therapies, including motivational interviewing and enhancement therapy, (Higgins et al., 2007; Hofmann et al., 2012; Miller, 1983; Miller et al., 1992) have been demonstrated to be effective in treating SUDs as well as the community reinforcement approach (CRA) treatments which combine aspects of these therapies (see Table 5.1).

Self-help groups, such as Alcoholics Anonymous, have been either a standard component of treatment or may be the only treatment available. A recent meta-analysis indicates that self-help is at least as effective as other evidence-based treatments (Kelly et al., 2020). Research has also demonstrated that Alcoholics Anonymous is as effective for women as it is for men, but the specific mediators of effectiveness for women are different and not measured in existing research (Kelly & Hoeppner, 2013). Although new treatments, such as mobile phone-based recovery support (Gustafson et al., 2014), automation of CBT in computer-based programs (Carroll et al., 2008), and virtual reality (Segawa et al., 2020) show efficacy, they are not yet widely used outside of the research setting and pay little attention to gender-based differences in effect.

Disease Progression/Resolution

SUDs, particularly those characterized as mild or moderate, often resolve without treatment. People who meet diagnostic criteria for mild AUDs in late adolescence or early adulthood often become asymptomatic once work and family responsibilities require them to maintain a healthier lifestyle. Studies also have demonstrated marriage is a marker for decreased alcohol use for both men and women (Power et al., 1999). Longitudinal studies have found, in general, alcohol and drug use decrease with age. In untreated populations, 25–70% of those who once met diagnostic criteria for SUD achieved recovery. Differences in the rates between studies are due to differences in definition of recovery, the time period examined, and whether the study population was community-based or treatment-seeking (Spinelli & Thyer, 2017). Treatment increases the probability of achieving remission and sustained recovery (Moos & Moos, 2006).

One exception to this general rule of remission with or without treatment is for people who have OUDs. While recovery, with or without treatment, is possible, most people with OUDs continue use for long periods of time or die before they achieve remission (Hser et al., 2007). Further, remission without medication is less common for people with OUDs than for other SUDs. Because of the high risk of death due to overdose or other injection drug use-related conditions, MOUD is the recommended treatment for people with OUDs.

Recent efforts have been made to define recovery using quality of life (QOL) measures rather than just abstinence or reduction in use of alcohol and drugs (White, 2007). With this broadened definition, the addiction recovery movement focuses on services that improve QOL over the long-term, rather than shorter-term behavioral treatments aimed at increasing abstinence from use. These recovery support services are often delivered by people in recovery and modeled on peer support services within the mental health system. There is a small body of evidence for the efficacy of these services that is still evolving (Bassuk et al., 2016; Ashford et al., 2020). The concept of addiction recovery has strong support in the United States, but the U. S.-based framework is not accepted in Europe or other parts of the world (Best & Hamer, 2021; Best et al., 2017).

Implications for Women's Behavioral Health

Despite an early research focus on women, particularly pregnant and parenting women with SUDs, research is only beginning to differentiate between sex as a biological factor and gender as a social/environmental factor. While there do not seem to be specific sex-linked genetic differences in SUD etiology or progression, there may be sex-linked gene-environment interactions that account for the apparent differences in disease rates, progression, and resolution.

Most research has been conducted in countries where women's roles have evolved and substance use has increased with growing equality, particularly in younger age cohorts. Cross-country research would help in understanding the effects of cultural expectations on substance use and the impacts on addiction etiology, progression, and treatment utilization. Multi-country studies would improve the understanding of the relationships between genetic and environmental risk and protection. Aside from continuing to require research on SUDs to include women and sex/gender-based analysis, additional policy considerations need to be highlighted. Women's roles as caretakers are factors to be taken into consideration in treatment delivery. Women are more likely to participate in treatment when childcare or eldercare services are provided and when their caretaker role is addressed in treatment. Increased efforts to provide gender-responsive treatment may reduce the treatment gap between men and women.

The child welfare system operates for women much as the criminal justice system does for men as a primary referrer and motivator for treatment. Children are removed to foster care solely because of a mother's SUD, regardless of her ability to care for them. Abstinence-based treatments, often required by the child welfare system instead of the more effective medication options, lead to poorer outcomes for women and their children, especially in permanency determinations for child placement. Alternatives to current child welfare and criminal justice practices should focus on gender issues to improve multigenerational outcomes, avoid family disruption, and disrupt intergenerational trauma and SUD cycles. These alternatives should include community-based family-oriented treatment that addresses multigenerational trauma. Better alignment between these systems would lead to improved outcomes for women and their children (Madden et al., 2022).

Internationally, trafficking in humans, weapons, and drugs is interlinked, so efforts to reduce drug use and illegal arms can also reduce modern slavery of women and children. UNODC efforts focus on protecting women and children or rescuing them from captors. Increased support and attention to the relationship between these crimes will improve women's mental health internationally and improve outcomes for multiple generations.

SUDs are complex conditions, intricately linked, both biologically and psychosocially, with anxiety and depression, especially for women. Understanding how women differ from men in SUD etiology, progression, and resolution is in the early stages of research. Considering the complexity of factors that may play roles in the prevention and treatment of SUDs may require research to incorporate social determinants of health and cultural factors in a more systematic manner.

References

Abbey, A. (2002). Alcohol-related sexual assault: A common problem among college students. *Journal of Studies on Alcohol, Suppl(s14)*, 118–128. https://doi.org/10.15288/jsas.2002.s14.118

Agabio, R., Pisanu, C., Luigi Gessa, G., & Franconi, F. (2017). Sex differences in alcohol use disorder. *Current Medicinal Chemistry, 24*(24), 2661–2670. https://doi.org/10.217 4/0929867323666161202092908

Agrawal, A., & Lynskey, M. T. (2008). Are there genetic influences on addiction: Evidence from family, adoption and twin studies. *Addiction, 103*(7), 1069–1081. https://doi.org/10.1111/j.1360-0443.2008.02213.x

Agrawal, A., Verweij, K., Gillespie, N., Heath, A., Lessov-Schlaggar, C., Martin, N., Nelson, E., Slutske, W., Whitfield, J., & Lynskey, M. (2012). The genetics of addiction – A translational perspective. *Translational Psychiatry, 2*(7), e140–e140. https://doi.org/10.1038/tp.2012.54

Amaro, H., Blake, S. M., Schwartz, P. M., & Flinchbaugh, L. J. (2001). Developing theory-based substance abuse prevention programs for young adolescent girls. *The Journal of Early Adolescence, 21*(3), 256–293. https://doi.org/10.1177/0272431601021003002

American Psychiatric Association. (2013). *Diagnostic and statistical manual of mental disorders (DSM-5)*. APA.

Andersen, S. L. (2003, Jan-Mar). Trajectories of brain development: Point of vulnerability or window of opportunity? *Neuroscience & Biobehavioral Reviews, 27*(1–2), 3–18. https://doi.org/10.1016/s0149-7634(03)00005-8

Annie E. Casey Foundation. (2020, April 13). *Black children continue to be disproportionately represented in foster care* [Web page]. https://datacenter.kidscount.org/updates/show/264-us-foster-care-population-by-race-and-ethnicity

Ashford, R. D., Bergman, B. G., Kelly, J. F., & Curtis, B. (2020). Systematic review: Digital recovery support services used to support substance use disorder recovery. *Human Behavior and Emerging Technologies, 2*(1), 18–32. https://doi.org/10.1002/hbe2.148

Babor, T. F., Kranzler, H. R., & Lauerman, R. J. (1989). Early detection of harmful alcohol consumption: Comparison of clinical, laboratory, and self-report screening procedures. *Addictive Behaviors, 14*(2), 139–157. https://doi.org/10.1016/0306-4603(89)90043-9

Bachman, J. G., Johnston, L. D., O'Malley, P. M., Schulenberg, J. E., & Miech, R. A. (2015). *The Monitoring the Future project after four decades: Design and procedures*. University of Michigan Institute for Social Research. https://deepblue.lib.umich.edu/bitstream/handle/2027.42/137908/mtf-occ82.pdf?sequence=1&isAllowed=y

Barbosa, C., Cowell, A. J., & Dowd, W. N. (2021). Alcohol consumption in response to the COVID-19 pandemic in the United States. *Journal of Addiction Medicine, 15*(4), 341–344. https://doi.org/10.1097/ADM.0000000000000767

Bassuk, E. L., Hanson, J., Greene, R. N., Richard, M., & Laudet, A. (2016). Peer-delivered recovery support services for addictions in the United States: A systematic review. *Journal of Substance Abuse Treatment, 63*, 1–9. https://doi.org/10.1016/j.jsat.2016.01.003

Bava, S., & Tapert, S. F. (2010, Dec). Adolescent brain development and the risk for alcohol and other drug problems. *Neuropsychology Review, 20*(4), 398–413. https://doi.org/10.1007/s11065-010-9146-6

Beayno, A., El Hayek, S., Noufi, P., Tarabay, Y., & Shamseddeen, W. (2019). The role of epigenetics in addiction: Clinical overview and recent updates. In F. H. Kobeissy (Ed.), *Psychiatric disorders: Methods and protocols* (Methods in Molecular Biology) (Vol. 2011, pp. 609–631). Springer. https://doi.org/10.1007/978-1-4939-9554-7_35

Beschner, G. M., Reed, B. G., & Mondanaro, J. (1981). *Treatment services for drug dependent women* (Report; DHHS-ADM-81-1177). National Institute on Drug Abuse. https://files.eric.ed.gov/fulltext/ED216255.pdf

Best, D., & Hamer, R. (2021). Addiction recovery in services and policy: An international overview. In N. El-Guebaly, G. Carrà, M. Galanter, & A. M. Baldacchino (Eds.), *Textbook of addiction treatment: International perspectives* (pp. 718–732). Springer.

Best, D., De Alwis, S. J., & Burdett, D. (2017). The recovery movement and its implications for policy, commissioning and practice. *Nordisk Alkohol Nark, 34*(2), 107–111. https://doi.org/10.1177/1455072517691058

Blake, S. M., Amaro, H., Schwartz, P. M., & Flinchbaugh, L. J. (2001). A review of substance abuse prevention interventions for young adolescent girls. *The Journal of Early Adolescence, 21*(3), 294–324. https://doi.org/10.1177/0272431601021003003

Blanco, C., & Volkow, N. D. (2019). Management of opioid use disorder in the USA: Present status and future directions. *The Lancet, 393*(10182), 1760–1772. https://doi.org/10.1016/S0140-6736(18)33078-2

Bobzean, S. A., DeNobrega, A. K., & Perrotti, L. I. (2014). Sex differences in the neurobiology of drug addiction. *Experimental Neurology, 259*, 64–74. https://doi.org/10.1016/j.expneurol.2014.01.022

Botvin, G. J., & Griffin, K. W. (2004). Life skills training: Empirical findings and future directions. *Journal of Primary Prevention, 25*(2), 211–232. https://doi.org/10.1023/B:JOPP.0000042391.58573.5b

Bradley, K. A., DeBenedetti, A. F., Volk, R. J., Williams, E. C., Frank, D., & Kivlahan, D. R. (2007). AUDIT-C as a brief screen for alcohol misuse in primary care. *Alcoholism: Clinical and Experimental Research, 31*(7), 1208–1217. https://doi.org/10.1111/j.1530-0277.2007.00403.x

Cadet, J. L. (2016). Epigenetics of stress, addiction, and resilience: Therapeutic implications. *Molecular Neurobiology, 53*(1), 545–560. https://doi.org/10.1007/s12035-014-9040-y

Carroll, M. E., & Smethells, J. R. (2016). Sex differences in behavioral dyscontrol: Role in drug addiction and novel treatments. *Frontiers in Psychiatry, 6*, 175. https://doi.org/10.3389/fpsyt.2015.00175

Carroll, M. E., Lynch, W. J., Roth, M. E., Morgan, A. D., & Cosgrove, K. P. (2004). Sex and estrogen influence drug abuse. *Trends in Pharmacological Sciences, 25*(5), 273–279. https://doi.org/10.1016/j.tips.2004.03.011

Carroll, K. M., Ball, S. A., Martino, S., Nich, C., Babuscio, T. A., Nuro, K. F., Gordon, M. A., Portnoy, G. A., & Rounsaville, B. (2008). Computer-assisted delivery of Cognitive-Behavioral Therapy for addiction: A randomized trial of CBT4CBT. *American Journal of Psychiatry, 165*(7), 881–888. https://doi.org/10.1176/appi.ajp.2008.07111835

Casey, B., & Jones, R. M. (2010). Neurobiology of the adolescent brain and behavior: Implications for substance use disorders. *Journal of the American Academy of Child and Adolescent Psychiatry, 49*(12), 1189–1201. https://doi.org/10.1016/j.jaac.2010.08.017

Castillo-Carniglia, A., Keyes, K. M., Hasin, D. S., & Cerdá, M. (2019). Psychiatric comorbidities in alcohol use disorder. *The Lancet Psychiatry, 6*(12), 1068–1080. https://doi.org/10.1016/S2215-0366(19)30222-6

Chang, G. (2001). Alcohol-screening instruments for pregnant women. *Alcohol Research & Health, 25*(3), 204. https://www.ncbi.nlm.nih.gov/pmc/articles/PMC6707175/

Chasnoff, I., Wells, A., McGourty, R., & Bailey, L. (2007). Validation of the 4P's Plus© screen for substance use in pregnancy validation of the 4P's Plus. *Journal of Perinatology, 27*(12), 744–748. https://doi.org/10.1038/sj.jp.7211823

Chassin, L., Pitts, S. C., DeLucia, C., & Todd, M. (1999). A longitudinal study of children of alcoholics: Predicting young adult substance use disorders, anxiety, and depression. *Journal of Abnormal Psychology, 108*(1), 106. https://doi.org/10.1037//0021-843x.108.1.106

Cherpitel, C. J. (1995, Aug). Screening for alcohol problems in the Emergency Department. *Annals of Emergency Medicine, 26*(2), 158–166. https://doi.org/10.1016/s0196-0644(95)70146-x

Cleveland, M. J., Feinberg, M. E., Bontempo, D. E., & Greenberg, M. T. (2008). The role of risk and protective factors in substance use across adolescence. *Journal of Adolescent Health, 43*(2), 157–164. https://doi.org/10.1016/j.jadohealth.2008.01.015

Collins, R. L., & Marlatt, G. A. (1983). Psychological correlates and explanations of alcohol use and abuse. In B. Tabakoff, P. B. Sutker, & C. L. Randall (Eds.), *Medical and social aspects of alcohol abuse* (pp. 273–308). Springer. https://doi.org/10.1007/978-1-4684-4436-0_10

Comprehensive Alcohol Abuse and Alcoholism Prevention, Treatment, and Rehabilitation Act of 1970, Pub. L. No. 91-616 [The Hughes Act]. (1972). https://www.govinfo.gov/content/pkg/STATUTE-84/pdf/STATUTE-84-Pg1848.pdf#page=6

Compton, W. M., Flannagan, K. S., Silveira, M. L., Creamer, M. R., Kimmel, H. L., Kanel, M., et al. (2023). Tobacco, alcohol, cannabis, and other drug use in the us before and during the early phase of the COVID-19 pandemic. *JAMA Network Open, 6*(1), e2254566–e2254566. https://doi.org/10.1001/jamanetworkopen.2022.54566

Covington, S. (1997). Women, addiction, and sexuality. In S. L. A. Straussner & E. Zelvin (Eds.), *Gender and addictions: Men and women in treatment* (pp. 71–95). Jason Aronson.

Covington, S. S. (1999). *Helping women recover: A program for treating substance abuse, special edition for use in the criminal justice system* (Program manual, NCJ Number 181142). Jossey-Bass Publishers.

Covington, S. S. (2008). Women and addiction: A trauma-informed approach. *Journal of Psychoactive Drugs, 40*(sup5), 377–385. https://doi.org/10.1080/02791072.2008.10400665

Datta, U., Schoenrock, S. E., Bubier, J. A., Bogue, M. A., Jentsch, J. D., Logan, R. W., Tarantino, L. M., & Chesler, E. J. (2020). Prospects for finding the mechanisms of sex differences in addiction with human and model organism genetic analysis. *Genes, Brain and Behavior, 19*(3), e12645. https://doi.org/10.1111/gbb.12645

Dawson, D. A., Grant, B. F., Stinson, F. S., & Zhou, Y. (2005). Effectiveness of the derived Alcohol Use Disorders Identification Test (AUDIT-C) in screening for alcohol use disorders and risk drinking in the US general population. *Alcoholism: Clinical and Experimental Research, 29*(5), 844–854. https://doi.org/10.1097/01.alc.0000164374.32229.a2

Degenhardt, L., Charlson, F., Ferrari, A., Santomauro, D., Erskine, H., Mantilla-Herrara, A., Whiteford, H., Leung, J., Naghavi, M., & Griswold, M. (2018, Dec). The global burden of disease attributable to alcohol and drug use in 195 countries and territories, 1990–2016: A systematic analysis for the Global Burden of Disease Study 2016. *The Lancet Psychiatry, 5*(12), 987–1012. https://doi.org/10.1016/S2215-0366(18)30337-7

Dennis, M. L., Titus, J. C., White, M. K., Unsicker, J. I., & Hodgkins, D. (2003). Global Appraisal of Individual Needs (GAIN). In J. P. Allen & V. B. Wilson (Eds.), *Assessing alcohol problems: A guide for clinicians and researchers* (2nd ed.). National Institute on Alcohol Abuse and Alcoholism. https://pubs.niaaa.nih.gov/publications/assessingalcohol/InstrumentPDFs/37_GAIN.pdf [From Report Appendix]

Des Jarlais, D. C., Feelemyer, J. P., Modi, S. N., Arasteh, K., & Hagan, H. (2012). Are females who inject drugs at higher risk for HIV infection than males who inject drugs: An international systematic review of high seroprevalence areas. *Drug and Alcohol Dependence, 124*(1–2), 95–107. https://doi.org/10.1016/j.drugalcdep.2011.12.020

DeWit, D. J., Adlaf, E. M., Offord, D. R., & Ogborne, A. C. (2000). Age at first alcohol use: A risk factor for the development of alcohol disorders. *American Journal of Psychiatry, 157*(5), 745–750. https://doi.org/10.1176/appi.ajp.157.5.745

Dhalla, S., & Kopec, J. A. (2007). The CAGE questionnaire for alcohol misuse: A review of reliability and validity studies. *Clinical and Investigative Medicine, 30*(1), 33–41. https://doi.org/10.25011/cim.v30i1.447

Duncan, D. F., Nicholson, T., White, J. B., Bradley, D. B., & Bonaguro, J. (2010). The baby boomer effect: Changing patterns of substance abuse among adults ages 55 and older. *Journal of Aging & Social Policy, 22*(3), 237–248. https://doi.org/10.1080/08959420.2010.485511

Edenberg, H. J., Gelernter, J., & Agrawal, A. (2019). Genetics of alcoholism. *Current Psychiatry Reports, 21*(4), 26. https://doi.org/10.1007/s11920-019-1008-1

Ellinwood, E. H., Smith, W. G., & Vaillant, G. E. (1966). Narcotic addiction in males and females: A comparison. *International Journal of the Addictions, 1*(2), 33–45. https://doi.org/10.3109/10826086609026750

Emiliussen, J., Nielsen, A. S., & Andersen, K. (2017). Identifying risk factors for late-onset (50+) alcohol use disorder and heavy drinking: A systematic review. *Substance Use and Misuse, 52*(12), 1575–1588. https://doi.org/10.1080/10826084.2017.1293102

Enoch, M.-A., & Goldman, D. (2001). The genetics of alcoholism and alcohol abuse. *Current Psychiatry Reports, 3*(2), 144–151. https://doi.org/10.1007/s11920-001-0012-3

Evans, E. A., Grella, C. E., & Upchurch, D. M. (2017). Gender differences in the effects of childhood adversity on alcohol, drug, and polysubstance-related disorders. *Social Psychiatry and Psychiatric Epidemiology, 52*(7), 901–912. https://doi.org/10.1007/s00127-017-1355-3

Ewing, J. A. (1984). Detecting alcoholism: The CAGE questionnaire. *JAMA, 252*(14), 1905–1907. https://doi.org/10.1001/jama.252.14.1905

Fattore, L., Altea, S., & Fratta, W. (2008). Sex differences in drug addiction: A review of animal and human studies. *Women's Health, 4*(1), 51–65. https://doi.org/10.2217/17455057.4.1.51

Felitti, V. J., Anda, R. F., Nordenberg, D., Williamson, D. F., Spitz, A. M., Edwards, V., & Marks, J. S. (1998). Relationship of childhood abuse and household dysfunction to many of the leading causes of death in adults: The Adverse Childhood Experiences (ACE) Study. *American Journal of Preventive Medicine, 14*(4), 245–258. https://doi.org/10.1016/s0749-3797(98)00017-8

Finkelstein, N. (1996). Using the relational model as a context for treating pregnant and parenting chemically dependent women. *Journal of Chemical Dependency Treatment, 6*(1–2), 23–44. https://doi.org/10.1300/J034v06n01_02

Gable, R. S. (1993). Toward a comparative overview of dependence potential and acute toxicity of psychoactive substances used nonmedically. *The American Journal of Drug and Alcohol Abuse, 19*(3), 263–281. https://doi.org/10.3109/00952999309001618

Gilligan, C. (1993). *In a different voice: Psychological theory and women's development.* Harvard University Press.

Gordon, J., & Robert, S. (1983). An operational classification of disease prevention. *Public Health Reports, 98*(2), 107–109. https://www.ncbi.nlm.nih.gov/pmc/articles/PMC1424415/pdf/pubhealthrep00112-0005.pdf

Grant, B. F., Goldstein, R. B., Saha, T. D., Chou, S. P., Jung, J., Zhang, H., Pickering, R. P., Ruan, W. J., Smith, S. M., & Huang, B. (2015). Epidemiology of DSM-5 alcohol use disorder: Results from the National Epidemiologic Survey on Alcohol and Related Conditions III. *JAMA Psychiatry, 72*(8), 757–766. https://doi.org/10.1001/jamapsychiatry.2015.0584

Greenfield, S. F., Brooks, A. J., Gordon, S. M., Green, C. A., Kropp, F., McHugh, R. K., Lincoln, M., Hien, D., & Miele, G. M. (2007). Substance abuse treatment entry, retention, and outcome in women: A review of the literature. *Drug and Alcohol Dependence, 86*(1), 1–21. https://doi.org/10.1016/j.drugalcdep.2006.05.012

Greenfield, S. F., Back, S. E., Lawson, K., & Brady, K. T. (2010). Substance abuse in women. *Psychiatric Clinics, 33*(2), 339–355. https://doi.org/10.1016/j.psc.2010.01.004

Grekin, E. R., Svikis, D. S., Lam, P., Connors, V., LeBreton, J. M., Streiner, D. L., Smith, C., & Ondersma, S. J. (2010). Drug use during pregnancy: Validating the Drug Abuse Screening Test against physiological measures. *Psychology of Addictive Behaviors, 24*(4), 719. https://doi.org/10.1037/a0021741

Grella, C. E. (2008). From generic to gender-responsive treatment: Changes in social policies, treatment services, and outcomes of women in substance abuse treatment. *Journal of Psychoactive Drugs, 40*(sup5), 327–343. https://doi.org/10.1080/02791072.2008.10400661

Grigsby, T. J., Howard, K., Howard, J. T., & Perrotte, J. (2023). COVID-19 concerns, perceived stress, and increased alcohol use among adult women in the United States. *Clinical Nursing Research, 32*(1), 84–93. https://doi.org/10.1177/10547738221136678

Guinle, M. I. B., & Sinha, R. (2020). The role of stress, trauma, and negative affect in alcohol misuse and alcohol use disorder in women. *Alcohol Research: Current Reviews, 40*(2), 05. https://doi.org/10.35946/arcr.v40.2.05

Gustafson, D. H., McTavish, F. M., Chih, M.-Y., Atwood, A. K., Johnson, R. A., Boyle, M. G., Levy, M. S., Driscoll, H., Chisholm, S. M., & Dillenburg, L. (2014). A smartphone application to support recovery from alcoholism: A randomized clinical trial. *JAMA Psychiatry, 71*(5), 566–572. https://doi.org/10.1001/jamapsychiatry.2013.4642

Haggerty, R. J., & Mrazek, P. J. (1994). *Reducing risks for mental disorders: Frontiers for preventive intervention research*. National Academies Press. https://www.nap.edu/catalog/2139/reducing-risks-for-mental-disorders-frontiers-for-preventive-intervention-research

Han, B. H., Moore, A. A., Sherman, S., Keyes, K. M., & Palamar, J. J. (2017). Demographic trends of binge alcohol use and alcohol use disorders among older adults in the United States, 2005–2014. *Drug and Alcohol Dependence, 170*, 198–207. https://doi.org/10.1016/j.drugalcdep.2016.11.003

Harris, A. H. S., Oliva, E., Bowe, T., Humphreys, K. N., Kivlahan, D. R., & Trafton, J. A. (2012). Pharmacotherapy of alcohol use disorders by the Veterans Health Administration: Patterns of receipt and persistence. *Psychiatric Services, 63*(7), 679–685. https://doi.org/10.1176/appi.ps.201000553

Hasin, D. S., & Grant, B. F. (2015). The National Epidemiologic Survey on Alcohol and Related Conditions (NESARC) Waves 1 and 2: Review and summary of findings. *Social Psychiatry and Psychiatric Epidemiology, 50*(11), 1609–1640. https://doi.org/10.1007/s00127-015-1088-0

Hasin, D. S., Van Rossem, R., McCloud, S., & Endicott, J. (1997). Differentiating DSM-IV alcohol dependence and abuse by course: Community heavy drinkers. *Journal of Substance Abuse, 9*, 127–135. https://doi.org/10.1016/s0899-3289(97)90011-0

Hatoum, A. S., Colbert, S. M. C., Johnson, E. C., et al. (2023). Multivariate genome-wide association meta-analysis of over 1 million subjects identifies loci underlying multiple substance use disorders. *Nature Mental Health, 1*(3), 210–223. https://doi.org/10.1038/s44220-023-00034-y

Hawkins, J. D., Catalano, R. F., & Miller, J. Y. (1992). Risk and protective factors for alcohol and other drug problems in adolescence and early adulthood: Implications for substance abuse prevention. *Psychological Bulletin, 112*(1), 64. https://doi.org/10.1037/0033-2909.112.1.64

Hawkins, E. J., Baer, J. S., & Kivlahan, D. R. (2008). Concurrent monitoring of psychological distress and satisfaction measures as predictors of addiction treatment retention. *Journal of Substance Abuse Treatment, 35*(2), 207–216. https://doi.org/10.1016/j.jsat.2007.10.001

Hien, D. A., Cohen, L. R., Miele, G. M., Litt, L. C., & Capstick, C. (2004). Promising treatments for women with comorbid PTSD and substance use disorders. *American Journal of Psychiatry, 161*(8), 1426–1432. https://doi.org/10.1176/appi.ajp.161.8.1426

Higgins, S. T., Silverman, K., & Heil, S. H. (2007). *Contingency management in substance abuse treatment*. Guilford Press.

Hofmann, S. G., Asnaani, A., Vonk, I. J., Sawyer, A. T., & Fang, A. (2012). The efficacy of cognitive behavioral therapy: A review of meta-analyses. *Cognitive Therapy and Research, 36*(5), 427–440. https://doi.org/10.1007/s10608-012-9476-1

Hser, Y.-I., Evans, E., Huang, D., & Anglin, D. M. (2004). Relationship between drug treatment services, retention, and outcomes. *Psychiatric Services, 55*(7), 767–774. https://doi.org/10.1176/appi.ps.55.7.767

Hser, Y.-I., Longshore, D., & Anglin, M. D. (2007). The life course perspective on drug use: A conceptual framework for understanding drug use trajectories. *Evaluation Review, 31*(6), 515–547. https://doi.org/10.1177/0193841X07307316

Humeniuk, R., Dennington, V., & Ali, R. on behalf of the WHO ASSIST Phase III Study Group. (2008). *The effectiveness of a brief intervention for illicit drugs linked to the alcohol, smoking and substance involvement screening test (ASSIST) in primary health care settings: A technical report of phase III findings of the WHO ASSIST randomized controlled trial* (Report). World Health Organization. https://www.who.int/substance_abuse/activities/assist_technical-report_phase3_final.pdf

Humeniuk, R. E., Henry-Edwards, S., Ali, R. L., Poznyak, V., & Monteiro, M. (2010). *The Alcohol, Smoking and Substance Involvement Screening Test (ASSIST) manual for use in primary care*. World Health Organization. https://apps.who.int/iris/rest/bitstreams/52736/retrieve

International Society of Substance Use Professionals. (2020, April). *The Colombo Plan Drug Advisory Programme (DAP) Training Series Universal Prevention Curriculum for Substance Use (UPC) Managers and Supervisors Series, Course 5: School based prevention interventions participant manual*. International Society of Substance Use Professionals. https://www.issup.net/training/universal-prevention-curriculum/upc-5-school-based-prevention-interventions

Iversen, J., Page, K., Madden, A., & Maher, L. (2015). HIV, HCV and health-related harms among women who inject drugs: Implications for prevention and treatment. *Journal of Acquired Immune Deficiency Syndromes, 69*(01), S176–S181. https://doi.org/10.1097/QAI.0000000000000659

Jang, S.-K., Saunders, G., Liu, M., Jiang, Y., Liu, D. J., Vrieze, S., & Team, A. R. (2020). Genetic correlation, pleiotropy, and causal associations between substance use and psychiatric disorder. *Psychological Medicine*, 1–11. https://doi.org/10.1017/S003329172000272X

Jellinek, E. M. (1947). Recent trends in alcoholism and in alcohol consumption. *Quarterly Journal of Studies on Alcohol, 8*(1), 1–42. https://doi.org/10.15288/qjsa.1947.8.1

Jellinek, E. M. (1952). Phases of alcohol addiction. *Quarterly Journal of Studies on Alcohol, 13*(4), 673–684. https://doi.org/10.15288/qjsa.1952.13.673

Johnson, K., Jones, C., Compton, W., Baldwin, G., Fan, J., Mermin, J., & Bennett, J. (2018). Federal response to the opioid crisis. *Current HIV/AIDS Reports, 15*(4), 293–301. https://doi.org/10.1007/s11904-018-0398-8

Johnson, K., Hills, H., Ma, J., Brown, C. H., & McGovern, M. (2020a). Treatment for opioid use disorder in the Florida Medicaid population: Using a cascade of care model to evaluate quality. *The American Journal of Drug and Alcohol Abuse*, 1–9. https://doi.org/10.1080/00952990.2020.1824236

Johnson, K., Rigg, K. K., & Eyles, C. H. (2020b). Receiving addiction treatment in the US: Do patient demographics, drug of choice, or substance use disorder severity matter? *International Journal of Drug Policy, 75*, 102583. https://doi.org/10.1016/j.drugpo.2019.10.009

Jozkowski, K. N., Marcantonio, T. L., & Hunt, M. E. (2017). College students' sexual consent communication and perceptions of sexual double standards: A qualitative investigation. *Perspectives on Sexual & Reproductive Health, 49*(4), 237–244. https://doi.org/10.1363/psrh.12041

Kandall, S. R. (2010). Women and drug addiction: A historical perspective. *Journal of Addictive Diseases, 29*(2), 117–126. https://doi.org/10.1080/10550881003684491

Kelly, J. F., & Hoeppner, B. B. (2013). Does Alcoholics Anonymous work differently for men and women? A moderated multiple-mediation analysis in a large clinical sample. *Drug and Alcohol Dependence, 130*(1–3), 186–193. https://doi.org/10.1016/j.drugalcdep.2012.11.005

Kelly, J. F., Abry, A., Ferri, M., & Humphreys, K. (2020). Alcoholics Anonymous and 12-step facilitation treatments for alcohol use disorder: A distillation of a 2020 Cochrane review for clinicians and policy makers. *Alcohol and Alcoholism, 55*(6), 641–651. https://doi.org/10.1093/alcalc/agaa050

Kessler, R. C. (2003). Epidemiology of women and depression. *Journal of Affective Disorders, 74*(1), 5–13. https://doi.org/10.1016/s0165-0327(02)00426-3

Keyes, K. M., Martins, S. S., Blanco, C., & Hasin, D. S. (2010). Telescoping and gender differences in alcohol dependence: New evidence from two national surveys. *American Journal of Psychiatry, 167*(8), 969–976. https://doi.org/10.1176/appi.ajp.2009.09081161

Keyes, K. M., Li, G., & Hasin, D. S. (2011, Dec). Birth cohort effects and gender differences in alcohol epidemiology: A review and synthesis. *Alcoholism: Clinical and Experimental Research, 35*(12), 2101–2112. https://doi.org/10.1111/j.1530-0277.2011.01562.x

Kilpatrick, D. G., Acierno, R., Resnick, H. S., Saunders, B. E., & Best, C. L. (1997). A 2-year longitudinal analysis of the relationships between violent assault and substance use in women. *Journal of Consulting and Clinical Psychology, 65*(5), 834. https://doi.org/10.1037/0022-006x.65.5.834

Kim, D. R., Bale, T. L., & Epperson, C. N. (2015). Prenatal programming of mental illness: Current understanding of relationship and mechanisms. *Current Psychiatry Reports, 17*(2), 5. https://doi.org/10.1007/s11920-014-0546-9

Kirk, D. S., & Wakefield, S. (2018). Collateral consequences of punishment: A critical review and path forward. *Annual Review of Criminology, 1*(1), 171–194. https://doi.org/10.1146/annurev-criminol-032317-092045

Knott, C. S., Coombs, N., Stamatakis, E., & Biddulph, J. P. (2015). All cause mortality and the case for age specific alcohol consumption guidelines: Pooled analyses of up to 10 population based cohorts. *BMJ, 350*. https://doi.org/10.1136/bmj.h384

Ko, J. Y., Patrick, S. W., Tong, V. T., Patel, R., Lind, J. N., & Barfield, W. D. (2016). Incidence of neonatal abstinence syndrome – 28 states, 1999–2013. *Morbidity and Mortality Weekly Report, 65*(31), 799–802. https://doi.org/10.15585/mmwr.mm6531a2

Koob, G. F., & Le Moal, M. (1997). Drug abuse: Hedonic homeostatic dysregulation. *Science, 278*(5335), 52–58. https://doi.org/10.1126/science.278.5335.52

Kumar, P. C., Cleland, C. M., Gourevitch, M. N., Rotrosen, J., Strauss, S., Russell, L., & McNeely, J. (2016). Accuracy of the Audio Computer Assisted Self Interview version of the Alcohol, Smoking and Substance Involvement Screening Test (ACASI ASSIST) for identifying unhealthy substance use and substance use disorders in primary care patients. *Drug and Alcohol Dependence, 165*, 38–44. https://doi.org/10.1016/j.drugalcdep.2016.05.030

Lange, S., Probst, C., Gmel, G., Rehm, J., Burd, L., & Popova, S. (2017). Global prevalence of fetal alcohol spectrum disorder among children and youth: A systematic review and meta-analysis. *JAMA Pediatrics, 171*(10), 948–956. https://doi.org/10.1001/jamapediatrics.2017.1919

Leavell, H. R., & Clark, E. G. (1958). *Textbook of preventive medicine* (3rd ed.). McGraw-Hill.

Li, M. D., & Burmeister, M. (2009). New insights into the genetics of addiction. *Nature Reviews Genetics, 10*(4), 225–231. https://doi.org/10.1038/nrg2536

Lorenz, K., & Ullman, S. E. (2016). Alcohol and sexual assault victimization: Research findings and future directions. *Aggression and Violent Behavior, 31*, 82–94. https://doi.org/10.1016/j.avb.2016.08.001

Lupien, S. J., McEwen, B. S., Gunnar, M. R., & Heim, C. (2009). Effects of stress throughout the lifespan on the brain, behaviour and cognition. *Nature Reviews Neuroscience, 10*(6), 434–445. https://doi.org/10.1038/nrn2639

Lynch, W. J. (2018). Modeling the development of drug addiction in male and female animals. *Pharmacology Biochemistry and Behavior, 164*, 50–61. https://doi.org/10.1016/j.pbb.2017.06.006

Lynskey, M. T., Nelson, E. C., Neuman, R. J., Bucholz, K. K., Madden, P. A., Knopik, V. S., Slutske, W., Whitfield, J. B., Martin, N. G., & Heath, A. C. (2005). Limitations of DSM-IV operationalizations of alcohol abuse and dependence in a sample of Australian twins. *Twin Research and Human Genetics, 8*(6), 574–584. https://doi.org/10.1375/183242705774860178

MacKillop, J. (2020). Is addiction really a chronic relapsing disorder? Commentary on Kelly et al. "How many recovery attempts does it take to successfully resolve an alcohol or drug problem? Estimates and correlates from a national study of recovering US adults". *Alcoholism: Clinical and Experimental Research, 44*(1), 41–44. https://doi.org/10.1111/acer.14246

Madden, L. M., Oliva, J., Eller, A., DiDomizio, E., Roosa, M., Blanchard, L., et al. (2022). Pregnant women and opioid use disorder: Examining the legal landscape for controlling women's reproductive health. *American Journal of Law & Medicine, 48*(2–3), 209–222. https://doi.org/10.1017/amj.2022.26

Marlatt, G. A., Baer, J. S., Donovan, D. M., & Kivlahan, D. R. (1988). Addictive behaviors: Etiology and treatment. *Annual Review of Psychology, 39*(1), 223–252. https://doi.org/10.1146/annurev.ps.39.020188.001255

Mason, B. J. (2022). Looking back, looking forward: Current medications and innovative potential medications to treat alcohol use disorder. *Alcohol Research: Current Reviews, 42*(1), 11. https://doi.org/10.35946/arcr.v42.1.11

McEwen, B. S., Eiland, L., Hunter, R. G., & Miller, M. M. (2012). Stress and anxiety: Structural plasticity and epigenetic regulation as a consequence of stress. *Neuropharmacology, 62*(1), 3–12. https://doi.org/10.1016/j.neuropharm.2011.07.014

McHugh, R. K., Votaw, V. R., Sugarman, D. E., & Greenfield, S. F. (2018). Sex and gender differences in substance use disorders. *Clinical Psychology Review, 66*, 12–23. https://doi.org/10.1016/j.cpr.2017.10.012

McLellan, A. T., Luborsky, L., Woody, G. E., & O'Brien, C. P. (1980). An improved diagnostic evaluation instrument for substance abuse patients: The Addiction Severity Index. *The Journal of Nervous and Mental Disease, 168(1), 26–33*.

McLellan, A. T., Luborsky, L., Cacciola, J., Griffith, J., Evans, F., Barr, H. L., & O'Brien, C. P. (1985). New Data from the Addiction Severity Index reliability and validity in three centers. *The Journal of Nervous and Mental Disease, 173(7), 412–423*.

McLellan, A. T., Cacciola, J. C., Alterman, A. I., Rikoon, S. H., & Carise, D. (2006). The Addiction Severity Index at 25: Origins, contributions and transitions. *American Journal on Addictions, 15*(2), 113–124. https://doi.org/10.1080/10550490500528316

Mellins, C. A., Walsh, K., Sarvet, A. L., Wall, M., Gilbert, L., Santelli, J. S., Thompson, M., Wilson, P. A., Khan, S., Benson, S., Bah, K., Kaufman, K. A., Reardon, L., & Hirsch, J. S. (2017). Sexual assault incidents among college undergraduates: Prevalence and factors associated with risk. *PLoS One, 12*(11), e0186471. https://doi.org/10.1371/journal.pone.0186471

Melo, J. A., Shendure, J., Pociask, K., & Silver, L. M. (1996). Identification of sex–specific quantitative trait loci controlling alcohol preference in C57BL/6 mice. *Nature Genetics, 13*(2), 147–153. https://doi.org/10.1038/ng0696-147

Milic, J., Glisic, M., Voortman, T., Borba, L. P., Asllanaj, E., Rojas, L. Z., Troup, J., Kiefte-de Jong, J. C., van Beeck, E., & Muka, T. (2018). Menopause, ageing, and alcohol use disorders in women. *Maturitas, 111*, 100–109. https://doi.org/10.1016/j.maturitas.2018.03.006

Miller, W. R. (1983). Motivational interviewing with problem drinkers. *Behavioural and Cognitive Psychotherapy, 11*(2), 147–172. https://doi.org/10.1017/S0141347300006583

Miller, W. R., Zweben, A., DiClemente, C. C., & Rychtarik, R. G. (1992). *Motivational enhancement therapy manual: A clinical research guide for therapists treating individuals with alcohol abuse and dependence* [Report] (NIH Publication No. 94-3723). (Project MATCH Monograph Series, Issue). National Institute on Alcohol Abuse and Alcoholism. https://pubs.niaaa.nih.gov/publications/projectmatch/match02.pdf

Moeller, F. G., Barratt, E. S., Dougherty, D. M., Schmitz, J. M., & Swann, A. C. (2001). Psychiatric aspects of impulsivity. *American Journal of Psychiatry, 158*(11), 1783–1793. https://doi.org/10.1176/appi.ajp.158.11.1783

Moos, R. H., & Moos, B. S. (2006). Rates and predictors of relapse after natural and treated remission from alcohol use disorders. *Addiction, 101*(2), 212–222. https://doi.org/10.1111/j.1360-0443.2006.01310.x

Najavits, L. M., Weiss, R. D., & Shaw, S. R. (1997). The link between substance abuse and post-traumatic stress disorder in women: A research review. *American Journal on Addictions, 6*(4), 273–283. https://doi.org/10.1111/j.1521-0391.1997.tb00408.x

National Academies of Sciences, Engineering, & Medicine. (2020). *Promoting positive adolescent health behaviors and outcomes: Thriving in the 21st century*. The National Academies Press. https://doi.org/10.17226/25552

National Center for Health Statistics. (2021). *Provisional drug overdose deaths by quarter and demographics – 2019 to 2020*. https://www.cdc.gov/nchs/data/health_policy/Provisional-Drug-Overdose-Deaths-by-Quarter-and-Demographic-Characteristics-2019-to-2020.pdf

National Institute on Drug Abuse Division of Epidemiology Prevention Research. (1996). *National Pregnancy and Health Survey. Drug Use among Women Delivering Livebirths: 1992* (Report; NIH Publication No. 96–3819). National Institutes of Health. https://ntrl.ntis.gov/NTRL/dashboard/searchResults/titleDetail/PB96175658.xhtml#

National Institutes of Health. (2015, June 9). *NOT-OD-15-102: Consideration of sex as a biological variable in NIH-funded research* [Web page]. https://orwh.od.nih.gov/sites/orwh/files/docs/NOT-OD-15-102%20Guidance.pdf

Navas, J. F., Martin-Perez, C., Petrova, D., Verdejo-Garcia, A., Cano, M., Sagripanti-Mazuquin, O., Perandres-Gomez, A., Lopez-Martin, A., Cordovilla-Guardia, S., Megias, A., Perales, J. C., & Vilar-Lopez, R. (2019). Sex differences in the association between impulsivity and driving under the influence of alcohol in young adults: The specific role of sensation seeking. *Accident Analysis and Prevention, 124*, 174–179. https://doi.org/10.1016/j.aap.2018.12.024

Novier, A., Diaz-Granados, J. L., & Matthews, D. B. (2015). Alcohol use across the lifespan: An analysis of adolescent and aged rodents and humans. *Pharmacology Biochemistry and Behavior, 133*(Jun), 65–82. https://doi.org/10.1016/j.pbb.2015.03.015

Oga, E. A., Mark, K., Peters, E. N., & Coleman-Cowger, V. H. (2020). Validation of the NIDA-modified ASSIST as a screening tool for prenatal drug use in an urban setting in the United States. *Journal of Addiction Medicine, 14*(5), 423–430. https://doi.org/10.1097/ADM.0000000000000614

Ondersma, S. J., Chang, G., Blake-Lamb, T., Gilstad-Hayden, K., Orav, J., Beatty, J. R., Goyert, G. L., & Yonkers, K. A. (2019). Accuracy of five self-report screening instruments for substance use in pregnancy. *Addiction, 114*(9), 1683–1693. https://doi.org/10.1111/add.14651

Patnode, C., Perdue, L., Rushkin, M., & O'Connor, E. (2020). *Screening for unhealthy use in primary care in adolescents and adults, Including pregnant persons: Updated systematic review for the U.S. Preventive Services Task Force*. U.S. Preventive Services Task Force. https://www.ncbi.nlm.nih.gov/books/NBK558174/

Peacock, A., Leung, J., Larney, S., Colledge, S., Hickman, M., Rehm, J., Giovino, G. A., West, R., Hall, W., Griffiths, P., Ali, R., Gowing, L., Marsden, J., Ferrari, A. J., Grebely, J., Farrell, M., & Degenhardt, L. (2018). Global statistics on alcohol, tobacco and illicit drug use: 2017 status report. *Addiction, 113*(10), 1905–1926. https://doi.org/10.1111/add.14234

Peltier, M. R., Verplaetse, T. L., Mineur, Y. S., Petrakis, I. L., Cosgrove, K. P., Picciotto, M. R., & McKee, S. A. (2019). Sex differences in stress-related alcohol use. *Neurobiology of Stress, 10*, 100149. https://doi.org/10.1016/j.ynstr.2019.100149

Petersen, N., & London, E. D. (2018). Addiction and dopamine: Sex differences and insights from studies of smoking. *Current Opinion in Behavioral Sciences, 23*, 150–159. https://doi.org/10.1016/j.cobeha.2018.07.002

Potterat, J. J., Rothenberg, R. B., Muth, S. Q., Darrow, W. W., & Phillips-Plummer, L. (1998). Pathways to prostitution: The chronology of sexual and drug abuse milestones. *Journal of Sex Research, 35*(4), 333–340. https://doi.org/10.1080/00224499809551951

Power, C., Rodgers, B., & Hope, S. (1999, Oct). Heavy alcohol consumption and marital status: Disentangling the relationship in a national study of young adults. *Addiction, 94*(10), 1477–1487. https://doi.org/10.1046/j.1360-0443.1999.941014774.x

Poznyak, V., Fleischmann, A., Rekve, D., Rylett, M., Rehm, J., & Gmel, G. (2013). The world health organization's global monitoring system on alcohol and health. *Alcohol Research: Current Reviews, 35*(2), 244. https://pubs.niaaa.nih.gov/publications/arcr352/244-249.htm

Prison Policy Initiative. (2019). *Policing women: Race and gender disparities in police stops, searches, and use of force* [Web page]. https://www.prisonpolicy.org/blog/2019/05/14/policingwomen/

Reed, G. M., First, M. B., Kogan, C. S., Hyman, S. E., Gureje, O., Gaebel, W., Maj, M., Stein, D. J., Maercker, A., Tyrer, P., Claudino, A., Garralda, E., Salvador-Carulla, L., Ray, R., Saunders, J. B., Dua, T., Poznyak, V., Medina-Mora, M. E., Pike, K. M., Ayuso-Mateos, J. L., Kanba, S., Keeley, J. W., Khoury, B., Krasnov, V. N., Kulygina, M., Lovell, A. M., de Jesus Mari, J., Maruta, T., Matsumoto, C., Rebello, T. J., Roberts, M. C., Robles, R., Sharan, P., Zhao, M., Jablensky, A., Udomratn, P., Rahimi-Movaghar, A., Rydelius, P. A., Bahrer-Kohler, S., Watts, A. D., & Saxena, S. (2019). Innovations and changes in the ICD-11 classification of mental, behavioural and neurodevelopmental disorders. *World Psychiatry, 18*(1), 3–19. https://doi.org/10.1002/wps.20611

Regier, D. A., Kuhl, E. A., & Kupfer, D. J. (2013). The DSM-5: Classification and criteria changes. *World Psychiatry, 12*(2), 92–98. https://doi.org/10.1002/wps.20050

Rehm, J., & Shield, K. D. (2019). Global burden of alcohol use disorders and alcohol liver disease. *Biomedicine, 7*(4), 99. https://doi.org/10.3390/biomedicines7040099

Roerecke, M., & Rehm, J. (2013). Alcohol use disorders and mortality: A systematic review and meta-analysis. *Addiction, 108*(9), 1562–1578. https://doi.org/10.1111/add.12231

Romero-Daza, N., Weeks, M., & Singer, M. (2003). "Nobody gives a damn if I live or die": Violence, drugs, and street-level prostitution in inner-city Hartford, Connecticut. *Medical Anthropology, 22*(3), 233–259. https://doi.org/10.1080/01459740306770

Sanchis-Segura, C., & Becker, J. B. (2016). Why we should consider sex (and study sex differences) in addiction research. *Addiction Biology, 21*(5), 995–1006. https://www.ncbi.nlm.nih.gov/pmc/articles/PMC5585537/

Saunders, J. B. (2017). Substance use and addictive disorders in DSM-5 and ICD 10 and the draft ICD 11. *Current Opinion in Psychiatry, 30*(4), 227–237. https://doi.org/10.1097/YCO.0000000000000332

Schuckit, M., Pitts, F. N., Reich, T., King, L. J., & Winokur, G. (1969). Alcoholism: I. Two types of alcoholism in women. *Archives of General Psychiatry, 20*(3), 301–306. https://doi.org/10.1001/archpsyc.1969.01740150045007

Schwartz, J. (2008). Gender differences in drunk driving prevalence rates and trends: A 20-year assessment using multiple sources of evidence. *Addictive Behaviors, 33*(9), 1217–1222. https://doi.org/10.1016/j.addbeh.2008.03.014

Segawa, T., Baudry, T., Bourla, A., Blanc, J.-V., Peretti, C.-S., Mouchabac, S., & Ferreri, F. (2020). Virtual reality (VR) in assessment and treatment of addictive disorders: A systematic review. *Frontiers in Neuroscience, 13*, 1409. https://doi.org/10.3389/fnins.2019.01409

Selzer, M. L. (1971). The Michigan Alcoholism Screening Test: The quest for a new diagnostic instrument. *American Journal of Psychiatry, 127*(12), 1653–1658. https://doi.org/10.1176/ajp.127.12.1653

Seventy-Second World Health Assembly. (2019, April 11). *Provisional agenda item 12.7: Eleventh revision of the International Classification of Diseases* (Report, A72/29 Add.1). https://apps.who.int/gb/ebwha/pdf_files/WHA72/A72_29Add1-en.pdf

Shepard, R. D., & Nugent, F. S. (2023). Epigenetics of drug addiction: The new molecular and medical genetics. In T. O. Tollefsbol (Ed.), *Handbook of epigenetics* (3rd ed., pp. 625–637). Elsevier. https://doi.org/10.1016/C2021-0-00437-5

Skeer, M. R., McCormick, M. C., Normand, S.-L. T., Mimiaga, M. J., Buka, S. L., & Gilman, S. E. (2011). Gender differences in the association between family conflict and adolescent substance use disorders. *Journal of Adolescent Health, 49*(2), 187–192. https://doi.org/10.1016/j.jadohealth.2010.12.003

Skinner, H. A. (1982). The drug abuse screening test. *Addictive Behaviors, 7*(4), 363–371. https://doi.org/10.1016/0306-4603(82)90005-3

Sloboda, Z., Glantz, M. D., & Tarter, R. E. (2012). Revisiting the concepts of risk and protective factors for understanding the etiology and development of substance use and substance use disorders: Implications for prevention. *Substance Use and Misuse, 47*(8–9), 944–962.

Socías, M. E., Volkow, N., & Wood, E. (2016). Adopting the 'cascade of care' framework: An opportunity to close the implementation gap in addiction care? *Addiction, 111*(12), 2079–2081. https://doi.org/10.1111/add.13479

Socías, M. E., Wood, E., Kerr, T., Nolan, S., Hayashi, K., Nosova, E., Montaner, J., & Milloy, M.-J. (2018). Trends in engagement in the cascade of care for opioid use disorder, Vancouver, Canada, 2006–2016. *Drug and Alcohol Dependence, 189*, 90–95. https://doi.org/10.1016/j.drugalcdep.2018.04.026

Spinelli, C., & Thyer, B. A. (2017). Is recovery from alcoholism without treatment possible? A review of the literature. *Alcoholism Treatment Quarterly, 35*(4), 426–444. https://doi.org/10.1080/07347324.2017.1355219

Strang, J., Volkow, N. D., Degenhardt, L., Hickman, M., Johnson, K., Koob, G. F., Marshall, B. D. L., Tyndall, M., & Walsh, S. L. (2020). Opioid use disorder. *Nature Reviews Disease Primers, 6*(1), 3. https://doi.org/10.1038/s41572-019-0137-5

Substance Abuse Mental Health Services Administration. (2019). *Key substance use and mental health indicators in the United States: Results from the 2018 National Survey on Drug Use and Health* [Report] (PEP19-5068). https://www.samhsa.gov/data/

The Management of Substance Use Disorders Work Group. (2015). *VA/DoD clinical practice guideline for the management of substance use disorders, version 3.0* (Report). Department of Veterans Affairs, Department of Defense. https://www.healthquality.va.gov/guidelines/mh/sud/vadodsudcpgrevised22216.pdf

The MITRE Corporation. (2020, June 22). *Alcohol and other substance use screening using the National Institute on Drug Use Quick Screen and USAUDIT (Alcohol Use Disorders Identification Test, Adapted for Use in the United States): Implementation Guide, Version 1.0*. Centers for Disease Control and Prevention. https://cds.ahrq.gov/sites/default/files/cds/artifact/1171/NIDA_QS_to_USAUDIT_Alcohol_Screening_IG.pdf

The Sentencing Project. (2020). *Incarcerated women and girls* [Web page]. https://www.sentencingproject.org/publications/incarcerated-women-and-girls/

Thomasson, H. R. (2002). Gender differences in alcohol metabolism. In M. Galanter (Ed.), *Recent developments in alcoholism* (pp. 163–179). Springer.

Tiffany, S. T., Friedman, L., Greenfield, S. F., Hasin, D. S., & Jackson, R. (2012). Beyond drug use: A systematic consideration of other outcomes in evaluations of treatments for substance use disorders. *Addiction, 107*(4), 709–718. https://doi.org/10.1111/j.1360-0443.2011.03581.x

Tuchman, E. (2010). Women and addiction: The importance of gender issues in substance abuse research. *Journal of Addictive Diseases, 29*(2), 127–138. https://doi.org/10.1080/10550881003684582

U. S. Department of Justice. (2020). *2019 Crime in the United States: Table 42: Arrests by Sex, 2019* [Web page]. https://ucr.fbi.gov/crime-in-the-u.s/2019/crime-in-the-u.s.-2019/topic-pages/tables/table-42

U. S. General Accounting Office. (1990, June 28). *Drug-exposed infants: A generation at risk: Report to the Chairman, Committee on Finance, U.S. Senate* [Report] (HRD-90-138). https://www.gao.gov/assets/hrd-90-138.pdf

U. S. Government Accountability Office. (2007, July 11). *African American children in foster care: Additional hhs assistance needed to help states reduce the proportion in care* [Report] (GAO-07-816). Author. https://www.gao.gov/assets/gao-07-816.pdf

United Nations Office on Drugs and Crime. (2018). *International standards on drug use prevention*. https://www.unodc.org/documents/prevention/UNODC-WHO_2018_prevention_standards_E.pdf

United Nations Office on Drugs and Crime. (2020). *World drug report, 2020* (Report). https://wdr.unodc.org/wdr2020/index.html

Valente, T. W. (2010). *Social networks and health: Models, methods, and applications*. Oxford University Press.

Vigna-Taglianti, F., Vadrucci, S., Faggiano, F., Burkhart, G., Siliquini, R., Galanti, M. R., & Group, E.-D. S. (2009). Is universal prevention against youths' substance misuse really universal? Gender-specific effects in the EU-Dap school-based prevention trial. *Journal of Epidemiology and Community Health, 63*(9), 722–728. https://doi.org/10.1136/jech.2008.081513

Vigna-Taglianti, F. D., Galanti, M. R., Burkhart, G., Caria, M. P., Vadrucci, S., & Faggiano, F. (2014). "Unplugged," A European school-based program for substance use prevention among adolescents: Overview of results from the EU-Dap trial. *New Directions for Youth Development, 2014*(141), 67–82. https://doi.org/10.1002/yd.2008

Volkow, N. D., Koob, G. F., & McLellan, A. T. (2016). Neurobiologic advances from the brain disease model of addiction. *New England Journal of Medicine, 374*(4), 363–371. https://doi.org/10.1056/NEJMra1511480

Weinstock, M. (2008). The long-term behavioural consequences of prenatal stress. *Neuroscience & Biobehavioral Reviews, 32*(6), 1073–1086. https://doi.org/10.1016/j.neubiorev.2008.03.002

White, W. L. (1998). *Slaying the dragon: The history of addiction treatment and recovery in America*. Chestnut Health Systems/Lighthouse Institute.

White, W. L. (2007). Addiction recovery: Its definition and conceptual boundaries. *Journal of Substance Abuse Treatment, 33*(3), 229–241. https://doi.org/10.1016/j.jsat.2007.04.015

White, A. M. (2020). Gender differences in the epidemiology of alcohol use and related harms in the United States. *Alcohol Research: Current Reviews, 40*(2), 01. https://doi.org/10.35946/arcr.v40.2.01

White, A. M., Castle, I. J. P., Powell, P. A., Hingson, R. W., & Koob, G. F. (2022). Alcohol-related deaths during the COVID-19 pandemic. *JAMA, 327*(17), 1704–1706.

Wilke, D. (1994). Women and alcoholism: How a male-as-norm bias affects research, assessment, and treatment. *Health and Social Work, 19*(1), 29–35. https://doi.org/10.1093/hsw/19.1.29

Wills, T. A., Vaccaro, D., & McNamara, G. (1994). Novelty seeking, risk taking, and related constructs as predictors of adolescent substance use: An application of Cloninger's theory. *Journal of Substance Abuse, 6*(1), 1–20. https://doi.org/10.1016/s0899-3289(94)90039-6

Winkelman, T. N., Villapiano, N., Kozhimannil, K. B., Davis, M. M., & Patrick, S. W. (2018). Incidence and costs of neonatal abstinence syndrome among infants with Medicaid: 2004–2014. *Pediatrics, 141*(4) https://www.ncbi.nlm.nih.gov/pmc/articles/PMC5869343/pdf/PEDS_20173520.pdf

Wong, C. C., Mill, J., & Fernandes, C. (2011). Drugs and addiction: An introduction to epigenetics. *Addiction, 106*(3), 480–489. https://doi.org/10.1111/j.1360-0443.2010.03321.x

Wood, H. P., & Duffy, E. L. (1966, Sep). Psychological factors in alcoholic women. *American Journal of Psychiatry, 123*(3), 341–345. https://doi.org/10.1176/ajp.123.3.341

World Health Organization. (1993). *The ICD-10 classification of mental and behavioural disorders: Diagnostic criteria for research* (Vol. 2). WHO. https://apps.who.int/iris/bitstream/handle/10665/37108/9241544554.pdf?sequence=1&isAllowed=y

World Health Organization. (1999). *Global status report on alcohol, 1999* (Report). WHO. https://www.who.int/substance_abuse/publications/en/GlobalAlcohol_overview.pdf?ua=1

World Health Organization. (2019). *Global status report on alcohol and health 2018* (Report). WHO. https://www.who.int/publications/i/item/9789241565639

World Health Organization. (2020, September). *International classification of diseases* (11th ed.). [Web page]. WHO. https://icd.who.int/browse11/l-m/en

Yap, M. B., Cheong, T. W., Zaravinos-Tsakos, F., Lubman, D. I., & Jorm, A. F. (2017). Modifiable parenting factors associated with adolescent alcohol misuse: A systematic review and meta-analysis of longitudinal studies. *Addiction, 112*(7), 1142–1162. https://doi.org/10.1111/add.13785

Yonkers, K. A., Gotman, N., Kershaw, T., Forray, A., Howell, H. B., & Rounsaville, B. J. (2010). Screening for prenatal substance use: Development of the Substance Use Risk Profile-Pregnancy scale. *Obstetrics and Gynecology, 116*(4), 827. https://doi.org/10.1097/AOG.0b013e3181ed8290

Young, N. K. (2016, February 23). *Examining the opioid epidemic: Challenges and opportunities. Hearing before the Committee on Finance, United States Senate, 114th Congress, 2nd session* [Testimony, pp. 8–10] (S. HRG. 114–529). U.S. Government Publishing Office. https://www.finance.senate.gov/imo/media/doc/23291.pdf

Part II
Selected At-Risk Populations

Chapter 6
Behavioral Health Disorders and HIV Incidence and Treatment Among Women

Vickie A. Lynn, Fern J. Webb, Crystal Joerg, and Kayla Nembhard

Introduction

Behavioral health disorders play a critical role in the acquisition and transmission of HIV. Behavioral health disorders, defined as mental health and substance use disorders, are common, recurring, and often serious yet treatable conditions (Substance Abuse and Mental Health Services Administration, 2013). These disorders are broadly characterized as unusual shifts in energy, concentration, and/or behaviors (mental disorders) or the inability to control the use of substances (substance use disorders) which limits or impairs functioning in major life activities (Merikangas et al., 2010). While women of all ages, races, ethnicities, sexual orientation, geographical locations, and backgrounds are at risk for acquiring HIV, women diagnosed with behavioral disorders (e.g., mental, substance use) are at higher risk for acquiring HIV and have worse health outcomes compared to women without these disorders (Cook et al., 2018). Insights into the definition, mechanisms, and clinical presentation of behavioral health disorders have increased over the last two decades, resulting in a better understanding of how these disorders play a vital role in influencing women's risk, access to treatment, and health outcomes as they relate to HIV incidence, prevalence, and mortality.

This chapter discusses the general risks associated with behavioral health disorders which undermine women's ability to prevent the acquisition, transmission, and

V. A. Lynn (✉) · C. Joerg · K. Nembhard
University of South Florida, Tampa, FL, USA
e-mail: vlynn@usf.edu; Cjoerg@usf.edu; knembhar@usf.edu

F. J. Webb
University of Florida, Jacksonville, FL, USA
e-mail: Fern.Webb@jax.ufl.edu

A. Hanson, B. L. Levin (eds.), *Women's Behavioral Health*,
https://doi.org/10.1007/978-3-031-58293-6_6

progression of HIV/AIDS (human immunodeficiency virus/acquired immunodeficiency syndrome) and complications concerning access to treatment and care. This chapter also focuses on the most prevalent mental health (i.e., depression, anxiety, schizophrenia) and substance use disorders (i.e., injection drug use) associated with HIV incidence and treatment among women. Sociodemographic characteristics and social determinants of health (SDOH) factors which influence the association between mental health and substance use disorders and HIV incidence and treatment among women are also summarized to provide a fuller context. The chapter concludes with examples of evidence-based and structural interventions that can potentially lessen the negative impact of mental health and substance use disorders on HIV prevention and treatment among women.

Incidence and Prevalence of HIV Among Women

Although the HIV pandemic is far from over from a global perspective, the early notion that HIV is a death sentence has, to some extent, been changed but only for individuals, communities, and countries who have access to viable and affordable prevention and treatment approaches (Teeraananchai et al., 2017). The risk of acquiring HIV is mainly through sexual intercourse, or by sharing infected drug use materials with someone living with HIV (Centers for Disease Control and Prevention [CDC], 2021b, January). In 2019, 38 million people were living with HIV globally (amFAR, 2020). Women accounted for 53% of all people living with HIV (LHIV), an estimated 19.2 million people (amFAR, 2020). In 2018, of the estimated 1.2 million people living in the United States (U.S.) who had HIV, 258,000 (23%) were women (CDC, 2019b, May). In addition, an estimated 36,400 new HIV cases were diagnosed during 2018, of which 18% were women (CDC, 2019b, May).

Disparities by Sociodemographic Characteristics

HIV incidence and mortality rates among the general population of women in the U.S. continue to decrease with relatively stable prevalence rates from 2014 through 2018. However, HIV continues to disproportionately affect women by sociodemographic characteristics (e.g., age, race/ethnicity, transmission mode, gender identity) (CDC, 2019a, April 29). Although incidence and mortality rates are decreasing, prevention remains a public health priority. It is estimated more than 90% of new HIV infections are attributable to people LHIV (Living with HIV) who are unaware of their status or not in care and treatment (Skarbinski et al., 2015).

Age

Young adults aged 20–24 remain at the highest risk of acquiring HIV (Pandey & Galvani, 2019). In 2019, the global incidence of HIV was two times higher among women between the ages of 10 and 24 years old compared to similarly aged men, or to women of other ages (UNAIDS, 2019). However, women aged 20–24 years old also remain at a high risk of acquiring HIV given their global population size of approximately 4%, while accounting for approximately 10% of all new HIV infections (UNAIDS, 2017). The population of women aged 13–24 living in the U.S. has the lowest incidence rate, while women between the ages of 25 and 34 had the highest HIV incidence rate compared to women of other ages (CDC, 2020, May). Women between 25 and 34 years of age also comprised 27% of all newly diagnosed cases, followed by women aged 35–44 (23%), women aged 45–54 (19%), and women aged 55 and older (16%) (CDC, 2020, May). In 2019, the percentage of women who died from HIV was highest among women aged 55+ (51%), followed by women aged 45–54 (28%) (CDC, 2020, May). Moreover, women aged 45–54 had the highest mortality rate at 5.2%, indicating women in this age group were dying faster compared to women dying in other age groups (CDC, 2020, May).

Race/Ethnicity

Data from several national studies indicate HIV disproportionately affects Black women (McCree et al., 2017, 2020; Nwangwu-Ike et al., 2021). In 2019, Black women had the highest HIV incidence, prevalence, and mortality rates compared to women of other races and/or ethnicities. In terms of percentages, Black women constituted 56% of all newly diagnosed HIV cases among women in the U.S., followed by White (22%) and then Hispanic (16%) women (see Table 6.1). Among all women, Black women accounted for 59% of all prevalent cases in 2018, followed by 16% of White women and 18% of Hispanic. Among women, Black women comprised 53% of all 2018 deaths due to HIV and had the highest mortality rate of 12.2. Further, Black women experience HIV 15 times more than White women, five times more than that of Hispanic women, and account for more than half of all new HIV infections among women (CDC, 2019b, May).

Mode of Transmission

The two most prevalent modes of HIV transmission among women are through heterosexual interaction and injection drug use (IDU, CDC, 2019a, April 29). Approximately 84% of all cases of HIV transmission were found to be through heterosexual interaction (see Table 6.1). Further, 16% of women contracted HIV via

Table 6.1 HIV rates by age, race/ethnicity and transmission

	Demographics	Incidence (2019)		Prevalence (2018)		Mortality (2018)	
		Cases	Rate per 100,000	Cases	Rate per 100,000	Cases	Rate per 100,000
Age group	13–24	933	3.7	6749	26.9	29	0.1
	25–34	1870	8.3	27,474	122.2	207	0.9
	35–44	1639	7.9	51,352	248.2	529	2.6
	45–54	1.280	6.2	71,304	338.1	1088	5.2
	55+	1108	2.1	83,122	163.0	1925	3.8
Race/ethnicity	American Indian/ Alaska Native	45	4.1	799	19.0	13	1.3
	Asian	98	1.1	2621	30.8	9	0.1
	Black/African American	3840	21.4	141,755	797.5	2163	12.2
	Hispanic	1142	4.9	43,787	790.8	561	2.4
	Native Hawaiian/ Other Pacific Islander	8	3.3	138	57.7	1	0.4
	White	1502	1.7	39,863	45.6	772	0.9
	Multiple races	193	7.8	11,038	456.1	259	10.7
			(Total %)		(Total %)		(Total %)
Modes of transmission	Heterosexual contact	5712	83.4	183,827	76.6	2460	65.1
	Injection drug user	1091	15.9	48,841	20.4	1258	33.3
	Other	25	<1	7333	3	60	1.6

Reference to specific commercial products, manufacturers, companies, or trademarks does not constitute its endorsement or recommendation by the U.S. Government, Department of Health and Human Services, or Centers for Disease Control and Prevention
CDC NCHHSTP AtlasPlus Diseases, 2019, April 29; Generated table, July 24, 2021
This material is available on the CDC website for no charge

IDU. One-third of all HIV deaths in women were among women who were injection drug users, indicating a disproportionate percentage of deaths among women who contract HIV via IDU (CDC, 2019a, April 29).

Gender Identity

Transgender women are defined as men whose assigned gender at birth was male but who identify (i.e., gender identity) as female. Transgender women are at increased risk for HIV infection compared to women who identify with their assigned gender at birth (Lake & Clark, 2019). In addition, there are differences between transgendered groups. Becasen et al. (2019) found 14% of transgendered women were HIV positive compared to 3.2% of transgendered men. Becasen et al. (2019) also found Black and Hispanic transgender women were particularly vulnerable to HIV infection.

Disparities by Social Determinants of Health (SDOH)

The risk of HIV and access to treatment among women are also affected by social determinants of health (SDOH), defined as "conditions in the social, physical, and economic environments in which people are born, live, learn, work, play, worship, and age" (Secretary's Advisory Committee …, July 26, 2010, para. 7). The increased vulnerability of women and girls to HIV is closely linked to economic and social inequalities, thus warranting further review (CDC, 2018, October). For example, living in poverty decreases one's ability to negotiate safer sex situations with partners, increases stress and the likelihood of being victimized, and limits access to physical and mental health care, factors associated with HIV incidence (Logan et al., 2002; Chop et al., 2017). More recently, findings show the transgender population is particularly vulnerable to HIV infection given their increased likelihood to work as sex workers, experience physical, mental, and sexual abuse; be socially discriminated against and treated unjustly, and be unemployed (Becasen et al., 2019). The intersection of gender and social inequities substantially increases the risk for HIV among women in the U.S.

Economic Stability and Education

Women with a higher socioeconomic status (SES) tend to communicate more often about safer sex and HIV or sexually transmitted disease prevention, putting them at a lower risk of acquiring HIV (Muchomba et al., 2015). Friedman et al. (2018) reported people of higher SES are often more likely to adhere to HIV medication/treatment regimens than individuals of lower SES, resulting in better HIV outcomes. Findings have been mixed regarding the association of education and HIV incidence. Hallfors et al. (2015) found no evidence of higher education associated with HIV prevention. However, a CDC (2018, October) analysis of SDOH among adults diagnosed with HIV infection found women with less than a high school education were more likely to have HIV compared with women with higher education levels.

Food Insecurity

Hunger and food insecurity have been found to increase the risk of HIV. Further, they have been identified as barriers to retention in health care, as well as the use of and adherence to antiretroviral therapy (ART). Chop et al. (2017) found food insecurity was associated with high sexual risk through transactional sex and the inability to negotiate safer sex practices with their partners, thus increasing women's risk for HIV infection. Aibibula et al. (2017) found people who experience food insecurity had 29% lower odds of achieving viral suppression. Although food insecurity is sometimes based on perceptions of gender inequality, it also gives an insight as to how poverty and poor quality of life increase the risk of HIV for women compared to men.

Violence

Violence, manifested through community violence, gender-based violence (GBV), or intimate partner violence (IPV), is independently associated with HIV incidence and mental disorders among women. On a societal level, community violence increases women's risk of contracting HIV by reducing the ability for some women to negotiate safer sex or avoid substance use (Frew et al., 2016). Women involved in the criminal justice system, especially those who were victims of crimes, were found to be at a higher risk of acquiring and transmitting HIV (Sprague et al., 2017).

Internationally, women living with HIV (LHIV) experience higher rates of GBV and/or IPV. Mental disorders among women with HIV coupled with GBV include depression, anxiety, traumatic stress symptoms, and suicidal thoughts (Zunner et al., 2015). It is estimated 50–90% of survivors of GBV develop mood and anxiety disorders (Zunner et al., 2015), which puts them at higher risk for HIV and other mental disorders. The World Health Organization (WHO) estimates 30% of all women experience physical or sexual violence from their intimate partners during their lifetime (Toskin et al., 2020). Although IPV is a global phenomenon occurs across SES, women in poverty-stricken communities are much more likely to experience IPV than women with higher SES (Gibbs et al., 2017). IPV independently predicts poor outcomes as it negatively impacts the biological outcomes as well as care for the HIV-infected individual (Schafer et al., 2012).

Behavioral Health Disorders Among Women

In light of the association between sociodemographic characteristics and SDOH factors with HIV incidence, prevalence, and mortality, women with behavioral health disorders are at significantly higher risks for HIV infection and poor health outcomes (Cook et al., 2004; CDC, 2019b, May). Women who experience poverty and trauma (including sexual abuse, child abuse, IPV, physical and/or mental abuse) often have an increased risk of negative mental, behavioral, and social consequences and are extremely vulnerable to HIV infection, regardless of their socio-cultural, economic, and political statuses (Machtinger et al., 2012). A review of the Women Interagency HIV Study data (Cook et al., 2018) revealed 50% of the participants had documented behavioral health disorders, including mood, anxiety, and substance use disorders. The women also met the criteria for depression and reported high rates of alcohol and substance use based on poverty, trauma, housing instability, caregiving demands, stigma, discrimination, and other health and social needs (Cook et al., 2018).

Mental Disorders and HIV Among Women

Research shows there is a reciprocal effect between HIV and mental health. women LHIV experience higher rates of depression, anxiety, and posttraumatic stress disorders compared with their male counterparts or HIV-unaffected women (Waldron et al., 2021). Mental disorders can be further exacerbated by stress, leaving women more susceptible to acquiring HIV, testing positive for HIV, and having negative health outcomes during HIV care and treatment (Yehia et al., 2014). Although the temporal relationship between mental and substance use disorders and HIV infection is often unclear, research shows women with HIV experience more than 3 times as many mental health conditions post-HIV diagnosis compared to pre-diagnosis (Orza et al., 2015).

Depression

Globally, more than 264 million people live with depression (GBD 2017 Disease and Injury Incidence and Prevalence Collaborators, 2018). HIV and depression are common comorbidities (Rubin & Maki, 2019). Depression is also the leading cause of neurobehavioral health complications in people LHIV next to substance use (Munjal et al., 2017). Among people LHIV, depression has long been recognized as an indicator of negative clinical outcomes, including poor quality of life, reduced medication adherence, worsened progression of the disease, and increased mortality rates (Nanni et al., 2015).

Childhood Trauma/Posttraumatic Stress Disorder

Women who experience childhood trauma, also known as adverse childhood experiences (ACEs), are at an increased risk for trauma as adults (Illangasekare et al., 2013). More specifically, childhood trauma has been associated with increased engagement in high-risk behaviors (Rodriguez et al., 2019). Further, individuals with HIV have higher rates of childhood trauma and poverty than those experienced by the larger population (Golin et al., 2016; LeGrand et al., 2015). Rodriguez et al. (2019) estimated more than 50% of persons living with HIV have experienced childhood trauma compared to 20–33% of uninfected individuals experiencing childhood trauma. Childhood trauma was significantly associated with anxiety and poorer mental health quality of life in persons infected with HIV (Young-Wolff et al., 2019). Thus, understanding the intersectionality of childhood trauma and mental health disorders among women infected with and living with HIV is important (for more about girls, see Chap. 2 in this volume).

Substance Use Disorders and HIV Among Women

Substance use among women (e.g., alcohol, opioids, methamphetamine, and cocaine) is associated with health-risk behaviors which increase the risk of HIV acquisition and transmission (El-Bassel et al., 2014). Women who use substances face increased vulnerability to HIV due to engagement in condomless vaginal or anal sex with partners or as work associated with the exchange of sex acts for drugs or money (Ramsey et al., 2010). Research shows a strong association between mental disorders, substance use, and HIV. In the Women's Interagency HIV Study (Cook et al., 2018), 3 out of 4 women (76%) reported having a mental disorder and/or a substance use disorder. Almost a third (32%) of the women were diagnosed with a mental disorder, 9% were diagnosed with a substance use disorder, and over a third (35%) were diagnosed with both mental and substance use disorders (Cook et al., 2018). In addition, mental health issues have been reported to lead to increased substance use and poor health outcomes (Melaku et al., 2015).

Injection Drug Use (IDU)

Globally, approximately one-third of an estimated 3.5 million women in the world who inject drugs are living with HIV (Azim et al., 2015; Iversen et al., 2015). Similar efforts are reported for IDU among women in the U.S., however, a demographic shift of use is observed. More women are using injectable drugs rather than prescription medications (El-Bassel & Strathdee, 2015a), which is of high relevance to HIV transmission.

The risk of acquiring or transmitting HIV is greater when injection equipment is shared/used with someone who is living with HIV. Needles, syringes, or other injection equipment may have blood in them. Since blood can carry HIV and HIV can survive in a used syringe for up to 42 days, the greater the risk with IDU. The CDC (2021a, April) reports one in every 10 HIV diagnoses is directly related to IDU. Women who inject drugs are more likely to have sex partners who also inject drugs and who may engage in sex work to help fund drug habits (El-Bassel & Strathdee, 2015b) (for more about substance abuse issues for women, see Chap. 5 in this volume).

Effective Treatments to Manage HIV Among Women

Medical advances in HIV treatment are increasing the life expectancies of people LHIV. The benefits of biomedical treatment in improving positive health outcomes and reducing HIV transmission risk among women are well documented, as people LHIV can expect to live a normal lifespan (Persson et al., 2016). Significant progress has been made since the beginning of the AIDS pandemic in the understanding of the disease itself, the factors which affect its transmission, and the efforts to continue its eradication (Kalidasan & Theva Das, 2020; Thomas et al., 2020). What remains clear is the increased incidence and prevalence of HIV, along with behavioral health disorders, may contribute to poor treatment and medication adherence (Waldron et al., 2021). Prioritizing behavioral health screening and treatment along with HIV treatment can have positive outcomes regarding HIV prevention and care also improve access to global mental health care (Remien et al., 2019).

Women diagnosed with HIV today, who are in care and treatment, and who achieve and maintain an undetectable viral load for longer than 6 months, have no risk of sexually transmitting HIV to their sex partners (Katz & Jha, 2019). Science has conclusively proven undetectable viral load = untransmittable HIV (U = U) (Calabrese & Mayer, 2019; Okoli et al., 2021). It is now possible for people living with HIV to have a life where they do not have to compromise on their quality of life (Dutta et al., 2021; Andersson et al., 2020). This has a great psychological impact which provides the necessary motivation to fight the disease.

Biomedical Treatments and Interventions

There has been significant progress in the biomedical treatment and prevention of HIV and to reduce HIV-related mortality. The first drug with potential was azido-thymidine (AZT), which was originally developed for the treatment of cancer (Fischl et al., 1987). Currently, ART makes HIV-1 infection a chronic and manageable disease (Rivera-Rivera et al., 2016). However, AIDS and non-AIDS comorbid conditions, such as mental disorders, persist even with the use of ART. Current ART drugs and those in development focus on different steps in the infection cycle (Saag et al., 2018). Integrase inhibitors, entry inhibitors, capsid inhibitors, maturation inhibitors, monoclonal antibodies, nukes, non-nukes, and many other categories of drugs with specific targets are in different stages of development. The U.S. Food and Drug Administration recently approved the use of Cabenuva (cabotegravir and rilpivirine), which is a monthly injectable treatment option for adults living with HIV (Hodge et al., 2021; Markham, 2020).

Biomedical interventions are key tools used in the prevention of HIV (Toskin et al., 2020). The transmission of HIV can be controlled (to a large extent) by using biomedical prevention strategies, such as pre-exposure prophylaxis (PrEP) and post-exposure prophylaxis (PEP) (Kamaara et al., 2019). The use of PrEP is an important strategy in reducing the transmission of HIV and, with high levels of adherence, has been proven to work (Baeten et al., 2014). The CDC Truvada study, one of the first studies to examine the use of PrEP in women, showed a 49% reduction in HIV incidence among the 557 females in the study (Thigpen et al., 2012). Drugs, such as Islatravir by Merck, are already in phases 2/3 and are considered as low, effective doses for PrEP.

Treatment approaches aim to ensure early biomedical intervention for all people living with HIV. Connecting people to biomedical treatment as soon as a diagnosis is confirmed helps to control the progression of the virus (Horter et al., 2020). Although previous studies have shown the uptake of PrEP for women is limited, few women are aware of PrEP and how it can help prevent the acquisition of HIV (Flash et al., 2017; Smith et al., 2015). Social marketing and public health awareness campaigns are needed to educate women, as well as providers and other public health professionals, on the use and success of PrEP (Flash et al., 2017).

Evidence-Based Informed (EBI) Behavioral Health Treatments

Given the impact of living with an HIV diagnosis and a behavioral health disorder on increased mortality among women, having evidence-based, informed treatments tailored to this population of women is crucial. More recently, psychopharmacological treatments have been used to treat mental illness among women LHIV. For example, mental health counseling and psychopharmacological treatment in combination with HIV treatment have been found to improve mental health functioning, increase CD4 counts (immune system function), and increase medication adherence (Reif et al., 2012). Studies have suggested the best way to address prevention and treatment needs is to combine biomedical and behavioral strategies (Bekker et al., 2012; Martinez et al., 2016). Successful strategies include incorporating psychosocial approaches and activities to improve HIV medication adherence or overall health rather than focusing on improving mental health (van Luenen et al., 2018), or using risk reduction methods to improve sexual health communication among adolescents and young adults experiencing homelessness (Craddock et al., 2020).

Cognitive-Behavioral Interventions (CBI)

At the start, HIV prevention methods used in the behavioral health field among women living with a behavioral health disorder predominantly existed within a clinical context and focused on cognitive-behavioral approaches within a small group setting (Kloos et al., 2005). For almost 20 years, CBI has included interpersonal effectiveness skills, supportive interventions, and mindfulness and relaxation developed to specifically assist women with HIV improve their mental health. Since the early 2000s, studies show the effectiveness of cognitive behavior to reduce stress, a key predictor of mental and substance use disorders (Waldron et al., 2021). The Stress Management and Relaxation Techniques/Expressive Supportive Therapy (SMART/EST, Ironson et al., 2005) was among the first to show how CBIs could improve quality of life, improve cognitive function, and decrease health-related distress among study participants. In addition to teaching tailored stress management techniques and relaxation, support groups also were found to significantly improve HIV medication adherence along with emotion-focused coping (Jones et al., 2007).

Supportive Interventions

Early diagnosis, linkage to care, and retention in care are important strategies for reducing the progression and transmission of HIV. Given the incidence, prevalence, and mortality of HIV among women of color (WOC), coupled with the high incidence and prevalence of mental disorders, interventions specifically designed for WOC are needed. The UNITY, for example, is an effective, supportive intervention developed to reduce HIV-related stigma for Black WLHV (Rao et al., 2018). Participants reported lower illness-related stigma compared to non-participants (Rao et al., 2018). The Sisters Informing Sisters on Topics about AIDS (SISTA) intervention was designed using a womanist perspective grounded in racial and gender pride (DiClemente & Wingood, 1995) as an evidence-based intervention (EBI) for women aged 18–45 who are sexually active. Given its effectiveness in Black women, the SISTA program has been modeled for women who are heterosexual, cis, and trans-Black women and WOC with behavioral health disorders (Perry-Mitchell & Davis-Maye, 2017; Owczarzak et al., 2016). Due to the effectiveness of SISTA and similar interventions, incidence rates of HIV decreased among Black women by at least 20% between 2008 and 2017 (Perry-Mitchell & Davis-Maye, 2017).

HIV Risk Reduction Models

HIV risk reduction models and strategies tend to inform intervention design and dissemination. Risk reduction is taught through individual skills-building around appropriate condom use, sexual assertiveness training, reframing attitudes, and beliefs regarding various risky sexual behaviors, problem-solving, and negotiation (Kloos et al., 2005; Kalichman et al., 2005; Marhefka et al., 2014; & Pandor et al., 2015). The CDC's Effective Interventions website (CDC, 2021c, March 5) maintains a website of scientifically proven treatment and prevention approaches that work to reduce new HIV infections. The CDC works closely with national partners and states to scale up the use of these interventions in local communities.

Psychopharmacological Treatments

Relatively few studies have tested the effectiveness of psychopharmacological treatments to improve mental health outcomes among individuals living with HIV (Waldron et al., 2021), resulting in significant knowledge gaps about effective treatments in this population. Furthermore, even less is known about effective pharmacotherapy to treat mental disorders, specifically among women LHIV. Goodlet (2019) describes gaps that include, but are not limited to, unknown interactions between medications commonly used to treat HIV (e.g., antiretrovirals), medications used to treat mental and substance use disorders (e.g., antidepressants, antipsychotics, mood stabilizers), and the inability to create effective, personalized treatment plans.

Evidence-Based Interventions and Approaches for Population Health

The research to help women LHIV and behavioral health disorders point to several evidence-based interventions (EBI) and approaches targeting the broader population of women. These interventions include the provision of prevention and education on their use of condoms, HIV testing, and treatment, with a focus on trauma-informed care, support groups, and programs designed to reduce stigma, increase engagement in care, and improve health and wellness (Coates et al., 2008; Kennedy et al., 2010; Sales et al., 2016; Horter et al., 2020). Collectively, these EBIs help to prevent HIV disease and behavioral health disorders by educating individuals and communities about ways to reduce risks, increase engagement in care, and improve health and wellness for key populations.

Challenges to Implementation of EBIs

During the past 40 years, a significant amount of progress has been made in the development of evidence-based prevention and treatment interventions focused on mental health, substance abuse, HIV, and women and girls. However, these EBIs are often siloed, with few examples offering a comprehensive approach to mental health, substance use, and HIV prevention and treatment across populations (Collins et al., 2021). In addition, implementing EBIs is also a challenge due to stigma, lack of therapeutic skill sets of professionals, and system-level factors which fail to support the programs proven to work.

Mental Health and HIV Stigma Despite decades of public health and awareness campaigns, the larger population still hold fears and negative attitudes toward mental health and HIV which directly affect an individual's willingness to seek prevention and treatment. For example, stigma associated with mental health and HIV prohibit people from seeking prevention or treatment needs. Research on help-seeking behaviors and mental health-related stigma found *self-stigma* and *help-seeking stigma* had negative effects on help-seeking behaviors. People, who perceive high levels of HIV related stigma, are 2.4 times more likely to delay seeking care (Clement et al., 2015; Gesesew et al., 2017). Likewise, high perception of stigma remains a barrier for individuals seeking HIV prevention and treatment. UNAIDS (2017) highlights stigma and discrimination and how it creates multiple barriers to

HIV prevention, testing, and treatment across the HIV continuum, The report also provides best practices in confronting HIV stigma and discrimination in health care and community settings. Reducing both HIV and mental health stigma plays a key role in strengthening the public health approach to care and treatment for at-risk populations.

Challenges to Implementing Therapeutic Interventions Profound barriers to effective HIV prevention for women with behavioral health disorders include stigma and subjective beliefs, values, and attitudes about sex and sexuality. These beliefs, values, and attitudes can be attributed to socially normed thinking about HIV and sex, ranging from norms constructed by various social groups to larger societal norms. For some cultures, the words and implied actions around *sex* and *sexuality* are offensive. Clinician beliefs and attitudes around sex/sexuality, women LHIV, and behavioral health disorders have been noted as a more subtle barrier that influences HIV prevention efforts within clinical settings (Agenor & Collins, 2013; Collins, 2006). Clinicians may assume individuals with behavioral health disorders are sexually undesirable, have cognitive or intellectual limitations, or be unable to engage in sexual activities responsibly (Collins, 2006). Depending on global, national, regional, or local socio-cultural contexts, clinicians may find it challenging to objectively center the needs of women LHIV as paramount in mental health care. Consequently, clinicians who align with such cultural values may have a difficult time reconciling HIV prevention efforts and mental health care (Collins, 2006).

System-Level Barriers to Implementation We now have a body of evidence which demonstrates people at-risk for and living with HIV benefit from behavioral health interventions (Sherr et al., 2011; van Luenen et al., 2018; Sikkema et al., 2015). However, system-level and structural barriers continue to impede the adoption and implementation of EBIs. As mentioned above, socially normed beliefs, values, and attitudes can pervade therapeutic settings with disastrous consequences. Within systems, providers lack effective therapeutic skillsets and treat patients based on inaccurate knowledge for the treatment of co-occurring HIV and behavioral health disorders (Agenor & Collins, 2013). At the institutional/facility level, there is poor prioritizing of service delivery specific to HIV prevention, as seen in terms of funding, training, and time (Agenor & Collins, 2013; Collins, 2006). Both affect delivery of private and public sector care. Kegeles et al. (2015) found funders would not support implementation of core intervention elements of multilevel HIV prevention interventions even though this impacts the ability of community-based organizations to adopt and adapt EBIs for the populations they serve. Bach-Mortensen et al. (2018) determined *resources limitations* was the most reported barrier to implementing EBIs in public, social, and health services in many high-income countries.

Implications for Women's Behavioral Health

Women LHIV are more likely to experience mental and/or substance use disorders, which further increase the burden of disease on their quality of life. Multi-modal approaches with tailored interventions based on risk factors due to SES and SDOH have been shown to significantly improve outcomes for women LHIV.

Research The existing literature suggests women living with behavioral health disorders are at higher risk of HIV compared to women not living with behavioral health disorders. Further research is needed to explore and understand behavioral health and women's risk of HIV and how intersecting vulnerabilities, such as poverty, gender, sexual identify, and racism, exacerbate risk. Research is needed to understand the implementation of HIV prevention health strategies in mental health services and other community-based settings. Four questions researchers should ask include: (1) what types of HIV prevention interventions are effective; (2) with whom they are effective; (3) what mode of delivery is best; and (4) how effective uptake and implementation in mental health and community settings can be increased.

Practice HIV prevention and behavioral health treatments are complex and multi-faceted, requiring the use of multiple prevention strategies. Given the risk of HIV among women living with behavioral health disorders and the risk of transmitting HIV for women currently diagnosed with HIV, it is essential women receive prevention education and screening for HIV, other sexually transmitted infections (STIs), substance use, and access to syringe service programs to help reduce women's risk. EBIs need to be offered not only in mental health treatment settings but also in integrated care settings, as many women LHIV often are first seen by a medical provider.

Public health educational interventions must include information about the risk of injecting drugs, safer sex strategies, and the use of biomedical prevention practice (i.e., PrEP). Education should also focus on changing attitudes toward the use of prevention methods and increase communication and negotiation skills in safer sex practices. Women living with behavioral health disorders should also be screened for HIV and other STIs on a routine basis regarding sexual behavior, substance use, and other HIV risk reduction strategies.

Since social stigmas associated with risk behaviors and HIV diagnosis prevent groups, especially women, from seeking prevention and treatment services, disease prevention and health promotion practices need to be integrated with chronic disease management practices. Interventions focused on providing comprehensive safer sex education are required to prevent disease as well as to remove the prejudice and social stigma associated with HIV as well as mental and substance abuse disorders. There is growing evidence educational interventions and public health campaigns can overcome many barriers to access, increase safer sex practices, and educate populations on the risks involved (Leung et al., 2020).

Another powerful tool is social media, which is used by a large percentage of the global population (Tanner et al., 2018). Social media interventions play an important role in community and individual health by providing a platform for education, in addition to having the ability to track and identify risk for both HIV and mental disorders as well as improve HIV services (Cao et al., 2017; Tso et al., 2016). However, one of the primary challenges to implementing social media interventions involves ethical issues including privacy and confidentiality and ensuring participant autonomy (Chiu et al., 2015).

Policy Today we have powerful tools to prevent the transmission of and control the progression of HIV and ending the HIV pandemic is within reach. In 2019, a new national initiative was announced to end the HIV epidemic in the U.S. by 2030 (Fauci et al., 2019). The *Ending the HIV Epidemic in the U.S. (EHE)* initiative plans to (1) reduce the number of new HIV infections by at least 90 percent by 2030, and (2) decrease the number of new HIV infections to fewer than 3000 per year (Health Resources & Services Administration, 2021, July). Although the initiative is focused on the geographical areas in the U.S. which comprise 50% of all new HIV diagnoses in the U.S. and not specifically key populations, such as WOC with HIV, the authors of this chapter suggest a broader more focused response is needed to address risk and protective factors for women.

Policy guidelines need to incorporate routine screening for HIV in health care and community settings where women are more likely to receive health and social services. Policies are needed to support the funding, implementation, and evaluation of EBI and practices specifically focused on women LHIV at-risk for and living with a mental health diagnosis.

References

Agenor, M., & Collins, P. Y. (2013). Preventing HIV among U.S. women of color with severe mental illness: Perceptions of mental health care providers working in urban community clinics. *Health Care for Women International, 34*(3–4), 281–302. https://doi.org/10.1080/0739933 2.2012.755983

Aibibula, W., Cox, J., Hamelin, A. M., McLinden, T., Klein, M. B., & Brassard, P. (2017). Association between food insecurity and HIV viral suppression: A systematic review and meta-analysis. *AIDS and Behavior, 21*(3), 754–765. https://doi.org/10.1007/s10461-016-1605-5

amFAR. (2020). *Statistics: Worldwide* [Website]. https://www.amfar.org/About-HIV-and-AIDS/Facts-and-Stats/Statistics%2D%2DWorldwide/

Andersson, G. Z., Reinius, M., Eriksson, L. E., Svedhem, V., Esfahani, F. M., Deuba, K., Rao, D., Lyatuu, G. W., Giovenco, D., & Ekström, A. M. (2020). Stigma reduction interventions in people living with HIV to improve health-related quality of life. *The Lancet HIV, 7*(2), e129–e140. https://doi.org/10.1016/S2352-3018(19)30343-1

Azim, T., Bontell, I., & Strathdee, S. A. (2015). Women, drugs and HIV. *International Journal of Drug Policy., 26*(Suppl 1), S16–S21. https://doi.org/10.1016/j.drugpo.2014.09.003

Bach-Mortensen, A. M., Lange, B. C., & Montgomery, P. (2018). Barriers and facilitators to implementing evidence-based interventions among third sector organisations: A systematic review. *Implementation Science, 13*(1), 1–19. https://doi.org/10.1186/s13012-018-0789-7

Baeten, J. M., Donnell, D., Mugo, N. R., Ndase, P., Thomas, K. K., Campbell, J. D., et al. (2014). Single-agent tenofovir versus combination emtricitabine plus tenofovir for pre-exposure prophylaxis for HIV-1 acquisition: An update of data from a randomised, double-blind, phase 3 trial. *The Lancet Infectious Diseases, 14*(11), 1055–1064. https://doi.org/10.1016/S1473-3099(14)70937-5

Becasen, J. S., Denard, C. L., Mullins, M. M., Higa, D. H., & Sipe, T. A. (2019). Estimating the prevalence of HIV and sexual behaviors among the US transgender population: A systematic review and meta-analysis, 2006–2017. *American Journal of Public Health, 109*(1), e1–e8. https://doi.org/10.2105/AJPH.2018.304727

Bekker, L. G., Beyrer, C., & Quinn, T. C. (2012). Behavioral and biomedical combination strategies for HIV prevention. *Cold Spring Harbor Perspectives in Medicine, 2*(8), a007435. https://doi.org/10.1101/cshperspect.a007435

Calabrese, S. K., & Mayer, K. H. (2019). Providers should discuss U= U with all patients living with HIV. *The Lancet HIV, 6*(4), e211–e213. https://doi.org/10.1016/S2352-3018(19)30030-X

Cao, B., Gupta, S., Wang, J., Hightow-Weidman, L. B., Muessig, K. E., Tang, W., et al. (2017). Social media interventions to promote HIV testing, linkage, adherence, and retention: Systematic review and meta-analysis. *Journal of Medical Internet Research, 19*(11), e394. https://doi.org/10.2196/jmir.7997

Centers for Disease Control and Prevention. (2018). Social determinants of health among adults with diagnosed HIV infection, 2016. *HIV Surveillance Supplemental Report, 23*(6), 1–103. https://www.cdc.gov/hiv/pdf/library/reports/surveillance/cdc-hiv-surveillance-supplemental-report-vol-23-6.pdf

Centers for Disease Control and Prevention. (2019a, April 29). *NCHHSTP AtlasPlus* [Dataset; National Center for HIV/AIDS, Viral Hepatitis, STD, and TB Prevention; Generated table, Diseases, July 24, 2021]. https://www.cdc.gov/nchhstp/atlas/index.htm

Centers for Disease Control and Prevention. (2019b). Diagnoses of HIV infection in the United States and dependent areas, 2018. *HIV Surveillance Report, 31*, 1–119. https://www.cdc.gov/hiv/pdf/library/reports/surveillance/cdc-hiv-surveillance-report-2018-updated-vol-31.pdf

Centers for Disease Control and Prevention. (2020). Estimated HIV incidence and prevalence in the United States, 2014–2018. *HIV Surveillance Supplemental Report, 25*(1), 1–78. https://www.cdc.gov/hiv/pdf/library/reports/surveillance/cdc-hiv-surveillance-supplemental-report-vol-25-1.pdf

Centers for Disease Control and Prevention. (2021a, April). *HIV and injection drug use* [Web page]. https://www.cdc.gov/hiv/risk/idu.html

Centers for Disease Control and Prevention. (2021b). HIV infection, risk, prevention, and testing behaviors among heterosexually active adults at increased risk for HIV infection: National HIV Behavioral Surveillance, 23 U.S. cities, 2019. *HIV Surveillance Special Report, 26*, 1–31. https://www.cdc.gov/hiv/pdf/library/reports/surveillance/cdc-hiv-surveillance-special-report-number-26.pdf

Centers for Disease Control and Prevention. (2021c, March 5). *HIV: Effective interventions* [Website]. Author. https://www.cdc.gov/hiv/effective-interventions/index.html

Chiu, C. J., Menacho, L., Fisher, C., & Young, S. D. (2015). Ethics issues in social media–based HIV prevention in low-and middle-income countries. *Cambridge Quarterly of Healthcare Ethics, 24*(3), 303–310. https://doi.org/10.1017/S0963180114000620

Chop, E., Duggaraju, A., Malley, A., Burke, V., Caldas, S., Yeh, P. T., Narasimhan, M., Amin, A., & Kennedy, C. E. (2017). Food insecurity, sexual risk behavior, and adherence to antiretroviral therapy among women living with HIV: A systematic review. *Health Care for Women International, 38*(9), 927–944. https://doi.org/10.1080/07399332.2017.1337774

Clement, S., Schauman, O., Graham, T., Maggioni, F., Evans-Lacko, S., Bezborodovs, N., Morgan, C., Rüsch, N., Brown, J. S., & Thornicroft, G. (2015). What is the impact of mental health-related stigma on help-seeking? A systematic review of quantitative and qualitative studies. *Psychological Medicine, 45*(1), 11–27. https://doi.org/10.1017/S0033291714000129

Coates, T. J., Richter, L., & Caceres, C. (2008). Behavioural strategies to reduce HIV transmission: How to make them work better. *The Lancet, 372*(9639), 669–684. https://doi.org/10.1016/S0140-6736(08)60886-7

Collins, P. Y. (2006). Challenges to HIV prevention in psychiatric settings: Perceptions of South African mental health care providers. *Social Science & Medicine, 63*(4), 979–990. https://doi.org/10.1016/j.socscimed.2006.03.003

Collins, P. Y., Velloza, J., Concepcion, T., Oseso, L., Chwastiak, L., Kemp, C. G., Simoni, J., & Wagenaar, B. H. (2021). Intervening for HIV prevention and mental health: A review of global literature. *Journal of the International AIDS Society, 24*(S2), e25710. https://doi.org/10.1002/jia2.25710

Cook, J. A., Grey, D., Burke, J., Cohen, M. H., Gurtman, A. C., Richardson, J. L., Wilson, T. E., Young, M. A., & Hessol, N. A. (2004). Depressive symptoms and AIDS-related mortality among a multisite cohort of HIV-positive women. *American Journal of Public Health, 94*(7), 1133–1140. https://doi.org/10.2105/AJPH.94.7.1133

Cook, J. A., Burke-Miller, J. K., Steigman, P. J., Schwartz, R. M., Hessol, N. A., Milam, J., Merenstein, D. J., Anastos, K., Golub, E. T., & Cohen, M. H. (2018). Prevalence, comorbidity, and correlates of psychiatric and substance use disorders and associations with HIV risk behaviors in a multisite cohort of women living with HIV. *AIDS and Behavior, 22*(10), 3141–3154. https://doi.org/10.1007/s10461-018-2051-3

Craddock, J. B., Barman-Adhikari, A., Combs, K. M., Fulginiti, A., & Rice, E. (2020). Individual and social network correlates of sexual health communication among youth experiencing homelessness. *AIDS and Behavior, 24*(1), 222–232. https://doi.org/10.1007/s10461-019-02646-x

DiClemente, R. J., & Wingood, G. M. (1995). A randomized controlled trial of an HIV sexual risk-reduction intervention for young African American women. *JAMA, 274*(16), 1271–1276. https://doi.org/10.1001/jama.1995.03530160023028

Dutta, R. K., Chinnapaiyan, S., Santiago, M. J., Rahman, I., & Unwalla, H. J. (2021). Gene-specific MicroRNA antagonism protects against HIV tat and TGF-β-mediated suppression of CFTR mRNA and function. *Biomedicine & Pharmacotherapy, 142*, 112090. https://doi.org/10.1016/j.biopha.2021.112090

El-Bassel, N., & Strathdee, S. A. (2015a). Bringing female substance users to the center of the global HIV response. *Journal of Acquired Immune Deficiency Syndromes, 69*, S94–S95. https://doi.org/10.1097/QAI.0000000000000625

El-Bassel, N., & Strathdee, S. A. (2015b). Women who use or inject drugs: An action agenda for women-specific, multilevel, and combination HIV prevention and research. *Journal of Acquired Immune Deficiency Syndromes (1999), 69*(Suppl 2), S182–S190. https://doi.org/10.1097/QAI.0000000000000628

El-Bassel, N., Gilbert, L., Goddard-Eckrich, D., Chang, M., Wu, E., Hunt, T., Epperson, M., Shaw, S. A., Rowe, J., Almonte, M., & Witte, S. (2014). Efficacy of a group-based multimedia HIV prevention intervention for drug-involved women under community supervision: Project WORTH. *PLoS One, 9*(11), e111528. https://doi.org/10.1371/journal.pone.0111528

Fauci, A. S., Redfield, R. R., Sigounas, G., Weahkee, M. D., & Giroir, B. P. (2019). Ending the HIV epidemic: A plan for the United States. *JAMA, 321*(9), 844–845. https://doi.org/10.1001/jama.2019.1343

Fischl, M. A., Richman, D. D., Grieco, M. H., Gottlieb, M. S., Volberding, P. A., Laskin, O. L., Leedom, J. M., Groopman, J. E., Mildvan, D., Schooley, R. T., Jackson, G. G., Durack, D. T., King, D., & The AZT Collaborative Working Group. (1987). The efficacy of azidothymidine (AZT) in the treatment of patients with AIDS and AIDS-related complex. *New England Journal of Medicine, 317*(4), 185–191. https://doi.org/10.1001/jama.1987.03390050066020

Flash, C. A., Dale, S. K., & Krakower, D. S. (2017). Pre-exposure prophylaxis for HIV prevention in women: Current perspectives. *International Journal of Women's Health, 9*, 391–401. https://doi.org/10.2147/IJWH.S113675

Frew, P. M., Parker, K., Vo, L., Haley, D., O'Leary, A., Diallo, D. D., Golin, C. E., Kuo, I., Soto-Torres, L., Wang, J., Adimora, A., Randall, L., del Rio, C., Hodder, S., & The HIV Prevention

Trials Network 064 (HTPN) Study Team. (2016). Socioecological factors influencing women's HIV risk in the United States: Qualitative findings from the women's HIV SeroIncidence study (HPTN 064). *BMC Public Health, 16*(1), 803. https://doi.org/10.1186/s12889-016-3364-7

Friedman, E. E., Dean, H. D., & Duffus, W. A. (2018). Incorporation of social determinants of health in the peer-reviewed literature: A systematic review of articles authored by the National Center for HIV/AIDS, Viral Hepatitis, STD, and TB Prevention. *Public Health Reports., 133*(4), 392–412. https://doi.org/10.1177/0033354918774788

GBD 2017 Disease and Injury Incidence and Prevalence Collaborators. (2018). Global, regional, and national incidence, prevalence, and years lived with disability for 354 diseases and injuries for 195 countries and territories, 1990–2017: A systematic analysis for the Global Burden of Disease Study 2017. *The Lancet, 392*(10159), 1789–1858. https://doi.org/10.1016/S0140-6736(18)32279-7

Gesesew, H. A., Tesfay Gebremedhin, A., Demissie, T. D., Kerie, M. W., Sudhakar, M., & Mwanri, L. (2017). Significant association between perceived HIV related stigma and late presentation for HIV/AIDS care in low and middle-income countries: A systematic review and meta-analysis. *PLoS One, 12*(3), e0173928. https://doi.org/10.1371/journal.pone.0173928

Gibbs, A., Jacobson, J., & Kerr Wilson, A. (2017). A global comprehensive review of economic interventions to prevent intimate partner violence and HIV risk behaviours. *Global Health Action, 10*(Sup pl 2), 1290427. https://doi.org/10.1080/16549716.2017.1290427

Golin, C. E., Haley, D. F., Wang, J., Hughes, J. P., Kuo, I., Justman, J., Adimora, A., Soto-Torres, L., O'Leary, A., & Hodder, S. (2016). Post-traumatic stress disorder symptoms and mental health over time among low-income women at increased risk of HIV in the US. *Journal of Health Care for the Poor and Underserved, 27*(2), 891–910. https://doi.org/10.1353/hpu.2016.0093

Goodlet, K. J., Zmarlicka, M. T., & Peckham, A. M. (2019). Drug-drug interactions and clinical considerations with co-administration of antiretrovirals and psychotropic drugs. *CNS Spectrum, 24*(3), 287–312. https://doi.org/10.1017/s109285291800113x

Hallfors, D. D., Cho, H., Rusakaniko, S., Mapfumo, J., Iritani, B., Zhang, L., Luseno, W., & Miller, T. (2015). The impact of school subsidies on HIV-related outcomes among adolescent female orphans. *The Journal of Adolescent Health: Official Publication of the Society for Adolescent Medicine, 56*(1), 79–84. https://doi.org/10.1016/j.jadohealth.2014.09.004

Health Resources & Services Administration. (2021, July). Ending the HIV Epidemic in the U. S. [Website]. https://www.hrsa.gov/ending-hiv-epidemic

Hodge, D., Back, D. J., Gibbons, S., Khoo, S. H., & Marzolini, C. (2021). Pharmacokinetics and drug–drug interactions of long-acting intramuscular cabotegravir and rilpivirine. *Clinical Pharmacokinetics, 60*(7), 1–19. https://doi.org/10.1007/s40262-021-01005-1

Horter, S., Seeley, J., Bernays, S., Kerschberger, B., Lukhele, N., & Wringe, A. (2020). Dissonance of choice: Biomedical and lived perspectives on HIV treatment-taking. *Medical Anthropology, 39*(8), 675-688-14. https://doi.org/10.1080/01459740.2020.1720981

Illangasekare, S., Burke, J., Chander, G., & Gielen, A. (2013). The syndemic effects of intimate partner violence, HIV/AIDS, and substance abuse on depression among low-income urban women. *Journal of Urban Health, 90*(5), 934–947. https://doi.org/10.1007/s11524-013-9797-8

Ironson, G., Weiss, S., Lydston, D., Ishii, M., Jones, D., Asthana, D., Tobin, J., Lechner, S., Laperriere, A., Schneiderman, N., & Antoni, M. (2005). The impact of improved self-efficacy on HIV viral load and distress in culturally diverse women living with AIDS: The SMART/EST Women's Project. *AIDS Care, 17*(2), 222–236. https://doi.org/10.1080/09540120512331326365

Iversen, J., Page, K., Madden, A., & Maher, L. (2015). HIV, HCV, and health-related harms among women who inject drugs: Implications for prevention and treatment. *Journal of Acquired Immune Deficiency Syndromes, 69*(Suppl 2), S176–S181. https://doi.org/10.1097/QAI.0000000000000659

Jones, D. L., McPherson-Baker, S., Lydston, D., Camille, J., Brondolo, E., Tobin, J. N., & Weiss, S. M. (2007). Efficacy of a group medication adherence intervention among HIV positive women: The SMART/EST Women's Project. *AIDS and Behavior, 11*(1), 79–86. https://doi.org/10.1007/s10461-006-9165-8

Kalichman, S., Malow, R., Dévieux, J., Stein, J. A., & Piedman, F. (2005). HIV risk reduction for substance using seriously mentally ill adults: Test of the information-motivation-behavior skills (IMB) model. *Community Mental Health Journal, 41*(3), 277–290. https://doi.org/10.1007/s10597-005-5002-1

Kalidasan, V., & Theva Das, K. (2020). Lessons learned from failures and success stories of HIV breakthroughs: Are we getting closer to an HIV cure? *Frontiers in Microbiology, 11,* 46. https://doi.org/10.3389/fmicb.2020.00046

Kamaara, E., Oketch, D., Chesire, I., Coats, C. S., Thomas, G., Ransome, Y., Willie, T. C., & Nunn, A. (2019). Faith and healthcare providers' perspectives about enhancing HIV biomedical interventions in Western Kenya. *Global Public Health, 14*(12), 1744–1756. https://doi.org/10.1080/17441692.2019.1647263

Katz, I., & Jha, A. K. (2019). HIV in the United States: Getting to zero transmissions by 2030. *Journal of the American Medical Association, 321*(12), 1153–1154. https://doi.org/10.1001/jama.2019.1817

Kegeles, S. M., Rebchook, G., Tebbetts, S., & Arnold, E. (2015). Facilitators and barriers to effective scale-up of an evidence-based multilevel HIV prevention intervention. *Implementation Science, 10*(1), 1–17. https://doi.org/10.1186/s13012-015-0216-2

Kennedy, C. E., Medley, A. M., Sweat, M. D., & O'Reilly, K. R. (2010). Behavioural interventions for HIV positive prevention in developing countries: A systematic review and meta-analysis. *Bulletin of the World Health Organization, 88,* 615–623. https://doi.org/10.2471/BLT.09.068213

Kloos, B., Gross, S. M., Meese, K. J., Meade, C. S., Doughty, J. D., Hawkins, D. D., Zimmerman, S. O., Snow, D. L., & Sikkema, K. J. (2005). Negotiating risk: Knowledge and use of HIV prevention by persons with serious mental illness living in supportive housing. *American Journal of Community Psychology, 36*(3–4), 357–372. https://doi.org/10.1007/s10464-005-8631-1

Lake, J. E., & Clark, J. L. (2019). Optimizing HIV prevention and care for transgender adults. *AIDS, 33*(3), 363–375. https://doi.org/10.1097/QAD.0000000000002095

LeGrand, S., Reif, S., Sullivan, K., Murray, K., Barlow, M. L., & Whetten, K. (2015). A review of recent literature on trauma among individuals living with HIV. *Current HIV/AIDS Reports, 12*(4), 397–405. https://doi.org/10.1007/s11904-015-0288-2

Leung, Y., Oates, J., Papp, V., & Chan, S. P. (2020). Speaking fundamental frequencies of adult speakers of Australian English and effects of sex, age, and geographical location. *Journal of Voice, 36*(3), 434.e1–434.e15. https://doi.org/10.1016/j.jvoice.2020.06.014

Logan, T. K., Cole, J., & Leukefeld, C. (2002). Women, sex, and HIV: Social and contextual factors, meta-analysis of published interventions, and implications for practice and research. *Psychological Bulletin, 128*(6), 851–885. https://doi.org/10.1037/0033-2909.128.6.851

Machtinger, E. L., Wilson, T. C., Haberer, J. E., & Weiss, D. S. (2012). Psychological trauma and PTSD in HIV-positive women: A meta-analysis. *AIDS Behavior, 16*(8), 2091–2100. https://doi.org/10.1007/s10461-011-0127-4

Marhefka, S. L., Buhi, E. R., Baldwin, J., Chen, H., Johnson, A., Lynn, V., & Glueckauf, R. (2014). Effectiveness of healthy relationships video-group – A videoconferencing group intervention for women living with HIV: Preliminary findings from a randomized controlled trial. *Telemedicine and e-Health, 20*(2), 128–134. https://doi.org/10.1089/tmj.2013.0072

Markham, A. (2020). Cabotegravir plus rilpivirine: First approval. *Drugs, 80*(9), 915–922. https://doi.org/10.1007/s40265-020-01326-8

Martinez, O., Wu, E., Levine, E. C., Muñoz-Laboy, M., Fernandez, M. I., Bass, S. B., Moya, E. M., Frasca, T., Chavez-Baray, S., Icard, L. D., Ovejero, H., Carballo-Dieguez, A., & Rhodes, S. D. (2016). Integration of social, cultural, and biomedical strategies into an existing couple-based behavioral HIV/STI prevention intervention: Voices of Latino male couples. *PLoS One, 11*(3), e0152361. https://doi.org/10.1371/journal.pone.0152361

McCree, D. H., Sutton, M., Bradley, E., & Harris, N. (2017). Changes in the disparity of HIV diagnosis rates among Black women – United States, 2010–2014. *Morbidity and Mortality Weekly Report, 66*(4), 104–106. https://doi.org/10.15585/mmwr.mm6604a3

McCree, D. H., Chesson, H., Bradley, E. L., Lima, A., & Fugerson, A. G. (2020). US regional changes in racial/ethnic disparities in HIV diagnoses among women in the United States, 2012 and 2017. *AIDS and Behavior, 24*(4), 1118–1123. https://doi.org/10.1007/s10461-019-02736-w

Melaku, L., Mossie, A., & Negash, A. (2015). Stress among medical students and its association with substance use and academic performance. *Journal of Biomedical Education*, 1–9. https://doi.org/10.1155/2015/149509

Merikangas, K. R., He, J. P., Burstein, M., Swanson, S. A., Avenevoli, S., Cui, L., Benjet, C., Georgiades, K., & Swendsen, J. (2010). Lifetime prevalence of mental disorders in US adolescents: Results from the National Comorbidity Survey Replication–Adolescent Supplement (NCS-A). *Journal of the American Academy of Child & Adolescent Psychiatry, 49*(10), 980–989. https://doi.org/10.1016/j.jaac.2010.05.017

Muchomba, F. M., Chan, C., & El-Bassel, N. (2015). Importance of women's relative socioeconomic status within sexual relationships in communication about safer sex and HIV/STI prevention. *Journal of Urban Health: Bulletin of the New York Academy of Medicine, 92*(3), 559–571. https://doi.org/10.1007/s11524-014-9935-y

Munjal, S., Ferrando, S. J., & Freyberg, Z. (2017). Neuropsychiatric aspects of infectious diseases: An update. *Critical Care Clinics, 33*(3), 681–712. https://doi.org/10.1016/j.ccc.2017.03.007

Nanni, M. G., Caruso, R., Mitchell, A. J., Meggiolaro, E., & Grassi, L. (2015). Depression in HIV infected patients: A review. *Current Psychiatry Reports, 17*(1), 530–541. https://doi.org/10.1007/s11920-014-0530-4

Nwangwu-Ike, N., Jin, C., Gant, Z., Johnson, S., & Balaji, A. B. (2021). An examination of geographic differences in social determinants of health among women with diagnosed HIV in the United States and Puerto Rico, 2017. *The Open AIDS Journal, 15*(1). https://doi.org/10.2174/1874613602115010010

Okoli, C., Van de Velde, N., Richman, B., Allan, B., Castellanos, E., Young, B., Brough, G., Eremin, A., Corbelli, G. M., McBritton, M., Hardy, W. D., & de Los Rios, P. (2021). Undetectable equals untransmittable (U= U): Awareness and associations with health outcomes among people living with HIV in 25 countries. *Sexually Transmitted Infections, 97*(1), 18–26. https://doi.org/10.1136/sextrans-2020-054551

Orza, L., Bewley, S., Logie, C. H., Crone, E. T., Moroz, S., Strachan, S., Vazquez, M., & Welbourn, A. (2015). How does living with HIV impact on women's mental health? Voices from a global survey. *Journal of the International AIDS Society, 18*(5 S). https://doi.org/10.7448/IAS.18.6.20289

Owczarzak, J., Broaddus, M., & Pinkerton, S. (2016). A qualitative analysis of the concepts of fidelity and adaptation in the implementation of an evidence-based HIV prevention intervention. *Health Education Research, 31*(2), 283–294. https://doi.org/10.1093/her/cyw012

Pandey, A., & Galvani, A. P. (2019). The global burden of HIV and prospects for control. *The Lancet HIV, 6*(12), e809–e811. https://doi.org/10.1016/S2352-3018(19)30230-9

Pandor, A., Kaltenthaler, E., Higgins, A., Lorimer, K., Smith, S., Wylie, K., & Wong, R. (2015). Sexual health risk reduction interventions for people with severe mental illness: A systematic review. *BMC Public Health, 15*(1), 1–13. https://doi.org/10.1186/s12889-015-1448-4

Perry-Mitchell, T., & Davis-Maye, D. (2017). Evidence-based African-centered HIV/AIDS prevention interventions: Best practice and opportunities. *Journal of Human Behavior in the Social Environment, 27*(1–2), 110–131. https://doi.org/10.1080/10911359.2016.1266861

Persson, A., Ellard, J., & Newman, C. E. (2016). Bridging the HIV divide: Stigma, stories and serodiscordant sexuality in the biomedical age. *Sexuality & Culture, 20*(2), 197–213. https://doi.org/10.1007/s12119-015-9316-z

Ramsey, S. E., Bell, K. M., & Engler, P. A. (2010). Human immunodeficiency virus risk behavior among female substance abusers. *Journal of Addictive Diseases, 29*(2), 192–199. https://doi.org/10.1080/10550881003684756

Rao, D., Kemp, C. G., Huh, D., Nevin, P. E., Turan, J., Cohn, S. E., Simoni, J. M., Andrasik, M., Molina, Y., Mugavero, M. J., & French, A. L. (2018). Stigma reduction among African American women with HIV: UNITY Health Study. *Journal of Acquired Immune Deficiency Syndrome, 78*(3), 269–275. https://doi.org/10.1097/QAI.0000000000001673

Reif, S. S., Pence, B. W., LeGrand, S., Wilson, E. S., Swartz, M., Ellington, T., & Whetten, K. (2012). In-home mental health treatment for individuals with HIV. *AIDS Patient Care and STDs, 26*(11), 655–661. https://doi.org/10.1089/apc.2012.0242

Remien, R. H., Stirratt, M. J., Nguyen, N., Robbins, R. N., Pala, A. N., & Mellins, C. A. (2019). Mental health and HIV/AIDS: The need for an integrated response. *AIDS, 33*(9), 1411–1420. https://doi.org/10.1097/QAD.0000000000002227

Rivera-Rivera, Y., Vázquez-Santiago, F. J., Albino, E., Sánchez, M. D., & Rivera-Amill, V. (2016). Impact of depression and inflammation on the progression of HIV disease. *Journal of Clinical & Cellular Immunology, 7*(3), 423–438. https://doi.org/10.4172/2155-9899.1000423

Rodriguez, V. J., Butts, S. A., Mandell, L. N., Weiss, S. M., Kumar, M., & Jones, D. L. (2019). The role of social support in the association between childhood trauma and depression among HIV-infected and HIV-uninfected individuals. *International Journal of STD & AIDS, 30*(1), 29–36. https://doi.org/10.1177/0956462418793736

Rubin, L. H., & Maki, P. M. (2019). HIV, depression, and cognitive impairment in the era of effective antiretroviral therapy. *Current HIV/AIDS Reports, 16*(1), 82–95. https://doi.org/10.1007/s11904-019-00421-0

Saag, M. S., Benson, C. A., Gandhi, R. T., Hoy, J. F., Landovitz, R. J., Mugavero, M. J., Sax, P. E., Smith, D. M., Thompson, M. A., Buchbinder, S. P., Del Rio, C., Eron, J. J., Jr., Fätkenheuer, G., Günthard, H. F., Molina, J. M., Jacobsen, D. M., & Volberding, P. A. (2018). Antiretroviral drugs for treatment and prevention of HIV infection in adults: 2018 recommendations of the International Antiviral Society-USA Panel. *JAMA, 320*(4), 379–396. https://doi.org/10.1001/jama.2018.8431

Sales, J. M., Swartzendruber, A., & Phillips, A. L. (2016). Trauma-informed HIV prevention and treatment. *Current HIV/AIDS Reports, 13*(6), 374–382. https://doi.org/10.1007/s11904-016-0337-5

Schafer, K. R., Brant, J., Gupta, S., Thorpe, J., Winstead-Derlega, C., Pinkerton, R., Laughon, K., Ingersol, K., & Dillingham, R. (2012). Intimate partner violence: A predictor of worse HIV outcomes and engagement in care. *AIDS Patient Care and STDs, 26*(6), 356–365. https://doi.org/10.1089/apc.2011.0409

Secretary's Advisory Committee on Health Promotion and Disease Prevention Objectives for 2020. (2010). *Healthy people 2020: An opportunity to address the societal determinants of health in the United States* [Website]. http://www.healthypeople.gov/2010/hp2020/advisory/SocietalDeterminantsHealth.htm

Sherr, L., Clucas, C., Harding, R., Sibley, E., & Catalan, J. (2011). HIV and depression: A systematic review of interventions. *Psychology, Health & Medicine, 16*(5), 493–527. https://doi.org/10.1080/13548506.2011.579990

Sikkema, K. J., Dennis, A. C., Watt, M. H., Choi, K. W., Yemeke, T. T., & Joska, J. A. (2015). Improving mental health among people living with HIV: A review of intervention trials in low-and middle-income countries. *Global Mental Health, 2*, e19. https://doi.org/10.1017/gmh.2015.17

Skarbinski, J., Rosenberg, E., Paz-Bailey, G., Hall, H. I., Rose, C. E., Viall, A. H., Fagin, J. L., Lansky, A., & Mermin, J. H. (2015). Human immunodeficiency virus transmission at each step of the care continuum in the United States. *JAMA Internal Medicine, 175*(4), 588–596. https://doi.org/10.1001/jamainternmed.2014.8180

Smith, D. K., Van Handel, M., Wolitski, R. J., Stryker, J. E., Hall, H. I., Prejean, J., Koenig, L. J., & Valleroy, L. A. (2015). Vital signs: Estimated percentages and numbers of adults with indications for preexposure prophylaxis to prevent HIV acquisition: United States, 2015. *Morbidity and Mortality Weekly Report, 64*(46), 1291–1295. https://www.jstor.org/stable/24856904

Sprague, C., Radhakrishnan, B., Brown, S., Sommers, T., & Pantalone, D. W. (2017). Southern women at risk: Narratives of familial and social HIV risk in justice-involved U.S. women in Alabama. *Violence and Victims, 32*(4), 728–753. https://doi.org/10.1891/0886-6708.VV-D-16-00077

Substance Abuse and Mental Health Services Administration. (2013). *Behavioral health, United States, 2012* (HHS Publication No. (SMA) 13–4797). Substance Abuse and Mental Health Services Administration. https://store.samhsa.gov/sites/default/files/d7/priv/sma13-4797.pdf

Tanner, A. E., Song, E. Y., Mann-Jackson, L., Alonzo, J., Schafer, K., Ware, S., Garcia, M., Hall, E., Bell, J., Van Dadm, C., & Rhodes, S. D. (2018). Preliminary impact of the weCare social media intervention to support health for young men who have sex with men and transgender women with HIV. *AIDS Patient Care and STDs, 32*(11), 450–458. https://doi.org/10.1089/apc.2018.0060

Teeraananchai, S., Kerr, S. J., Amin, J., Ruxrungtham, K., & Law, M. G. (2017). Life expectancy of HIV-positive people after starting combination antiretroviral therapy: A meta-analysis. *HIV Medicine, 18*(4), 256–266. https://doi.org/10.1111/hiv.12421

Thigpen, M. C., Kebaabetswe, P. M., Paxton, L. A., Smith, D. K., Rose, C. E., Segolodi, T. M., Henderson, F. L., Pathak, S. R., Soud, F. A., Chillag, K. L., Mutanhuaurwa, R., Chirwa, L. I., Kasonde, M., Abebe, D., Buliva, E., Gvetadze, R. J., Johnson, S., Sukalac, T., Thomas, V. T., Hart, C., Johnson, J. A., Malotte, C. K., Hendrix, C. W., & Brooks, J. T. (2012). Antiretroviral preexposure prophylaxis for heterosexual HIV transmission in Botswana. *New England Journal of Medicine, 367*(5), 423–434. https://doi.org/10.1056/NEJMoa1110711

Thomas, J., Ruggiero, A., Paxton, W. A., & Pollakis, G. (2020). Measuring the success of HIV-1 cure strategies. *Frontiers in Cellular and Infection Microbiology, 10*, 134. https://doi.org/10.3389/fcimb.2020.00134

Toskin, I., Bakunina, N., Gerbase, A. C., Blondeel, K., Stephenson, R., Baggaley, R., Mirandola, M., Aral, S. O., Laga, M., Holmes, K. K., Winkelmann, C., & Winkelmann, C. (2020). A combination approach of behavioral and biomedical interventions for prevention of sexually transmitted infections. *Bulletin of the World Health Organization, 98*(6), 431–434. https://doi.org/10.2471/BLT.19.238170

Tso, L. S., Tang, W., Li, H., Yan, H. Y., & Tucker, J. D. (2016). Social media interventions to prevent HIV: A review of interventions and methodological considerations. *Current Opinion in Psychology, 9*, 6–10. https://doi.org/10.1016/j.copsyc.2015.09.019

UNAIDS. (2017). *Confronting discrimination: Overcoming HIV-related stigma and discrimination in health-care settings and beyond.* Joint United Nations Program on HIV/AIDS 2017. http://www.unaids.org/sites/default/files/media_asset/confronting-discrimination_en.pdf

UNAIDS. (2019). *Women and HIV: Spotlight on adolescent girls and young women.* UNAIDS. https://www.unaids.org/sites/default/files/media_asset/2019_women-and-hiv_en.pdf

van Luenen, S., Garnefski, N., Spinhoven, P., Spaan, P., Dusseldorp, E., & Kraaij, V. (2018). The benefits of psychosocial interventions for mental health in people living with HIV: A systematic review and meta-analysis. *AIDS and Behavior, 22*(1), 9–42. https://doi.org/10.1007/s10461-017-1757-y

Waldron, E. M., Burnett-Zeigler, I., Wee, V., Ng, Y. W., Koenig, L. J., Pederson, A. B., Tomaszewski, E., & Miller, E. S. (2021). Mental health in women living with HIV: The unique and unmet needs. *Journal of the International Association of Providers of AIDS Care, 20*, 2325958220985665. https://doi.org/10.1177/2325958220985665

Yehia, B. R., Cui, W., Thompson, W. W., Zack, M. M., McKnight-Eily, L., DiNenno, E., Rose, C. E., & Blank, M. B. (2014). HIV testing among adults with mental illness in the United States. *AIDS Patient Care and STDs, 28*(12), 628–634. https://doi.org/10.1089/apc.2014.0196

Young-Wolff, K. C., Sarovar, V., Sterling, S. A., Leibowitz, A., McCaw, B., Hare, C. B., Silverberg, M. J., & Satre, D. D. (2019). Adverse childhood experiences, mental health, substance use, and HIV-related outcomes among persons with HIV. *AIDS Care, 31*(10), 1241–1249. https://doi.org/10.1080/09540121.2019.1587372

Zunner, B., Dworkin, S. L., Neylan, T. C., Bukusi, E. A., Oyaro, P., Cohen, C. R., Abwok, M., & Meffert, S. M. (2015). HIV, violence and women: Unmet mental health care needs. *Journal of Affective Disorders, 174*, 619–626. https://doi.org/10.1016/j.jad.2014.12.017

Chapter 7
Rural Behavioral Health Services

Bruce Lubotsky Levin and Ardis Hanson

Introduction

Globally, over the last 75 years, rural health care has been identified as a major public health problem. Considering that 3.4 billion (~43%) of the world's population live in rural, frontier, or remote areas of the world with unacceptable levels of poverty, rural health is a significant policy and services issue. In addition, rural women not only make up a quarter of the global population but 70% of the global population living in poverty are women. Hence, it is critical that international and national reforms in the design and provision of rural behavioral health care systems address the rising obstacles to accessing equitable and evidence-based health and behavioral health services (Farmer et al., 2010; Morales et al., 2020; Perkins et al., 2019). Nevertheless, significant challenges remain. This chapter addresses these obstacles by examining challenges to care faced by women with behavioral health disorders in rural, remote, and frontier areas, offers frameworks to better understand rural behavioral health, and contextualizes challenges rural women face.

Rural communities are increasingly heterogeneous, with substantial regional differences in ethnic, racial, immigrant, refugee, and native-born composition. Demographically, approximately 80% of the U.S. rural population is Caucasian, followed by Hispanic (9%), Black (8%), Native American (2%), individuals reporting being multiple races (1.8%), and Asian and Pacific Islander (1% and 0.1%

B. L. Levin (✉)
College of Behavioral & Community Sciences, College of Public Health, University of South Florida, Tampa, FL, USA
e-mail: levin@usf.edu

A. Hanson
USF Health Libraries and the College of Public Health, University of South Florida, Tampa, FL, USA
e-mail: hanson@usf.edu

   151
A. Hanson, B. L. Levin (eds.), *Women's Behavioral Health*,
https://doi.org/10.1007/978-3-031-58293-6_7

respectively). However, regional differences, such as long-settled Appalachian communities in the American Southeast, differ radically from Central Western rural communities with large immigrant African populations, such as the Sudanese, Somali, and Ethiopian communities in South Dakota.

There have been very few changes in the larger delivery of behavioral health services in rural, remote, and frontier areas. While we do have the resource of tele-health, states and providers are unwilling to ensure access and utilization of services are affordable and accessible to all persons with a behavioral or co-occurring disorder. Although emergency legislative and regulatory changes were implemented as the COVID-19 pandemic continued, there are cases where services and reimbursement for services have reverted to pre-public health emergency status. Thus, the delivery of behavioral health services is still a pressing and significant issue for billions of people living in rural, frontier, or remote areas. Hence, this chapter will examine issues and challenges for rural behavioral health from a practice and policy perspective.

Obstacles in obtaining rural health care services for any population begin with the lack of accessible services, social and geographic isolation, inhospitable climates, and a scarcity of resources. Rural health care systems often lack human service or support service infrastructures, have shortages of service providers, have services modeled on urban (metropolitan) delivery system models, and have poor communication due to linguistic, cultural, and literacy differences (Levin & Hanson, 2020). These challenges often result in inefficient coordination of care. Compounding these obstacles are historical and current issues specific to behavioral health, including stigma and discrimination (individual, family, and community), poor integration with physical (somatic) health services, non-integrated benefits and payer structures, and reliance on public sector funding. These obstacles are likely to affect the unique behavioral health needs of women living in rural areas.

Poverty, especially multidimensional poverty, also affects the access, delivery, and use of behavioral health. More than just monetary poverty (less than $2.15 per day international poverty line), multidimensional poverty also addresses measures of education and level of infrastructure indicators. Using the measure developed by the United Nations Development Programme and Oxford Poverty and Human Development Initiative (2020), of the 22% of the world's population (1.3 billion) who live in multi-dimensional poverty, approximately 85% live in rural, remote, or frontier areas across 107 developing countries (UNDP/OPHDI, 2020). Rural women and girls are affected disproportionately by multi-dimensional poverty (UNDP/OPHDI, 2020) as well as by repatriation and the reintegration of rural populations forced into resettlement areas or refugee status (Garnier et al., 2018; UNDP & OXPHDI, 2021).

Defining Rural, Remote, and Frontier Areas

According to the United Nations (UN, n.d.), the global rural population is now close to 3.4 billion. Africa and Asia have nearly 90% of the world's rural population. The countries with the largest rural populations are India (893 million) and China (578 million) (UN, n.d.). The United States has a rural population of 60 million, which covers 97% of its land area (Ratcliffe et al., 2016, December). Ten out of 50 states have 40 percent or more of their population living in rural or frontier areas, spread across almost 2500 counties.[1]

However, how the definition of rural, remote, and frontier areas varies by each individual country. In addition, countries often use a variety of mechanisms to define an area as rural, remote, or frontier. These mechanisms may be an administrative decision, a statistical definition (number of people per square mile), employment in a specific sector (agricultural), provision of infrastructure and services, or allocation of fiscal transfers based on locale or population. Since each nation has its own way of identifying these areas, these definitions affect international comparisons of countries.

Definitions matter, as determining types of services (behavioral health) for specific populations (women and girls) in geographical locations (urban, rural, or in between) may be dependent upon perception of priority based on data. Reclassing an area as urban may require significant outlay of public monies for added service delivery needs and new or enhanced infrastructures. Although the Global Monitoring Framework of the 2030 Agenda for Sustainable Development has indicators for urban and rural areas (UN, 2015, October 21), it remains difficult to compare rural areas across nations.

The UN Statistical Commission (2020, March 6) encourages the adoption of the "Degree of Urbanization" as a recommended method for international comparisons. Designed to monitor access to services and infrastructure in areas across population sizes and densities, the method allows for the use of geo-coded microdata and the aggregation of such data. This method can not only lead to better determining the needs of women and girls but also more equitably establishing or re-ranking priorities and goals across local, state, national, and international governments. Adoption of this standard may encourage nations to show progress toward the Sustainable Development Goals and to better address the effects of behavioral health disorders on women and girls across the lifespan.

Prevalence of Rural Behavioral Health Disorders

Globally, it is estimated that 970 million (1 in every 6) individuals have behavioral health disorders (Institute of Health Metrics and Evaluation, 2019). Since rural women make up over a quarter of the total world population (Chandra et al., 2020), behavioral health disorders potentially affect approximately 242 million rural women globally. In the United States, there are similar proportional estimates, with approximately 23% of rural women with diagnosable mental illnesses (American

---

[1](Maine (61%), Vermont (61%), West Virginia (51%), Mississippi (50%), Montana (44%), Arkansas (43%), South Dakota (43%), Kentucky (41%), Alabama (40%), and North Dakota (40%).

College of Obstetricians and Gynecologists, 2014) and upwards to 25% of older rural women having behavioral health disorders (Morales et al., 2020).

Rural adult populations also have higher risk and more severe consequences of health-related behaviors and chronic diseases and are less likely to receive mental health services (Chen et al., 2022; Matthews et al., 2017). Untreated mental and substance use disorders and at-risk behaviors do not resolve themselves and continue throughout the lifespan of girls and women. Further, co-occurring physical and/or mental disorders and the social determinants of health (SDOH) affect persistence of these behaviors and chronic diseases. General health disparities in women living in rural, remote, or frontier areas include self-reports of fair or poor overall health status, including higher incidences of alcohol, tobacco, or substance use; cerebrovascular disease deaths, certain types of cancers, ischemic heart disease, and overall higher rates of mortality (Centers for Disease Control and Prevention, 2022; Garcia et al., 2019; Monnat & Beeler Pickett, 2011; Turecamo et al., 2023; Walker & Brown, 2022). Other instances of disparities include difficulty with basic activities of daily activities, limitation of complex activities, obesity, suicide, and unintentional injury (Dahlhamer et al., 2018; Ivey-Stephenson et al., 2017; Monnat & Beeler Pickett, 2011).

In addition to the cumulative effects of ongoing economic and social challenges, the COVID-19 pandemic exacerbated rural women's behavioral health disorders and resulted in more challenges for the already over-taxed rural behavioral health delivery systems (Coley & Baum, 2022). Data also suggest the mental health sequelae of COVID-19 will likely mirror the sequelae of previous epidemics, such as increased depression and suicide rates over time (Han et al., 2020), two population health issues already problematic in rural, remote, and frontier areas.

For the first time in decades, life expectancy in the United States decreased in 2020 due to COVID-19 (Agency for Healthcare Research and Quality [AHRQ], 2022). As hospitalizations and mortality rates increased and the lockdowns continued, the prevalence rates of anxiety and depression rose significantly (37% and 29%, respectively), more than four times higher than the 2019 prevalence rates (Coley & Baum, 2022). More women and girls reported persistent feelings of sadness or hopelessness. Published studies and surveillance data not only show an increase in both alcohol and illicit drug use (with elevated risks of post-traumatic stress and suicide) (Kaniuka et al., 2021) but also show the inadequacy of treatment and recovery programs (AHRQ, 2022). Deaths related to opioids increased in rural areas. Closure of rural hospitals, already at a downward trend, also affected provision of behavioral health services (AHRQ, 2022). Other countries reported similar trends (Organisation for Economic Co-operation and Development, 2021, May 12). Mental health deteriorated during lockdown in France (Ramiz et al., 2021) and rural communities had poorer mental health outcomes due to depression, anxiety, and posttraumatic stress disorder (Diaz et al., 2021). In addition, individuals with "long COVID" faced higher incidence of mood disorders (Wulf Hanson et al., 2022) (for more on epidemiology of disorders, see Chaps. 3 and 5 in this volume).

Challenges Faced by Women in Rural, Remote, or Frontier Areas

Women living in rural, remote, or frontier areas often face greater public health challenges than in urban or suburban areas. Women are more likely to live in poverty, are less likely to have health insurance (especially insurance to cover behavioral health services), be sicker, and have very limited access to general health care (Cromartie, 2017, November). Many of the challenges mirror issues common with geographical isolation, such as transportation to basic or emergency services and providers, lack of trained health and behavioral health professionals in rural areas, transition from primary care to behavioral health providers, and limited social, educational, eldercare, and childcare resources and supports (Dolja-Gore et al., 2022; Handley et al., 2014; Perkins et al., 2013).

Women in rural areas also face a wide range of health disparities throughout their lifespan. These include higher disease burden, levels of obesity, mortality rates, and shorter life expectancy compared to women living in urban areas (Cosby et al., 2008; Yang et al., 2019). Furthermore, rural communities face a number of social risk factors, such as employment and educational opportunities (National Academies of Sciences & Medicine, 2021). In combination, these challenges are affected by population health crises, outbreaks of HIV transmission, or epidemics/pandemics.

The costs of rural health and behavioral health services affect and are affected by a lack of women-oriented behavioral health care services, the stigma associated with seeking behavioral health care, and behavioral health literacy (knowledge about behavioral health systems and treatment options). Layer in the frames of social determinants of health, intersectionality, and health as a human right to existing rural cultural frames, and the challenges in the provision of culturally appropriate behavioral health services, from prevention to intervention, seem almost insurmountable. Finally, considering the inherent invisibility of rural women and girls nationally and globally, it is essential to continue to address the importance of women's behavioral health incrementally.

Framing Women's Rural Behavioral Health Services

In addition to overarching global frames, such as the SDOH and the sustainable development goals (SDG), there are frames constructed specific to rural settings that address services access, system design, utilization, and outcomes. A place-based understanding addresses an important cultural frame for rural populations and may be key to understanding the contexts of how rural women use behavioral health services.

In Australia, where approximately 30% of the population lives in rural, remote, or frontier areas, Hart et al. (2011) created a "rural adversity" frame. Rural adversity addresses the relationship between adverse environmental events and social and economic capital in rural areas which affect the inception or life courses of mental illnesses. Bourke et al. (2012) use a six-factor model to understand the drivers of rural health outcomes across different rural contexts. The six factors highlight the differences between rural and urban settings: geographic locality, "rural locale," local health responses, broader health systems, social structures, and power relations (levels of government and community members). Lawrence-Bourne et al. (2020) offer another rural frame incorporating elements of both of these frames. Their rural diversity frame takes micro-, meso-, and macro perspectives to address how rural populations can plan effective preparedness, response, and recovery strategies to address rural communities and systemic events.

In the United States, Bushy (1997) created a four-factor model emphasizing availability, accessibility, affordability, and acceptability that is still relevant today for national US rural policy (McEwen et al., 2012). *Availability* examines staffing or service shortages which often limit receiving services. *Accessibility* looks at services coordination, including transportation, to health, behavioral health, and social services providers and facilities across public, private, and hybrid sectors. *Affordability* involves the costs of care, such as direct and indirect costs, and affordable insurance that covers individual needs. *Acceptability* addresses the persistent discrimination, perception, and stigma attached to utilizing behavioral health services (Bushy, 1997; McEwen et al., 2012). Similar to the Lawrence-Bourne and colleagues frame (2020), RAND created a multi-level framework mapping system-level mechanisms and elements that may affect outcomes in rural communities at the individual, household, and organizational levels (Ryan et al., 2019). RAND's model also attempts to anticipate the effects of change and the effects of interventions in the context of successful patient, provider, and system outcomes. See Table 7.1 for a review of rural population frames.

All four of these models attempt to emphasize the uniqueness of rural communities, including geographic context, economics, demographic characteristics, patterns of dispersion, social fabric, distinctness of local and regional space, and lifecycle. These types of frames not only provide models and contexts of care but also address the intersectionality and intersectoral approaches needed to address sex/gender, urban/rural, and health equity elements necessary to ensure the appropriate treatment of women with behavioral health disorders.

Availability

Nationally, non-metropolitan counties have a significantly smaller per capita supply of behavioral health providers than metropolitan counties (Andrilla et al., 2018; Larson et al., 2016, September). Not only is the supply of behavioral health workers not sufficient to meet the demand for mental health and substance use services nationally, but the demand in rural areas is far greater. To effectively serve women with behavioral health disorders in rural areas, we are looking at more than just

Table 7.1 Rural population frames

Country	Date	Title/Focus	Authors
United States	1997	Availability, Accessibility, Affordability, Acceptability	Busby
Australia	2011	Rural Adversity	Hart et al.
Australia	2012	Drivers of Rural Health Outcomes	Bourke et al.
United States	2019	RAND Multi-Level Framework	Ryan et al.
Australia	2020	Rural Diversity	Lawrence-Bourne et al.

psychiatrists. We are looking at behavioral health nurse practitioners; behavioral health physician assistants; clinical, counseling, and school psychologists; marriage and family therapists, mental health counselors; mental health and substance abuse social workers; school counselors; substance abuse and behavioral disorder counselors; and more. Rural populations have limited access to mental health care, whether it is through private or public sector institutional care or community-based care, shortages of behavioral health providers, infrastructure issues, or state and federal public policy.

Since there are few state-supported mental hospitals in the United States, rural hospitals may provide care and access for individuals with behavioral health disorders. However, since 2010, more than 130 rural hospitals have closed their doors. Currently, 25 percent of rural hospitals (354) across 40 states are at elevated risk for closure (Mosley et al., 2020, April). Eighty-one percent of rural hospitals (287 hospitals across 16 states) are considered critical resources to their communities based on their services to vulnerable populations, geographic isolation, economic impact, and their placement on the social vulnerability index (Mosley et al., 2020, April).

Factors affecting the rural hospital crisis include degradation of the payer mix, changing patient care benefit models, declining volume of patient care, health professional shortages, and lack of technology upgrades. The demographics of US rural communities (poverty and declining populations) often result in higher rates of uninsured, Medicaid, and Medicare patients, with more instances of under-compensated and uncompensated care. Budget-strapped rural hospitals also lack the capital to invest in electronic health records (EHRs), telehealth, and advanced imaging and diagnostic platforms and tools. When hospitals close, other health professional practices, such as private physician practices, pharmacies, and other medical services often follow, affecting access for rural residents.

Accessibility

When rural hospitals close, the number of health care providers in counties with rural hospital closures is lower, compared to those counties without closures, and the distance for residents to access general and specialty health care services increases after rural hospital closures (US GAO, 2020). In the United States, rural areas have 17 mental health providers per 10,000 population (Randolph et al., 2023, February) and as hospitals close, other providers and facilities are essential to fill the service gap. Access, however, is more than a provider-to-population ratio. Access is a critical component of an effective health care system, with its focus on the volume of services delivered and recipients' satisfaction with access to services. Access should also examine adequacy of access, for example, use and nonuse, as in services wanted by the recipient but not received. Although access to services is often framed in terms of structural, financial, and personal barriers, which influence service utilization (Institute of Medicine, 1993), access is also an interconnected and evolving process, especially when seen from the perspective of women who live in rural, remote, or frontier areas.

Workforce Shortages Since provider shortages and uneven distribution of providers are major factors in the delivery of rural health care services (Weinhold & Gurtner, 2014), there are significant mental health and addictions workforce shortages, particularly in rural, frontier, and remote areas. With a national median of 61 behavioral health providers per 100,000 residents, (Jain, 2022, September 25), the availability of health and behavioral health professional shortages in rural and frontier areas is very low.

Although 163 million Americans live in Health Professional Shortage Areas (HPSA), the majority of HPSAs are in rural America, with significant overlap across rural and southern counties. Looking at mental health HPSAs across geographic area, population, and facility, there were a total of 6528 HPSA designations in total. Of those 6528 HPSAs, 3936 were rural and 489 were partially rural (Bureau of Health Workforce, 2023). Rural areas also may be designated as Medically Underserved Areas/Populations (MUA/P). In 2023, there were 2166 rural medically underserved areas and 220 partially rural MUA/Ps. However, these shortages will be exacerbated based on workforce projections by the Health Resources and Services Administration (HRSA), which indicate the demand for the behavioral health workforce will continue to outstrip availability (HRSA, 2023).

Crisis Care Rural behavioral health crisis care is addressed by a variety of state strategies. Innovative programs include Alaska's Behavioral Health Aide (BHA) program, Oklahoma's transformation of all its CMHCs to CCBHCs, South Dakota's Virtual Crisis Care program, Utah's crisis stabilization initiatives, and Wyoming's statewide expansion of Mental Health First Aid. Post-crisis care is equally important, as shown by the Tennessee Department of Mental Health and Substance Use Services (2022, May) Project Recovery, which uses a unique mobile integrated primary, mental health, and substance use care program.

Community Mental Health and Certified Community Behavioral Health Clinics Community mental health centers (CMHCs) and community health centers (CHCs) are important safety net facilities for persons who are on Medicaid, dually eligible (Medicaid and Medicare), or under/uninsured. Between 2000 and

2019, access to behavioral health services saw a decrease in the number of CMHCs and an increase in the number of CHCs offering mental health services. The number of CMHCs decreased from 182 centers to 15 centers (a 91.8% decrease) while the number of CHCs increased from 184 to 573 centers (a 211.4% increase) (Borders et al., 2022, June). The increase in the provision of mental health services by CHCs was influenced by CHC's Federally Qualified Health Center (FQHC) designations, federal initiatives to integrate behavioral health services into primary care, and HRSA's Integrated Behavioral Health Services grant program.

However, there has been an uptick in the number of CMHCs with the implementation of the federally funded Certified Community Behavioral Health Clinic (CCBHC) Demonstration Program, funded by Section 223 of the Protecting Access to Medicare Act (PAMA, 2014; Public Law 113-93). All eight demonstration states have CCBHCs in areas designated as either a medically underserved area/population or a mental health professional shortage area. By 2019, 66 CCBHCs were established with 377 unique service locations, which improved access to a broader range of recovery, support, and treatment services across urban, rural, and frontier communities. Supported by SAMHSA, Medicaid (Section 223 Demonstration program), and independent state initiatives, such as Kansas' Rural Emergency Hospital Act, CCBHCs provide essential mental health and services use disorders, such as 24-hour mobile crisis teams, screening, and case management. Further, services are accessible to individuals who need care, regardless of ability to pay or payor. Studies have shown the CCBHC demonstration programs have been successful in reducing behavioral health emergency department visits, with some reductions in hospitalizations (Brown et al., 2023). New models of rural care coordination also are being used, such as the nurse navigator model and the medication addiction treatment (MAT) case management model.

Telebehavioral Health   While telebehavioral health has been touted as an alternative to the transportation needs and the geographical isolation of rural women, there are additional usage challenges (Lambert et al., 2013, December). These challenges include: 1) reimbursement for services, either mirroring patient cost-shifting, low reimbursement, or interstate commerce, credentialing, or licensing concerns; 2) telehealth-specific informed consent requirements; and 3) facility fee payments (Talbot et al., 2020). Identifying measures and developing data elements appropriate to rural telebehavioral health can assist in meeting some of these challenges, thereby providing better access to services (Ward et al., 2020, April).

Affordability

Since rural Americans have poorer overall health, lower incomes, and are more likely to be under- or uninsured, they face more cost barriers to health care especially rising health insurance premiums and deductibles. Even with the inception of the Affordable Care Act (ACA) and Medicaid expansion, uninsured rates in rural areas have been and continue to be higher than in urban areas. In states that did not adopt Medicaid expansion, rural uninsured rates were nearly twice as high (21%) as those in expansion-adopted states (12%) (Turrini et al., 2021, July).

Affordability of insurance plans for rural residents varies across provider networks, premiums, and cost sharing. Cheaper insurance policies, for example, may have service providers who are not likely to be geographically close. Health care plans are extremely variable when comparing discrete elements, such as benefit designs, copayments, deductibles, and costs of provider. Since rural enrollees have higher coinsurance for their mental health care than urban individuals, they also may have insufficient coverage and higher out-of-pocket costs, which often lead to continued utilization of services by enrollees (Chen et al., 2022; Ziller et al., 2010). Provisions and riders, such as preexisting conditions and lifetime limit clauses, further affect eligibility and coverage. Small business plans and individual insurance plans offer far fewer covered services for behavioral health disorders and even fewer trauma-focused or addiction services for women. Rural women also have problems paying medical bills. Because of the cost of care, women often delay or go without medical care, go without prescriptions, or reduce therapeutic dosages significantly to extend their medications (Ziller et al., 2023, March).

Affordability, however, also must address provider concerns. Current reimbursement offered by federal and private insurers to rural providers significantly affects the provision of behavioral health services. Since Medicare and other payers pay less than the actual costs to deliver services in rural areas, rural providers (private practice or clinic) may decide to limit or to not provide services. Patient cost-shifting due to high deductibles and co-payments (demanded by Medicare and commercial carriers) is a major concern for providers. In addition, high numbers of uninsured patients, and "no-show" rates among behavioral health clients are among the reasons providers may choose not to provide reimbursable services (for more about financing of services, see Chap. 11 in this volume).

Acceptability

Behaviors and disorders present differently across cultural contexts and may be interpreted or named differently within a community, a social group, a family, or by an individual. Therefore, addressing acceptability requires attention to how social interactions are conducted between patients and providers. "What is said" may not be as important as "how it is said" (Staton et al., 2019). Hence, it is important to address rural preferences and beliefs as well as the multi-faceted characteristics of rural populations.

Traditional or multi-generational beliefs play a role in individual and societal beliefs. These beliefs may affect the management of mental or substance use disorders. Attitudes, such as stoicism, or reactions, such as distress, may affect access to or the ability of women to seek behavioral health services (Burgess, 2016; Judd et al., 2006; Snell-Rood et al., 2017). Poverty also affects an individual's self-perception of power or social status, creates chronic stress, worsens feelings of distress, and is a major barrier to effective utilization of services by rural women.

Recognizing a woman has a mental health or substance use problem and deciding to seek treatment also may be influenced by perceptions of mental and substance use disorders and the provision of services. External stigma (societal) as well as internalized (individual) stigma often affect treatment outcomes, utilization of services, and provision of mental health services. Studies show that women living in rural areas have higher degrees of stigma compared to women living in urban areas (Ezell et al., 2021; Hailemariam et al., 2019; Mutiso et al., 2018; Nguyen et al., 2020; Rasmussen et al., 2019; Schroeder et al., 2021). These stigmas may affect life events, such as marriage, starting a family, employment, and other daily life activities. Stigma also affects behavioral health care workers (Gwaikolo et al., 2017), which may in turn affect workforce availability (*For more on stigma, see* Chap. 9 *on stereotypes, stigma, and social media*).

Rural Appalachia has some of the highest rates of disability, impaired quality of life, and morbidity in the United States, with extremely limited services and a number of social barriers which restrict treatment (Snell-Rood et al., 2017). A woman may know that depression is a treatable medical condition, but her community stigmatizes it as a mental illness. She may know depression is a normal reaction to the SDOH in her region but rationalizes not to seek treatment by calling it "distress." She then does not seek or utilize care based how she conceptualizes depression and her reaction to the stigma of a mental illness. To make seeking behavioral health care acceptable and legitimate for individuals and communities, it is critical to address the disparities and inequities of care that exist in rural, remote, and frontier areas.

Creating culturally acceptable ways to identify how mental illnesses may be "named" and perceived is central to developing culturally appropriate evidence-based interventions (Snell-Rood et al., 2019). However, culturally acceptable interactions should be less about recycling stereotypes and more about communicative strategies, language patterns, and styles of communication (Staton et al., 2019). Minimizing the perception of power differentials and increasing a woman's confidence she is understood in terms of how she describes her experience of her mental illness should increase help-seeking behaviors and utilization of services.

Finally, the stigma attached to behavioral health disorders and health behaviors, including drug and alcohol use, may be diminishing. For the first time, the latest *Rural Healthy People* survey found behavioral health disorders (mental and substance use disorders) were among the top three health priorities for survey participants (Callaghan et al., 2023). Culturally appropriate community-based rural education programs have proven effective in addressing access to and utilization of services (Okafor et al., 2022).

Rural Healthy People 2030 in its latest survey examined health conditions, health behaviors, populations, settings and systems, and the social determinants of health (Callaghan et al., 2023). Results of the survey provide critical information based on geographic regions and sociodemographic characteristics of the participants. More importantly, it illustrates changes and consistencies in priorities over time.

Consistently identified by women as barriers to care are (1) unaffordable services, (2) costly medications, (3) lack of insurance coverage or benefits, (4) inability to get an appointment with a provider, or (5) not knowing where or how to get help across services delivery systems. Hence, identifying and implementing policy recommendations is critical to improving care and increasing services utilization. A National Rural Health Association (2022) position paper suggested three policy recommendations to improve the behavioral health of rural populations: (1) strengthening the workforce; (2) increasing integration, coordination, and access to care; and (3) increasing the use of telehealth/telebehavioral services. These three policy recommendations should make behavioral health services, regardless of payer or ability, to pay accessible to all individuals.

Accessibility, availability, affordability, and acceptability of care remain significant concerns. Looking at the *Healthy People 2020* outcomes, approximately 24% of trackable targets were met or exceeded in rural areas (Office of the Assistant Secretary for Health, [2021]). However, rural residents identified "Health Care Access and Quality," "Mental Health and Mental Disorders," and "Addiction" as the top three Healthy People priorities (Callaghan et al., 2023). "Mental Health and Mental Disorders" and "Addiction" ranked as first and second in the Health Conditions category, with "Drug and Alcohol Use" ranking first in Health Behaviors category, and "Health Care Access and Quality" ranking first in the Social Determinants of Health category (Callaghan et al., 2023).

Implications for Women's Behavioral Health

In its assessment of the nation's ability to adequately treat behavioral health disorders, the U.S. Health Resources and Services Administration (HRSA, n.d., p. 4) recently noted, *"The baseline assumption that current levels of service are 'sufficient' does not address the evidence of high levels of unmet need for behavioral health services."* This is particularly true when addressing the needs of women with behavioral health disorders who live in rural, remote, or frontier areas. When making rural-urban comparisons due to the wide geographic variation across states, regions, and nations, it is critical to review how data are clustered. Effectively addressing populations, services, disparities, or epidemiology of disorders requires a more exact approach than current practice for data collection and analysis. For example, using averages as a starting point may also result in a skewed understanding of the challenges faced by rural women's behavioral health services provision.

The CCBHC demonstration programs have highlighted continuing challenges to the provision of services to rural populations, such as credentialing and licensure requirements, workforce shortages, inexperience in providing specific services to certain populations (e.g., youth), and billing and claims/encounter data (Office of the Assistant Secretary for Planning and Evaluation et al., 2019, September). However, the CCBHC demonstration programs and other state initiatives have also identified the need to implement innovative programs and policies with fidelity to ensure improvement in behavioral health services delivery and utilization. A major reason for programmatic or policy failure is the failure to implement an intervention or policy as intended. This results in poorer outcomes for women with behavioral health disorders living in rural areas, remote, or frontier areas. Addressing these challenges in a systematic and planful manner should improve services delivery for women living in rural, frontier, and remote areas.

References

Agency for Healthcare Research and Quality. (2022). *National healthcare quality and disparities report* [Report; AHRQ Publication No. 22(23)-0030]. AHRQ. https://www.ahrq.gov/sites/default/files/wysiwyg/research/findings/nhqrdr/2022qdr.pdf

American College of Obstetricians and Gynecologists. (2014). *ACOG Committee Opinion No. 586: Health disparities in rural women* [Report]. ACOG. https://www.acog.org/clinical/clinical-guidance/committee-opinion/articles/2014/02/health-disparities-in-rural-women

Andrilla, C. H. A., Patterson, D. G., Garberson, L. A., Coulthard, C., & Larson, E. H. (2018). Geographic variation in the supply of selected behavioral health providers. *American Journal of Preventive Medicine, 54*(6 Suppl 3), S199–s207. https://doi.org/10.1016/j.amepre.2018.01.004

Borders, T., Williams, T., Youngen, K., & Cecil, J. (2022, June). *Non-metropolitan and metropolitan trends in mental health treatment availability in community health and community mental health centers* [Policy Brief]. Rural & Underserved Health Research Center. https://uknowledge.uky.edu/ruhrc_reports/22/

Bourke, L., Humphreys, J. S., Wakerman, J., & Taylor, J. (2012). Understanding drivers of rural and remote health outcomes: A conceptual framework in action. *Australian Journal of Rural Health, 20*(6), 318–323. https://doi.org/10.1111/j.1440-1584.2012.01312.x

Brown, J. D., Stewart, K. A., Miller, R. L., Dehus, E., Rose, T., DeWitt, K., Chapman, R., Wishon, A., Breslau, J., Dey, J., & Jacobus-Kantor, L. (2023). Impacts of the Certified Community Behavioral Health Clinic Demonstration on emergency department visits and hospitalizations. *Psychiatric Services, 74*(9), 911–920. https://doi.org/10.1176/appi.ps.20220410

Bureau of Health Workforce. (2023). *Health Workforce Shortage Areas* [Dataset; variables Discipline: Mental Health, State/territory: All, Rural Status]. Health Resources and Services Administration, U.S. Department of Health and Human Services. https://data.hrsa.gov/topics/health-workforce/shortage-areas

Burgess, R. A. (2016). Policy, power, stigma and silence: Exploring the complexities of a primary mental health care model in a rural South African setting. *Transcultural Psychiatry, 53*(6), 719–742. https://doi.org/10.1177/1363461516679056

Bushy, A. (1997). Mental health and substance abuse: Challenges in providing services to rural clients. In Center for Substance Abuse Treatment (Ed.), *Bringing excellence to substance abuse services in rural and frontier America* (pp. 45–54). [Report; HHS Publication No. [SMA] 97–3134; TAP Series 20]. U.S. Department of Health and Human Services, Rural Information Center Health Service. http://adaiclearinghouse.net/downloads/TAP-20-Bringing-Excellence-to-Substance-Abuse-Services-in-Rural-and-Frontier-America-110.pdf

Callaghan, T., Kassabian, M., Johnson, N., Shrestha, A., Helduser, J., Horel, S., Bolin, J. N., & Ferdinand, A. O. (2023). Rural Healthy People 2030: New decade, new challenges. *Preventive Medicine Reports, 33*, 102176. https://doi.org/10.1016/j.pmedr.2023.102176

Centers for Disease Control and Prevention. (2022). Quickstats: Age-adjusted rates* of alcohol-induced deaths,(†) by urban-rural status(§) - United States, 2000-2020. *MMWR: Morbidity and Mortality Weekly Report, 71*(44), 1425. https://doi.org/10.15585/mmwr.mm7144a5

Chandra, P. S., Ross, D., & Agarwal, P. P. (2020). Mental health of rural women. In S. K. Chaturvedi (Ed.), *Mental health and illness in the rural world* (pp. 119–150). Springer.

Chen, Z., Roy, K., Khushalani, J. S., & Puddy, R. W. (2022). Trend in rural-urban disparities in access to outpatient mental health services among US adults aged 18-64 with employer-sponsored insurance: 2005–2018. *Journal of Rural Health, 38*(4), 788–794. https://doi.org/10.1111/jrh.12644

Coley, R. L., & Baum, C. F. (2022). Trends in mental health symptoms, service use, and unmet need for services among US adults through the first 8 months of the COVID-19 pandemic. *Translational Behavioral Medicine, 12*(2), 273–283. https://doi.org/10.1093/tbm/ibab133

Cosby, A. G., Neaves, T. T., Cossman, R. E., Cossman, J. S., James, W. L., Feierabend, N., Mirvis, D. M., Jones, C. A., & Farrigan, T. (2008). Preliminary evidence for an emerging nonmetropolitan mortality penalty in the United States. *American Journal of Public Health, 98*(8), 1470–1472. https://doi.org/10.2105/ajph.2007.123778

Cromartie, J. (2017, Nov). *Rural America at a glance, 2017 edition* [Report; Economic Information Bulletin No. EIB-182]. U.S. Census Bureau Economic Research Service. https://www.ers.usda.gov/webdocs/publications/85740/eib-182.pdf?v=43054

Dahlhamer, J., Lucas, J., Zelaya, C., Nahin, R., Mackey, S., DeBar, L., Kerns, R., Von Korff, M., Porter, L., & Helmick, C. (2018). Prevalence of chronic pain and high-impact chronic pain among adults - United States, 2016. *MMWR: Morbidity and Mortality Weekly Report, 67*(36), 1001–1006. https://doi.org/10.15585/mmwr.mm6736a2

Diaz, A., Baweja, R., Bonatakis, J. K., & Baweja, R. (2021). Global health disparities in vulnerable populations of psychiatric patients during the COVID-19 pandemic. *World Journal of Psychiatry, 11*(4), 94–108. https://doi.org/10.5498/wjp.v11.i4.94

Dolja-Gore, X., Loxton, D., D'Este, C., & Byles, J. E. (2022). Transitions in health service use among women with poor mental health: A 7-year follow-up. *Family Medicine and Community Health, 10*(2). https://doi.org/10.1136/fmch-2021-001481

Ezell, J. M., Walters, S., Friedman, S. R., Bolinski, R., Jenkins, W. D., Schneider, J., Link, B., & Pho, M. T. (2021). Stigmatize the use, not the user? Attitudes on opioid use, drug injection, treatment, and overdose prevention in rural communities. *Social Science and Medicine, 268*, 113470. https://doi.org/10.1016/j.socscimed.2020.113470

Farmer, J., Clark, A., & Munoz, S. A. (2010). Is a global rural and remote health research agenda desirable or is context supreme? *Australian Journal of Rural Health, 18*(3), 96–101. https://doi.org/10.1111/j.1440-1584.2010.01140.x

Garcia, M. C., Rossen, L. M., Bastian, B., Faul, M., Dowling, N. F., Thomas, C. C., Schieb, L., Hong, Y., Yoon, P. W., & Iademarco, M. F. (2019). Potentially excess deaths from the five leading causes of death in metropolitan and nonmetropolitan counties - United States, 2010-2017. *MMWR: Surveillance Summaries, 68*(10), 1–11. https://doi.org/10.15585/mmwr.ss6810a1

Garnier, A., Jubilut, L. L., & Bergtora Sandvik, K. (2018). *Refugee resettlement: Power, politics and humanitarian governance. Bergham.* https://doi.org/10.3167/9781785339448

Gwaikolo, W. S., Kohrt, B. A., & Cooper, J. L. (2017). Health system preparedness for integration of mental health services in rural Liberia. *BMC Health Services Research, 17*(1), 508. https://doi.org/10.1186/s12913-017-2447-1

Hailemariam, M., Ghebrehiwet, S., Baul, T., Restivo, J. L., Shibre, T., Henderson, D. C., Girma, E., Fekadu, A., Teferra, S., Hanlon, C., Johnson, J. E., & Borba, C. P. C. (2019). "He can send her to her parents": The interaction between marriageability, gender and serious mental illness in rural Ethiopia. *BMC Psychiatry, 19*(1), 315. https://doi.org/10.1186/s12888-019-2290-5

Han, R. H., Schmidt, M. N., Waits, W. M., Bell, A. K. C., & Miller, T. L. (2020). Planning for mental health needs during COVID-19. *Current Psychiatry Reports, 22*(12), 66. https://doi.org/10.1007/s11920-020-01189-6

Handley, T. E., Kay-Lambkin, F. J., Inder, K. J., Lewin, T. J., Attia, J. R., Fuller, J., Perkins, D., Coleman, C., Weaver, N., & Kelly, B. J. (2014). Self-reported contacts for mental health problems by rural residents: Predicted service needs, facilitators and barriers. *BMC Psychiatry, 14*, 249. https://doi.org/10.1186/s12888-014-0249-0

Hart, C. R., Berry, H. L., & Tonna, A. M. (2011). Improving the mental health of rural New South Wales communities facing drought and other adversities. *Australian Journal of Rural Health, 19*(5), 231–238. https://doi.org/10.1111/j.1440-1584.2011.01225.x

Health Resources and Services Administration. (2023). *Behavioral health workforce projections, 2017–2030* [Fact Sheet]. U. S. Department of Health & Human Services. https://bhw.hrsa.gov/sites/default/files/bureau-health-workforce/data-research/bh-workforce-projections-fact-sheet.pdf

Institute of Health Metrics and Evaluation. (2019). *Global Health Data Exchange (GHDx)* [Online; Mental disorders]. https://vizhub.healthdata.org/gbd-results/

Institute of Medicine. (1993). *Access to health care in America.* The National Academies Press. https://doi.org/10.17226/2009

Ivey-Stephenson, A. Z., Crosby, A. E., Jack, S. P. D., Haileyesus, T., & Kresnow-Sedacca, M. J. (2017). Suicide trends among and within urbanization levels by sex, race/ethnicity, age group, and mechanism of death - United States, 2001-2015. *Morbidity and Mortality Weekly Report. Surveillance Summaries, 66*(18), 1–16. https://doi.org/10.15585/mmwr.ss6618a1

Jain, S. (2022, Sept 25). *Geographic analysis reveals mismatch in supply of and demand for behavioral health providers and primary care physicians* [Report]. Trilliant Health. https://www.trillianthealth.com/hubfs/The%20Compass_09.25.22.pdf?utm_campaign

Judd, F., Jackson, H., Komiti, A., Murray, G., Fraser, C., Grieve, A., & Gomez, R. (2006). Help-seeking by rural residents for mental health problems: The importance of agrarian values. *The Australian and New Zealand Journal of Psychiatry, 40*(9), 769–776. https://doi.org/10.1080/j.1440-1614.2006.01882.x

Kaniuka, A. R., Cramer, R. J., Wilsey, C. N., Langhinrichsen-Rohling, J., Mennicke, A., Patton, A., Zarwell, M., McLean, C. P., Harris, Y. J., Sullivan, S., & Gray, G. (2021). COVID-19 exposure, stress, and mental health outcomes: Results from a needs assessment among low income adults in Central North Carolina. *Frontiers in Psychiatry, 12,* 790468. https://doi.org/10.3389/fpsyt.2021.790468

Lambert, D., Gale, J., Hansen, A. Y., Croll, Z., & Hartley, D. (2013, Dec). *Telemental health in today's rural health system* [Research & Policy Brief; PB-51]. Maine Rural Health Research Center. http://muskie.usm.maine.edu/Publications/MRHRC/Telemental-Health-Rural.pdf

Larson, E. H., Patterson, D. G., Garberson, L. A., & Andrilla, C. H. A. (2016, Sept). *Supply and distribution of the behavioral health workforce in rural America* [Data Brief #160]. http://depts.washington.edu/fammed/rhrc/wp-content/uploads/sites/4/2016/09/RHRC_DB160_Larson.pdf

Lawrence-Bourne, J., Dalton, H., Perkins, D., Farmer, J., Luscombe, G., Oelke, N., & Bagheri, N. (2020). What is rural adversity, how does it affect wellbeing and what are the implications for action? *International Journal of Environmental Research and Public Health, 17*(19). https://doi.org/10.3390/ijerph17197205

Levin, B. L., & Hanson, A. (2020). Rural behavioral health services. In B. L. Levin & A. Hanson (Eds.), *Foundations of behavioral health* (pp. 301–319). Springer Nature). https://doi.org/10.1007/978-3-030-18435-3

Matthews, K. A., Croft, J. B., Liu, Y., Lu, H., Kanny, D., Wheaton, A. G., Cunningham, T. J., Khan, L. K., Caraballo, R. S., Holt, J. B., Eke, P. I., & Giles, W. H. (2017). Health-related behaviors by urban-rural county classification - United States, 2013. *MMWR: Surveillance Summaries, 66*(5), 1–8. https://doi.org/10.15585/mmwr.ss6605a1

McEwen, B. S., Eiland, L., Hunter, R. G., & Miller, M. M. (2012). Stress and anxiety: Structural plasticity and epigenetic regulation as a consequence of stress. *Neuropharmacology, 62*(1), 3–12. https://www.ncbi.nlm.nih.gov/pmc/articles/PMC3196296/pdf/nihms314638.pdf

Monnat, S. M., & Beeler Pickett, C. (2011). Rural/urban differences in self-rated health: Examining the roles of county size and metropolitan adjacency. *Health & Place, 17*(1), 311–319. https://doi.org/10.1016/j.healthplace.2010.11.008

Morales, D. A., Barksdale, C. L., & Beckel-Mitchener, A. C. (2020). A call to action to address rural mental health disparities. *Journal of Clinical & Translational Science, 4*(5), 463–467. https://doi.org/10.1017/cts.2020.42

Mosley, D., DeBehnke, D., Gaskell, S., & Weil, A. (2020, April). *2020 Rural Hospital Sustainability Index: Trends in rural hospital financial viability, community essentiality, and patient outmigration.* [Web page]. Guidehouse. https://guidehouse.com/-/media/www/site/insights/healthcare/2020/guidehouse-navigant-2020-rural-analysis.pdf

Mutiso, V. N., Musyimi, C. W., Tomita, A., Loeffen, L., Burns, J. K., & Ndetei, D. M. (2018). Epidemiological patterns of mental disorders and stigma in a community household survey in urban slum and rural settings in Kenya. *International Journal of Social Psychiatry, 64*(2), 120–129. https://doi.org/10.1177/0020764017748180

National Academies of Sciences, Engineering, & Medicine. (2021). *Population health in rural America in 2020: Proceedings of a workshop* [Report]. The National Academies Press. https://doi.org/10.17226/25989.

National Rural Health Association. (2022, Jan). *Mental health in rural America* [Report]. Author. https://www.ruralhealth.us/NRHA/media/Emerge_NRHA/Advocacy/Government%20affairs/2022/2022-NRHA-Mental-Health-Position-Paper-Final.pdf

Nguyen, T., Tran, T., Green, S., Hsueh, A., Tran, T., Tran, H., & Fisher, J. (2020). Proof of concept of participant informed, psycho-educational, community-based intervention for people with severe mental illness in rural Vietnam. *International Journal of Social Psychiatry, 66*(3), 232–239. https://doi.org/10.1177/0020764019898234

Office of the Assistant Secretary for Health. (2021). *Healthy People 2020: An end of decade snapshot* [Report]. U. S. Department of Health and Human Services. https://health.gov/sites/default/files/2020-12/HP2020EndofDecadeSnapshot.pdf

Office of the Assistant Secretary for Planning and Evaluation, Office of Disability, Aging, & Long-Term Care Policy. (2019, Sept). *Certified community behavioral health clinics demonstration program: Report to Congress, 2018* [Report]. U. S. Department of Health & Human Services. https://aspe.hhs.gov/sites/default/files/migrated_legacy_files//191806/CCBHRptCong.pdf

Okafor, I. P., Oyewale, D. V., Ohazurike, C., & Ogunyemi, A. O. (2022). Role of traditional beliefs in the knowledge and perceptions of mental health and illness amongst rural-dwelling women in western Nigeria. *African Journal of Primary Health Care & Family Medicine, 14*(1), e1–e8. https://doi.org/10.4102/phcfm.v14i1.3547

Organisation for Economic Co-operation and Development. (2021, May 12). *Tackling the mental health impact of the COVID-19 crisis: An integrated, whole-of-society response.* [Web page]. OECD. https://read.oecd-ilibrary.org/view/?ref=1094_1094455-bukuf1f0cm&title=Tackling-the-mental-health-impact-of-the-COVID-19-crisis-An-integrated-whole-of-society-response

Perkins, D., Fuller, J., Kelly, B. J., Lewin, T. J., Fitzgerald, M., Coleman, C., Inder, K. J., Allan, J., Arya, D., Roberts, R., & Buss, R. (2013). Factors associated with reported service use for mental health problems by residents of rural and remote communities: Cross-sectional findings from a baseline survey. *BMC Health Services Research, 13*, 157. https://doi.org/10.1186/1472-6963-13-157

Perkins, D., Farmer, J., Salvador-Carulla, L., Dalton, H., & Luscombe, G. (2019). The Orange Declaration on rural and remote mental health. *Australian Journal of Rural Health, 27*(5), 374–379. https://doi.org/10.1111/ajr.12560

Protecting Access to Medicare Act (PAMA), Pub. L. No. 113–93, § 223. (2014, April 1). https://www.congress.gov/113/plaws/publ93/PLAW-113publ93.pdf

Ramiz, L., Contrand, B., Rojas Castro, M. Y., Dupuy, M., Lu, L., Sztal-Kutas, C., & Lagarde, E. (2021). A longitudinal study of mental health before and during COVID-19 lockdown in the French population. *Globalization and Health, 17*(1), 29. https://doi.org/10.1186/s12992-021-00682-8

Randolph, R. K., Holmes, G. M., Thompson, K., Thomas, S., Perry, J., John, R., Gurzenda, S., Ricks, K., & Andrew Maxwell, A. (2023, Feb). *Rural population health in the United States: A chartbook* [Report]. North Carolina Rural Health Research Program, Sheps Center, University of North Carolina. https://www.shepscenter.unc.edu/download/25553/

Rasmussen, J. D., Kakuhikire, B., Baguma, C., Ashaba, S., Cooper-Vince, C. E., Perkins, J. M., Bangsberg, D. R., & Tsai, A. C. (2019). Portrayals of mental illness, treatment, and relapse and their effects on the stigma of mental illness: Population-based, randomized survey experiment in rural Uganda. *PLoS Medicine, 16*(9), e1002908. https://doi.org/10.1371/journal. pmed.1002908

Ratcliffe, M., Burd, C., Holder, K., & Fields, A. (2016, Dec). *Defining rural at the U.S. Census Bureau* [Report; ACSGEO-1]. U.S. Census Bureau. https://www2.census.gov/geo/pdfs/reference/ua/Defining_Rural.pdf

Ryan, G. W., Ryan, G. W., Catt, D., Catt, D., Davis, L., Davis, L., Irwin, J. L., Irwin, J. L., Sohler Everingham, S. M., & Sohler Everingham, S. M. (2019). *A systemic framework for understanding the dynamics of rural communities in America* [Working Paper]. https://www.rand.org/pubs/working_papers/WR1327.html

Schroeder, S., Tan, C. M., Urlacher, B., & Heitkamp, T. (2021). The role of rural and urban geography and gender in community stigma around mental illness. *Health Education & Behavior, 48*(1), 63–73. https://doi.org/10.1177/1090198120974963

Snell-Rood, C., Hauenstein, E., Leukefeld, C., Feltner, F., Marcum, A., & Schoenberg, N. (2017). Mental health treatment seeking patterns and preferences of Appalachian women with depression. *American Journal of Orthopsychiatry, 87*(3), 233–241. https://doi.org/10.1037/ort0000193

Snell-Rood, C., Jenkins, R., Hudson, K., Frazier, C., Noble, W., & Feltner, F. (2019). Building interventions when distress is under debate: A case study from Appalachia. *Transcultural Psychiatry, 56*(5), 918–946. https://doi.org/10.1177/1363461519833580

Staton, M., Cramer, J., Walker, R., Snell-Rood, C., & Kheibari, A. (2019). The importance of shared language in rural behavioral health interventions: An exploratory linguistic analysis. *Rural Mental Health, 43*(4), 138–149. https://doi.org/10.1037/rmh0000117

Talbot, J. A., Jonk, Y. C., Burgess, A. R., Thayer, D., Ziller, E., Paluso, N., & Coburn, A. F. (2020). Telebehavioral health (TBH) use among rural Medicaid beneficiaries: Relationships with telehealth policies. *Journal of Rural Mental Health, 44*, 217–231. https://doi.org/10.1037/rmh0000160

Tennessee Department of Mental Health and Substance Use Services. (2022, May). *Project Rural Recovery: Delivering mobile integrated care where Tennesseans live, work, and recover: Year 1–2 annual report March 31, 2020 - March 30, 2022* [Report]. TDMHSUS. https://www.tn.gov/content/dam/tn/mentalhealth/documents/Project_Rural_Recovery_Annual_Report_May22.pdf

Turecamo, S. E., Xu, M., Dixon, D., Powell-Wiley, T. M., Mumma, M. T., Joo, J., Gupta, D. K., Lipworth, L., & Roger, V. L. (2023). Association of rurality with risk of heart failure. *JAMA Cardiology, 8*(3), 231–239. https://doi.org/10.1001/jamacardio.2022.5211

Turrini, G., Branham, D., Chen, L., Conmy, A., Chappel, A., De Lew, N., & Sommers, B. D. (2021, July). *Access to affordable care in rural America: Current trends and key challenges* [Report; Research Report No. HP-2021-16]. ASPE Office of Health Policy. https://aspe.hhs.gov/sites/default/files/2021-07/rural-health-rr.pdf

UN Statistical Commission. (2020, March 6). *A recommendation on the method to delineate cities, urban and rural areas for international statistical comparisons* [Report, Degree of Urbanisation]. European Commission, Eurostat and DG for Regional and Urban Policy, ILO, FAO, OECD, UN-Habitat, & World Bank. https://unstats.un.org/unsd/statcom/51st-session/documents/BG-Item3j-Recommendation-E.pdf

United Nations. (2015, Oct 21). *Transforming our world: the 2030 Agenda for Sustainable Development* [Report; A/RES/70/1]. United Nations. https://sdgs.un.org/sites/default/files/publications/21252030%20Agenda%20for%20Sustainable%20Development%20web.pdf

United Nations. (n.d.). *68% of the world population projected to live in urban areas by 2050, says UN*. [Web page]. United Nations, Department of Economic and Social Affairs,. https://www.un.org/en/desa/68-world-population-projected-live-urban-areas-2050-says-un

United Nations Development Programme, & Oxford Poverty and Human Development Initiative. (2020). *Global Multidimensional Poverty Index 2020: Charting pathways out of multidimensional poverty: Achieving the SDGs* [Report]. United Nations Development Programme & Oxford Poverty and Human Development Initiative. https://ophi.org.uk/wp-content/uploads/G-MPI_Report_2020_Charting_Pathways.pdf

United Nations Development Programme, & Oxford Poverty and Human Development Initiative. (2021). *Global Multidimensional Poverty Index 2021: Unmasking disparities by ethnicity, caste and gender* [Report]. UNDP & OPHDI. https://ophi.org.uk/wp-content/uploads/UNDP_OPHI_GMPI_2021_Report_Unmasking.pdf

United States Government Accountability Office. (2020, Dec). *Rural hospital closures: Affected residents had reduced access to health care services* [Report: GAO-21-93]. GAO. https://www.gao.gov/assets/gao-21-93.pdf

Walker, B. H., & Brown, D. C. (2022). Trends in lifespan variation across the spectrum of rural and urban places in the United States, 1990-2017. *SSM Population Health, 19*, 101213. https://doi.org/10.1016/j.ssmph.2022.101213

Ward, M., Fox, K., Merchant, K., Burgess, A., Ullrich, F., Parenteau, L., Talbot, J., Pearson, K., Mackenzie, J., Wiggins, W., & Miller, S. (2020, April). *Measure and data element identification for the HRSA Evidence-Based Tele-Behavioral Health Network Program and the HRSA Substance Abuse Treatment Telehealth Network Grant Program* [Research & Policy Brief]. Rural Telehealth Research Center. https://www.ruralhealthresearch.org/publications/1333

Weinhold, I., & Gurtner, S. (2014). Understanding shortages of sufficient health care in rural areas. *Health Policy, 118*(2), 201–214. https://doi.org/10.1016/j.healthpol.2014.07.018

Wulf Hanson, S., Abbafati, C., Aerts, J. G., Al-Aly, Z., Ashbaugh, C., Ballouz, T., Blyuss, O., Bobkova, P., Bonsel, G., Borzakova, S., Buonsenso, D., Butnaru, D., Carter, A., Chu, H., De Rose, C., Diab, M. M., Ekbom, E., El Tantawi, M., Fomin, V., Frithiof, R., Gamirova, A., Glybochko, P. V., Haagsma, J. A., Haghjooy Javanmard, S., Hamilton, E. B., Harris, G., Heijenbrok-Kal, M. H., Helbok, R., Hellemons, M. E., Hillus, D., Huijts, S. M., Hultström, M., Jassat, W., Kurth, F., Larsson, I. M., Lipcsey, M., Liu, C., Loflin, C. D., Malinovschi, A., Mao, W., Mazankova, L., McCulloch, D., Menges, D., Mohammadifard, N., Munblit, D., Nekliudov, N. A., Ogbuoji, O., Osmanov, I. M., Peñalvo, J. L., Petersen, M. S., Puhan, M. A., Rahman, M., Rass, V., Reinig, N., Ribbers, G. M., Ricchiuto, A., Rubertsson, S., Samitova, E., Sarrafzadegan, N., Shikhaleva, A., Simpson, K. E., Sinatti, D., Soriano, J. B., Spiridonova, E., Steinbeis, F., Svistunov, A. A., Valentini, P., van de Water, B. J., van den Berg-Emons, R., Wallin, E., Witzenrath, M., Wu, Y., Xu, H., Zoller, T., Adolph, C., Albright, J., Amlag, J. O., Aravkin, A. Y., Bang-Jensen, B. L., Bisignano, C., Castellano, R., Castro, E., Chakrabarti, S., Collins, J. K., Dai, X., Daoud, F., Dapper, C., Deen, A., Duncan, B. B., Erickson, M., Ewald, S. B., Ferrari, A. J., Flaxman, A. D., Fullman, N., Gamkrelidze, A., Giles, J. R., Guo, G., Hay, S. I., He, J., Helak, M., Hulland, E. N., Kereselidze, M., Krohn, K. J., Lazzar-Atwood, A., Lindstrom, A., Lozano, R., Malta, D. C., Månsson, J., Mantilla Herrera, A. M., Mokdad, A. H., Monasta, L., Nomura, S., Pasovic, M., Pigott, D. M., Reiner, R. C., Jr., Reinke, G., Ribeiro, A. L. P., Santomauro, D. F., Sholokhov, A., Spurlock, E. E., Walcott, R., Walker, A., Wiysonge, C. S., Zheng, P., Bettger, J. P., Murray, C. J. L., & Vos, T. (2022). Estimated global proportions of individuals with persistent fatigue, cognitive, and respiratory symptom clusters following symptomatic COVID-19 in 2020 and 2021. *JAMA, 328*(16), 1604–1615. https://doi.org/10.1001/jama.2022.18931

Yang, J. C., Roman-Urrestarazu, A., McKee, M., & Brayne, C. (2019). Demographic, socioeconomic, and health correlates of unmet need for mental health treatment in the United States, 2002-16: Evidence from the National Surveys on drug use and health. *International Journal for Equity in Health, 18*(1), 122. https://doi.org/10.1186/s12939-019-1026-y

Ziller, E. C., Anderson, N. J., & Coburn, A. F. (2010). Access to rural mental health services: Service use and out-of-pocket costs. *Journal of Rural Health, 26*(3), 214–224. https://doi.org/10.1111/j.1748-0361.2010.00291.x

Ziller, E., Milkowski, C., & Burgess, A. (2023, March). *Rural working-age adults report more cost barriers to health care* [Policy Brief; PB-80]. Maine Rural Health Research Center. https://digitalcommons.usm.maine.edu/insurance/90/

Chapter 8
Stereotypes, Stigma, and Social/Mass Media in Women's Behavioral Health

Bruce Lubotsky Levin and Ardis Hanson

Introduction

Persons with behavioral health disorders face two major challenges. First, they struggle with symptoms of behavioral health disorder, burden of disease, and impaired functioning that result from serious mental illnesses, substance use disorders, and complex comorbid disorders. Second, they must face and deal with the stereotypes and prejudice that result from individual and societal misconceptions about behavioral health disorders. Therefore, people with behavioral health disorder are denied opportunities for a good quality of life. This can include employment, housing, health care, and community integration. Although there has been extensive research to understand the effects of these disorders, research is just beginning to explain the roots of stigma in behavioral health disorder, especially for mental illness.

The vision of the World Health Organization (WHO) is that every individual should be able "to participate fully in society free from stigma and discrimination" (WHO, 2022, June 16, p. 248). This is reiterated by the Special Rapporteur of the United Nations who argues that human rights cannot be successfully addressed unless stigma is acknowledged as the root of discrimination. This discrimination often leads to human rights violations and the exclusion of entire groups nationally, regionally, and globally (de Albuquerque, 2012, July 2).

B. L. Levin
College of Behavioral & Community Sciences, College of Public Health, University of South Florida, Tampa, FL, USA
e-mail: levin@usf.edu

A. Hanson (✉)
USF Health Libraries and the College of Public Health, University of South Florida, Tampa, FL, USA
e-mail: hanson@usf.edu

The challenges facing people with behavioral health disorders are exacerbated by the societal consequences and beliefs surrounding mental illnesses and substance use disorders. Stigma, prejudice, discrimination, and trivialization of persons with behavioral health disorders continue in traditional media and on social media. Stigma and stereotypes are difficult to mitigate as they are socially constructed by individuals and communities at all levels. However, all media, particularly social and mass media, can be powerful tools to reduce these misperceptions and reactions using health education and health promotion initiatives to users of social/mass media.

This chapter will examine how the social construction of stigmas and stereotypes associated with behavioral health disorders affect and are affected by the physical and virtual societies in which they exist. The term "stigma" is used throughout this chapter to represent societal, group, and individual attitudes, beliefs, behaviors, and structures that comprise or influence the persistent discrimination and prejudice faced by individuals with behavioral health disorders. In this chapter, behavioral health disorders may be used interchangeably with mental illnesses or substance use disorders.

Understanding the Relationship Between Stigma and Behavioral Health

The social construction of stigma and stereotypes examines how these beliefs are created and perpetuated into individual, group, and societal behaviors. In addition, the implications of stigma generate significant direct and indirect costs on individuals, families, and communities. The psychological and physical burdens placed on persons who are singled out by society or laws are significant and extensive. Also, stigma is constantly changing targets. For example, the stigma surrounding epilepsy is over 4000 years old. The stigma surrounding mental illnesses has a history that is also millennial years old, while the stigma surrounding HIV/AIDS is approximately 40 years old. Public and private shaming and shunning, little or no protections under the law, and being seen as less than human are the legacies of stigma and stereotyping.

Conceptualizing Stigma

Stigma is the "most formidable obstacle" when returning to a productive and fulfilling life for persons with mental illnesses (U.S. Office of the Surgeon General, Office of Disability, 2005, p. 3). Every individual deserves "a life in the community, with meaningful employment, interpersonal relationships, and community participation" (President's New Freedom Commission on Mental Health, 2003, p. 1). However, stigma can be "invoked as a persistent and pernicious problem" (Mahajan et al., 2008).

The variability in manifestations of stigma across settings, across and within cultural and societal groups, and by types has led to difficulty in measuring the extent of stigma. For example, internal stigma (felt or self-stigmatization) refers to the expectation of discrimination or the shame that individuals feel about their illnesses; it stops them from seeking help or openly discussing their experiences of living and coping with their illnesses. External stigma (enacted or discrimination) refers to the unfair treatment which persons with behavioral health disorders experience in society or within families.

The most prevalent conceptualization of stigma in the United States is from the literature on serious mental illness. Goffman (1963, p. 3) defined stigma as "an attribute that is deeply discrediting" that reduces the individual "from a whole and usual person to a tainted, discounted one". He suggests society stigmatizes individuals based on a category or attribute that is seen as a "difference" or "deviance". That difference creates a notion of a "spoiled identity", that is, an identity gone wrong; hence, persons who are stigmatized are constantly striving to adjust their social identities to manage others' impressions of themselves (Goffman, 1961, 1963).

Stigmas of character traits encompass "blemishes of individual character" or perceived blemishes inferred from having mental illnesses or substance use disorders. Stigmas of character traits can easily translate into stigmas based on group identity. Two underlying social functions attributed to stigmatization include social control and theories of deviance. However, it is important to establish that stigma exists in the relationship between an attribute, such as mental illness, and an audience, such as an individual or a group (Goffman, 1963). Further, enacted stigma is discrimination, that is, opportunities are withheld from individuals who are considered by others to be different or individuals who are penalized or discriminated against in some societal or legislative way.

Building on Goffman's work, the WHO (2001, p. 16) defines stigma as "a mark of shame, disgrace or disapproval which results in an individual being rejected, discriminated against, and excluded from participating in a number of different areas of society". Parker and Aggleton (2003) suggest the classic view of stigma as a "significantly discrediting" attribute has evolved into the reproduction of social difference, not always viewed positively in society. Further, recognition of this "social difference" may lead to social and psychological issues for individuals perceived as "different", such as isolation, loss of self-esteem, or being afraid of strangers.

Social Distance, Identity, and Labelling

Since the social categorization of individuals is inevitable and ubiquitous, persons who are "different" are socially excluded. This is particularly true when they are perceived as a physical or moral threat (Lupton, 2003; Turner, 1987). Social distance, a core component of stigma, is the desire to avoid contact with a specific group of individuals. Stigmatized individuals are kept at a social distance, whether of their own choosing or through the eyes of others (Hogg & Abrams, 1988; Oakes et al., 1994). In their review of 50 years of the literature, Jorm and Oh (2009) found labelling a person as having a mental illness can increase social distance. However, the effect of the label varies depending how it is used (e.g., "person first" language versus "mentally ill") and how familiar the person who is doing the labelling is with mental disorders (media, provider, or general public). The general public, for example, is more likely to seek social distance if an individual has sought professional help. Conversely, family members and professionals may seek more social distance if the individual has not sought help.

Identity is considered an emergent and indexical concept (Hanson, 2014). Identity is emergent as it is seldom static as identity is (re)conceived as a person moves through their lifespan. Identity is indexical because a person may (re)categorize him- or herself numerous times over their lifetime for many reasons and, for many, because of chronic illnesses (Hanson, 2014). How individuals account for their identity and the language they use to describe their circumstances provide insights into how they conceptualize and engage in relationships, activities, and social groups. These situated "accountings-for" (Baker, 2004) also offer a way to better understand how persons categorize themselves and are categorized by others.

Labelling theory suggests the label itself activates stereotypes perpetuated in families, society, and the media. Early studies debated whether stigma arises from non-normative behaviors associated with mental illness or that prejudice is triggered from sociocultural perceptions attached to the label of mental illness (Baldwin et al., 1975; Bean, 1979; Caetano, 1974; Corrigan & Penn, 1999; Eisenberg, 1977; Gove, 1970, 1979, 1982; Grunebaum & Chasin, 1978; Murphy, 1977; Roman, 1971; Rotenberg, 1974; Scheff, 1966, 1974; Trice & Roman, 1968). In a study of deinstitutionalization in California, the use of labelling in California mental health policy contributed to a more negative assessment of persons with mental illnesses (Benson, 1980). This is particularly true in the areas of rehabilitation and reintegration, as well as in issues surrounding quality and continuity of care. The demedicalization of homosexuality and reframing it as a "suboptimal condition" may have created image issues for LGBTQA+ women in the health sciences literature, which may have subsequently contributed to lack of or poor utilization of behavioral health services due to provider bias (Schwanberg, 1985).

Labelling affects multiple domains of people's lives. Stigmatization has significant effects in numerous areas: criminal involvement, health, housing, income, and quality of life (Link & Phelan, 2001; Stickney et al., 2012). The literature also suggests biogenetic causal theories and diagnostic labelling affect perceptions of dangerousness and unpredictability, and as people's fear grow, so does their need for social distance (Read et al., 2006). Loss of an individual's previous identity as a "whole" or "normal" person and current labels regarding one's disease or disability status are hindrances in how individuals perceive themselves vis-à-vis their personal, social, and work identities.

There is also a cumulative effect of labelling and stigma. Stigmatizing an illness is the first step in creating both a continuum of illnesses and a layering of stigma

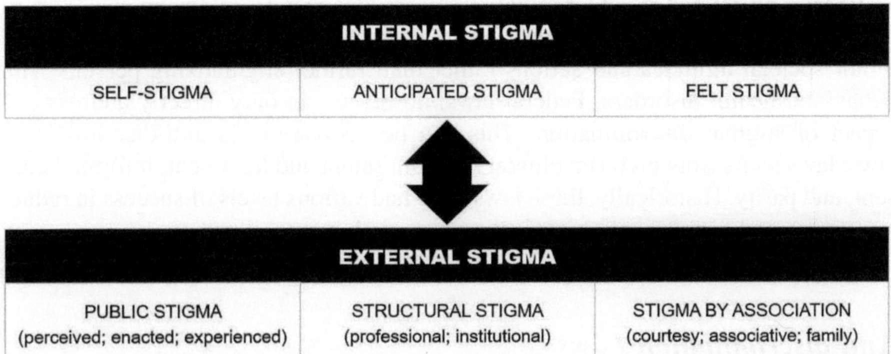

Fig. 8.1 Types of stigmas

(self, public, stigma by association) that further stigmatizes individuals with that illness. Three factors have been identified as major contributors to self-stigma: (1) little or no sense of identification with persons with mental illnesses, (2) the perceived legitimacy of that discrimination, and (3) an elevated level of perceived discrimination (Corrigan & Watson, 2002; Rüsch et al., 2006). Although there are many sub-categories of stigma, as shown in Fig. 8.1, stigma starts from internal (self-stigma) or external stigma (enacted stigma), and stigma is then enacted across institutions and society. Stigma, however it is named, results in persons with mental illnesses not seeking treatment. And, for women, the stigma of mental illness affects them not only as a "person with" but as "person caring for" themselves or others.

Socio-legal Aspects of Stigma

As Goffman (1963) reminds us, stigma is profoundly embedded and enacted in social relationships. Then, by extension, stigma is embodied in legislation. Such legislation has significant legal implications and consequences, particularly for women. Legislation codifies structural stigma into everyday life, affecting vulnerable populations, sometimes for decades (Goldberg et al., 2022). Regardless of intent, legal language can be stigmatizing as it can be created and driven by certain individuals or ideologies.

Legislation may be created using different agendas, such as agendas based on services or rights. A services agenda looks to increase access, utilization, and quality of behavioral health-care services. A rights agenda looks to eliminate discrimination and promote the civil rights of persons with behavioral health disorders. Although these agendas may be framed differently, the intent of these legislative agendas are to (1) address treatment; (2) promote self-efficacy, help-seeking, social inclusion, and recovery; and (3) reframe stigma as discrimination.

Reframing stigma as discrimination places it squarely in the intersection of human rights and other discrimination models. It also places the onus on larger unfair societal attitudes and actions rather than further stigmatizing persons with behavioral health disorders. Federal laws, however, can only directly address one aspect of stigma: discrimination. This can be addressed via anti-discrimination laws, laws addressing civil (involuntary) commitment and treatment, informed consent, and parity. Historically, these laws have had various levels of success in reducing stigma and discrimination against persons with mental illnesses.

Anti-discrimination Laws

There have been concerted efforts to address the discrimination that accompanies the stigma of mental and substance use disorders, starting with anti-discrimination laws, which ensure equal treatment under the law (Read et al., 2020; Shahwan et al., 2022). According to the WHO (2022, June 16), mental health services, policies, and laws are not priorities in most countries; hence, significant change to address the stigma of mental illness is complex. In India, for example, the legislative provisions of the Hindu Marriage Act do not mirror Indian societal value systems and attitudes towards marriage for women with mental illnesses. Societal norms often override the legal intent and provisions of the Act, leaving married women with behavioral health disorders at a major disadvantage (Sharma et al., 2015). In Liberia, the stigma of mental illness was identified as a major factor for services redesign in rural areas within the country. Recovering after nearly two decades of political violence and epidemics, stigma was directed not only at persons with mental illnesses but also their family members and mental health workers (Gwaikolo et al., 2017).

The intent of the Gender Equality Act in Korea in 2014 was to decrease the societal discrimination women faced and to increase women's participation and representation in society. In their longitudinal study, Kim et al. (2022) examined the relationship between the passage of the Act and depression among women. They found a moderate reduction in symptoms in women with depression. Anti-discrimination legislation targeted towards women, such as gender equality, could lead to greater improvements in public mental health (Kim et al., 2022).

In the United States, federal laws prohibit discrimination against and require accommodation for individuals with behavioral health disorders. The Americans with Disabilities Act in 1990 ensured everyone has equal opportunities for employment, accommodations for visible and "invisible" disabilities, and transportation, as well as access to and use of state and local government services. The Affordable Care Act of 2010 built upon the Americans with Disabilities Act by establishing special insurance protections to help persons with mental illnesses and substance use disorders.

In the European Union (EU), Chapter 3 of the EU Charter prohibits any discrimination based on "sex, race, colour, ethnic or social origin, genetic features, language, religion or belief, political or any other opinion, membership of a national minority, property, birth, disability, age or sexual orientation" (European Parliament et al., 2012, October 26, p. 400). These types of anti-discrimination initiatives are particularly important in the provision of public services and benefits programs, as well as other state-mandated actions, such as civil commitment.

Civil Commitment

Civil commitment (forced institutionalization), a legal process confining a person to a mental hospital or behavioral health unit against their wishes, is complex and varies by state and federal jurisdictions. In the United States, while state law generally governs civil commitment, there are constitutional (federal) concerns for persons with serious mental illnesses. These concerns fall under the *Due Process Clause* of the Fourteenth Amendment in the US Constitution (Rogers, 2023, May 24). The clause addresses procedural and substantive due process issues. Procedural requirements address burden of proof and right to counsel, expert witness, and jury trial. Substantive due process protections address dangerousness, right to safety, freedom from confinement, and right to receive or refuse treatment (Rogers, 2023, May 24).

Civil commitment is intended to balance the need for public safety with the rights of individuals with mental illnesses. However, how civil commitment is legislated and portrayed can mitigate or reinforce stigma. In the United States, discussions around the stigma and discrimination due to civil commitment became more prominent with the rise of the consumer/survivor/ex-psychiatric patient (c/s/x) rights movement in the late 1960s. Studies show that the stigma of involuntary commitment is formed by an individual's emotional and cognitive reactions to coercion as well as through actual coercive experiences of involuntary hospitalization (Rüsch et al., 2014; Xu et al., 2019).

A study in Norway by Wormdahl et al. (2021) examined individuals' trajectories into involuntary commitment. Four recurrent themes were as follows: (1) managing deterioration and deprivation more effectively, (2) difficulty in receiving help, (3) insufficient adaptation of available services, and (4) rethinking acute (crisis) care services and workflow. They also found significant gaps between policy and practice. How policies were implemented did not necessarily lead to a decrease in admissions. Policies also did not increase access to or utilization of less restrictive services for adults with severe mental illnesses at risk of involuntary commitment (Wormdahl et al., 2021).

How involuntary commitments are handled may also affect recovery, as self-stigma and empowerment are at the opposite ends of the services/treatment spectrum (Rüsch et al., 2009a, b). With the current emphases on centered care and shared decision-making, recovery and empowerment are integral to informed consent and legal competence.

Informed Consent and Legal Competence

Informed consent standards, from a legal perspective, protect the autonomy of individuals with mental illnesses and ensure individuals have the right to make their own treatment decisions. It also ensures individuals with behavioral health disorders retain their autonomy to make informed decisions about their choice to engage in treatment and/or research (Webb et al., 2022). To make those decisions, practitioners must provide accurate information about alternatives, benefits, potential risks, and likely outcomes if that specific treatment is or is not pursued. Consent must always be voluntary, not coerced. An individual also must be shown to be legally competent. The laws surrounding competence require mental capacity to be shown by one's ability to reason and deliberate, understand information pertinent to the decision, and communicate a choice.

Legal competence is seen as either a yes or no judicial decision. However, there are larger conversations on whether the amount of capacity required for legal competence should be higher based upon the gravity of the treatment decision (Brophy et al., 2018). This is particularly true for individuals under community treatment orders. A recent study in Norway examining the effects of new capacity-based legislation found positive changes for providers and patients (Wergeland et al., 2022). Behavioral health professionals had new awareness of the importance of the shared decision-making practice, particularly in the areas of autonomy and consent to treatment. Patients were assessed more often on their current conditions in the community and their ability to consent. Behavioral health professionals also wanted more flexible care, adjusting care and treatment according to the patient's current condition (Wergeland et al., 2022). Although this study illustrates positive changes, access to treatment still faces major barriers from economic, provider, or health systems infrastructure perspectives.

Parity

One of the most significant forms of stigma, as manifested by structural discrimination, is the lack of parity for mental health and addiction insurance coverage, when compared to the insurance coverage for physical health. In the United States, the Mental Health Parity and Addiction Equity Act in 2008 was passed after 20 plus years since its first introduction as a federal bill in 1996. Mental health parity laws require insurance companies to provide equal coverage for both behavioral health and physical health conditions. Although parity laws can help reduce the stigma associated with seeking treatment by ensuring individuals have easier access to care, inadequate enforcement of these laws remains a critical factor in the outcomes observed for persons with behavioral health conditions. This is particularly true when examining the social, political, and behavioral determinants of health and barriers vis-à-vis the fundamental rights of self-determination and redress of grievances. (For more information on insurance and financing, see Chap. 10, Financing Behavioral Health Services).

Behavioral health services are still significantly underfunded compared to physical health services. This lack of funding affects access to and utilization of care. For example, when only 1 in 5 people in high-income countries and only 1 in 27 people in low-/lower-income countries receive treatment for depression (Thornicroft et al., 2017), stigma and discrimination significantly affect behavioral health at a population level. Considering the burden of disease associated with behavioral health disorders, stigma (and its resulting discrimination) may be considered a primary "driver of morbidity and mortality" (Hatzenbuehler et al., 2013, p. 813).

Other Consequences of Stigma and Discrimination

Regardless of laws enacted to increase access to care and to reduce the stigma associated with behavioral health disorders, individuals often endure other consequences from stigma. "Anticipated discrimination" and/or "experienced discrimination" affect an individual's ability to engage in school, social activities, or work (Brohan et al., 2023; Uçok et al., 2012). Structural stigma affects services delivery and health systems. Bolster-Foucault et al. (2021) identified ten domains where structural stigma is manifested. These domains include (1) legal frameworks; (2–4) welfare, health, and economic policies; (5–6) social and built environments; (7) biomedical technology; (8) diagnostic frameworks; (9) media and marketing; and (10) health-care practices and interventions across both private and public sectors (Bolster-Foucault et al., 2021).

Illness concealment, a major coping mechanism, may also affect an individual's willingness to seek or receive care (Isaksson et al., 2018). In an examination of ten English-speaking countries by the Mental Health Million Project (2021), 58% of the population did not seek services for their diagnosable mental disorders. Twenty-two percent of individuals cited internal or external stigma as the reason for not seeking services. Fear of involuntary commitment deterred 13% of respondents (Mental Health Million Project, 2021). Discrimination experiences may also be due to the intersectoral/intersectional nature of the human experience (e.g. affiliative, cultural, identity, social, and/or geographical). Intersectorality and intersectionality compounds levels of discrimination based on other sociocultural characteristics or determinants of health (Azizpour et al., 2018; Moore et al., 2017; Rai et al., 2020; Schroeder et al., 2021).

Women with behavioral health disorders and female caregivers of persons with behavioral health disorders suffer more from stigma and discrimination than men, as shown in a number of country and global studies (Dubreucq et al., 2021; Ebuenyi et al., 2019; Farrelly et al., 2014; Koschorke et al., 2017). Women with behavioral health disorders who wish to become mothers, for example, not only must address the effects of illness on pregnancy but must also endure caregiver or provider reactions, including anger, abuse, or selective support (Banerjee et al., 2022). In Iran, for example, women who attempt suicide are not only labelled as "mentally ill" but are accused of other socially inappropriate actions, such as illicit sexual affairs (Azizpour et al., 2018).

Multiple factors across macro, meso, and micro levels, respectively, affect societal norms, political and service systems, and legislation and policy. Legal mechanisms addressing stigma and behavioral health disorders vary significantly from country to country or between jurisdictions. However, the currency of such laws and their enforcement need review and oversight by stakeholders interested in improving outcomes for persons with behavioral health disorders (Sugiura et al., 2020). Lack of resources, inflexible health-care practices, and lack of access to services in the early stages of deterioration can increase the risk of involuntary hospital admission.

Different approaches to conceptualizing stigma and the psychosocial consequences of stigma and discrimination could help inform legislation, policy, and practice. New ways of looking at stigma, such as "a science of stigma" (Keusch et al., 2006), and the development of cross-cutting measurement and intervention tools (van Brakel et al., 2019) could help researchers, policymakers, and practitioners to recognize and mitigate the intersectionality aspect of stigma. Integrating research from the behavioral, epidemiological, and neurological sciences would provide insights into the global burden of disease, etiology, and contributing factors (behavioral, social, and political determinants of health) of behavioral health disorders. Such insights could lead to effective evidence-based interventions and reduce the mortality and morbidity associated with these disorders. In addition, advocacy and public awareness campaigns could complement legal and judicial efforts to implement effective stigma mitigation interventions to reduce stigma and discrimination. However, examining how stigma is ameliorated or exacerbated due to the use of social media is an emerging area.

Social Media/Mass Media Relationship with Stereotypes and Stigma

Changing behavioral health-related public norms and behaviors is challenging since there are numerous structural, social, and psychological factors that influence an individual's or society's attitudes or beliefs. In the United State, the first publication on mental health from the US Office of the Surgeon General (1999), emphasized the importance of addressing stigma across cultural, sociopolitical, and community norms. In 2001, the international conference *Stigma and Global Health: Developing a Research Agenda* challenged the research community to examine the relationships between stigma and health at a global level. Of the 19 funded proposals, 10 focused on stigma of mental illnesses, drug use, and behavioral health disorders (Michels et al., 2006). More recent analyses of media and surveys show that there are clearly cross-national differences in how stigma is seen globally (Evans-Lacko et al., 2012; Olafsdottir & Pescosolido, 2011; Pescosolido et al., 2015; Stickney et al., 2012). Numerous studies also show the relationships between public perceptions of mental illnesses and the lived experiences of persons with mental illnesses (Manago et al., 2019; Olafsdottir & Pescosolido, 2009; Pescosolido et al., 2013, 2021).

The rise of social media as a preferred communication method began with the establishment of the first social media site in 1997 (boyd & Ellison, 2007) and the availability of mainstream internet access at home in the early 1990s. As telecommunication infrastructures and cell phone use continue to grow, media can be either an opportunity or a detriment in the struggle to de-stigmatize and reduce discrimination of mental illnesses and addictive disorders (Sharma et al., 2020). Hashtags, such as #MentalHealth and #anxiety, are used in millions of TikTok/X videos, totaling 20 billion views since their inception (Amato, 2022, January 5).

Patterns of social media use have been useful to identify population-level trends and informing public health responses. Content- and style-based language changes may be early indicators of relapse in schizophrenia (Birnbaum et al., 2019). Instagram photos may be predictive of the onset or worsening of depression (Reece & Danforth, 2017). Studies monitoring social media sites, such as Twitter and Reddit, during the COVID-19 pandemic saw increases in members' coping mechanisms (Low et al., 2020; Sarker et al., 2020). The use of curated and monitored social network sites has been shown to be effective as therapeutic interventions. Social media also has been increasingly used in health policymaking and health equity initiatives (Welch et al., 2016; Yeung, 2018). Reviews on the effectiveness of mass media and social media interventions for reducing mental health-related stigma are mixed (Clement et al., 2013). While some interventions have been shown to reduce prejudicial components of stigma, there is not enough evidence to determine if the interventions themselves are effective in reducing discrimination. However, innovative approaches are being implemented globally using a variety of tools.

Online Support Forums

Over the past 20 years, online mental health support forums have emerged as an important tool for improving mental health and well-being and have played a key role in peer support and recovery. Online forums mitigate the social and geographic isolation persons with behavioral health disorders experience. Forum members are able to connect socially with others who may be experiencing the same challenges to find and share information (Smith-Merry et al., 2019).

Perinatal mental illness is a global health concern. Internal stigma prevents many women from seeking and receiving treatment and also plays a significant role in illness concealment. A study conducted by Moore et al. (2017) found that although long-term forum users reported higher levels of internal stigma, users also reported more disclosure of their symptoms to health-care providers. Their findings suggest changes in provider practice. Providers recommending trustworthy and moderated online forums to their patients could potentially increase women's comfort levels for disclosing symptoms, thereby improving patient outcomes during pregnancy (Moore et al., 2017). (For more information on reproductive health issues for women with behavioral disorders, see Chap. 3)

Anonymity and ease of access to social media are particularly important for young persons with behavioral health disorders. A survey of 1300 youth found that 90% of teens and young adults (aged 14–22) turned to social media, blogs, and online forums to find information on mental health issues (Rideout & Fox, 2018). Ninety-one percent of the girls and young women reported seeking online resources, tools, and information related to health and mental health. However, 22% of persons with moderate to severe depressive symptoms reported that the use of social media made them feel worse (Rideout & Fox, 2018).

Having a sense of how stigma and stereotyping occur and are perceived by individuals is key in developing effective anti-stigma campaigns and effective health promotion and educational materials. However, representations and attitudes about these illnesses are not widely investigated at either a national or global level. Mobile technologies, platforms, and apps (applications) are used increasingly to combat stigma and stereotyping of mental illnesses. They provide accurate information on diagnosis and treatment, protest against discriminatory acts, and increase contact with other people.

#Campaigns

The Pan American Health Organization (PAHO, 2023) launched a mental health stigma reduction campaign *#DoYourShare to support mental health* to reduce stereotypes, prejudices, and discriminatory behaviors towards people with behavioral health disorders. The PAHO campaign has been embraced by a number of countries in South America and the Caribbean, including Suriname, Chile, Brazil, and Trinidad and Tobago, with additional campaigns in their countries. *#Do Your Share* ties into Goals 7 and 11 of PAHO's *Sustainable Health Agenda for the Americas 2018–2030* (Evidence and Knowledge in Health, and Health Inequalities and Inequities, respectively).

Apps

Researchers in the Institut du Cerveau et de la Moelle Epinière (ICM) and CERMES3 developed Crazy'App to assess public perceptions of persons with mental and substance use disorders and as an educational campaign (Morgiève et al., 2019). Crazy'App incorporated video testimony from individuals with mental illnesses, a series of questions to determine existing knowledge, and videos from psychiatrists discussing successful treatment and management of these disorders. Premiered in 2016 at *Mental désordre, changer le regard sur les trouble psychiques*, a Parisian exhibition, Crazy'App is the first survey of its type in France (Morgiève et al., 2019).

Integrated Platforms

Designed to help people with schizophrenia through recovery, the *Personalized Real-Time Intervention for Motivation Enhancement* (PRIME) app is a smartphone-based, social networking platform. It is designed to mitigate negative symptoms, using motivational coaching from trained therapists, and to create a community supporting self-determination (Schlosser et al., 2016). Participants reported positive experiences of social support from coaches and peers with significant increases in social engagement and reciprocal interactions with coaching (Schlosser et al., 2016).

The *Moderated Online Social Therapy* (MOST/MOST+) platform is another example of an innovation that offers personalized therapy and opportunities for social connections. It offers therapeutic content, activities and practical strategies, moderated online community discussions, and access to clinical and vocational experts and peers. Developed by Orygen, Australia's Centre of Excellence in Youth Mental Health, participants in MOST+ reported that they felt more socially connected and safe (Alvarez-Jimenez et al., 2020).

Adapting the MOST+ platform to the Netherlands, the *Engage Young people early* (ENYOY) is a clinical- and peer-moderated treatment platform to support young people (aged 16–25 years) (van Doorn et al., 2021). The intent of ENYOY is to bridge the gaps in treatment and services individuals face as they cross developmental stages from childhood to adolescence to adulthood. A recent evaluation of the platform found it to be user-friendly, safe, accessible, and inclusive (van Doorn et al., 2022).

Horyzons, an Australian moderated online social intervention for persons experiencing first-episode psychosis to move towards recovery, was designed to create a sense of community and inclusion and offer mutual support (Alvarez-Jimenez et al., 2019). Adapted for use in the United States, early results for Horyzons USA were significant. Participants noted improvements in living skills and increases in psychological well-being and reductions in depressive symptoms (Ludwig et al., 2021). A 2023 evaluation of Horyzons found that users felt more competent managing their mental health because of the familiarity, privacy, and perceived safety of the intervention (Pokowitz et al., 2023).

Caveats with the Use of Social Media

Social media has been touted as a way to increase engagement and utilization of services and decrease stigma and the discrimination associated with mental illnesses and substance use disorders. However, there are concerns regarding the use of self-disclosed information. In their study on Twitter use by persons with serious mental illnesses, Naslund and Aschbrenner (2019) found more than one-third of participants had concerns regarding privacy. Participants identified four risk areas: (1) employment, (2) personal relationships, (3) fear of stigma, and (4) hostility or harassment. Social media use has shown that individuals with behavioral health disorders may be targeted by shaming, cyberbullying, and harassment (Ge, 2020; Gupta et al., 2022).

Implications for Women's Behavioral Health

The US Surgeon General's report on disability established the health and wellness of persons with disabilities as an important public health concern (U.S. Office of the Surgeon General, Office of Disability, 2005, p. 21). Considering the complexity of stigma and the role it plays in return to work, we offer several recommendations for research and practice, grounded within the social determinants of health framework. First, research on stigma should change. It is not sufficient to determine if an individual accepts or denies the existence of stigma. We should be examining the applicability of stigma to each individual. Meisenbach (2010), for example, offers a typology of stigma communication management strategies that could help reshape how we as researchers and practitioners address stigma, as well as the effect of stigma on people's decisions to return to work. In addition, conceptual and context-specific empirical investigations can be strengthened by working with the *International Classification of Functioning, Disability and Health* vocabulary and frame (WHO, 2017). This would provide new understandings of functional disabilities in stigmatized populations with chronic illnesses. Context-specific research conducted in parallel with broader comparative work would illustrate the reproduction of social processes that create, perpetuate, or destroy stigma (Parker & Aggleton, 2003).

In addition, we need to reconceptualize research on disability issues, using frameworks and vocabulary that move it out of an "exclusion" frame and into an "inclusion" frame. Qualitative studies should be more than just the reporting of what people said. There is value in the discursive analysis of written and verbal communication (talk and text). This way of analysis can help uncover the issues and solutions that can and should be addressed and pulled into policy (Hanson, 2014). Community-based survey research should incorporate stigma concepts and measures to illustrate the linkages between stigma and outcomes at a more meso- or macro-level. Core outcome measures for stigma could be incorporated in research with persons with behavioral health disorders to inform the evidence base.

At the meso- or macro-level, research should address strategic and policy-oriented issues and outcomes on political and legal actions to reduce stigma at local, state, regional, national, and international levels. This could be important in assessing which stigma reduction interventions are successfully adopted and implemented within specific social, cultural, political, and economic contexts. The inclusion of behavioral health measures in research may help broaden our understanding of how stigma is expressed in social interaction (Crawford, 1996) as well as provide a "normative" voice that quantitative studies provide in policy to practice legislation and regulation. Finally, intervention research should consider incorporation of the community and social mobilization literature in its efforts to reduce stigma (Altman, 1994). To improve outcomes and quality of life for women with behavioral health disorders, we must address how acute and chronic mental illnesses may be reframed to reduce stigma and discrimination within social, cultural, political, and economic determinants of health.

References

Altman, D. (1994). *Power and community: Organizational and cultural responses to AIDS*. Taylor & Francis.

Alvarez-Jimenez, M., Bendall, S., Koval, P., Rice, S., Cagliarini, D., Valentine, L., D'Alfonso, S., Miles, C., Russon, P., Penn, D. L., Phillips, J., Lederman, R., Wadley, G., Killackey, E., Santesteban-Echarri, O., Mihalopoulos, C., Herrman, H., Gonzalez-Blanch, C., Gilbertson, T., Lal, S., Chambers, R., Daglas-Georgiou, R., Latorre, C., Cotton, S. M., McGorry, P. D., & Gleeson, J. F. (2019). HORYZONS trial: Protocol for a randomised controlled trial of a moderated online social therapy to maintain treatment effects from first-episode psychosis services. *BMJ Open, 9*(2), e024104. https://doi.org/10.1136/bmjopen-2018-024104

Alvarez-Jimenez, M., Rice, S., D'Alfonso, S., Leicester, S., Bendall, S., Pryor, I., Russon, P., McEnery, C., Santesteban-Echarri, O., Da Costa, G., Gilbertson, T., Valentine, L., Solves, L., Ratheesh, A., McGorry, P. D., & Gleeson, J. (2020). A novel multimodal digital service (Moderated Online Social Therapy+) for help-seeking young people experiencing mental ill-health: Pilot evaluation within a National Youth E-Mental Health Service. *Journal of Medical Internet Research, 22*(8), e17155. https://doi.org/10.2196/17155

Amato, M. (2022, Jan 5). TikTok is helping Gen Z with mental health. Here's what it can and can't do. *Los Angeles Times,* Online. https://www.latimes.com/lifestyle/story/2022-01-05/those-struggling-with-mental-health-have-found-validation-on-tiktok-heres-how#:~:text=TikTok%20videos%20with%20the%20hashtag,trendy%20dances%20and%20goofy%20humor.

Azizpour, M., Taghizadeh, Z., Mohammadi, N., & Vedadhir, A. (2018). Fear of stigma: The lived experiences of Iranian women after suicide attempt. *Perspectives in Psychiatric Care, 54*(2), 293–299. https://doi.org/10.1111/ppc.12237

Baker, C. (2004). Membership categorization and interview accounts. In D. Silverman (Ed.), *Qualitative research: Theory, method and practice*. Sage Publications.

Baldwin, B. A., Floyd, H. H., Jr., & McSeveney, D. R. (1975). Status inconsistency and psychiatric diagnosis: A structural approach to labeling theory. *Journal of Health and Social Behavior, 16*(3), 257–267. http://www.jstor.org/stable/pdfplus/2136875.pdf?acceptTC=true

Banerjee, D., Arasappa, R., Chandra, P. S., & Desai, G. (2022). "It seemed like my fault for wanting to become a mother ..." - Experiences and perceptions related to motherhood in women with severe mental illness. *Asia-Pacific Psychiatry, 14*(4), e12519. https://doi.org/10.1111/appy.12519

Bean, P. (1979). Psychiatrists' assessments of mental illness: A comparison of some aspects of Thomas Scheff's approach to labelling theory. *British Journal of Psychiatry, 135*(8), 122–128. https://doi.org/10.1192/bjp.135.2.122

Benson, P. R. (1980). Labeling theory and community care of the mentally ill in California: The relationship of social theory and ideology to public policy. *Human Organization, 39*(2), 134–141.

Birnbaum, M. L., Ernala, S. K., Rizvi, A. F., Arenare, E. A. R. V. M., De Choudhury, M., & Kane, J. M. (2019). Detecting relapse in youth with psychotic disorders utilizing patient-generated and patient-contributed digital data from Facebook. *NPJ Schizophrenia, 5*(1), 17. https://doi.org/10.1038/s41537-019-0085-9

Bolster-Foucault, C., Ho Mi Fane, B., & Blair, A. (2021). Structural determinants of stigma across health and social conditions: A rapid review and conceptual framework to guide future research and intervention. *Health Promotion and Chronic Disease Prevention in Canada: Research, Policy and Practice, 41*(3), 85–115. https://doi.org/10.24095/hpcdp.41.3.03

Boyd, D. M., & Ellison, N. B. (2007). Social network sites: Definition, history, and scholarship. *Journal of Computer-Mediated Communication, 13*(1), 210–230. https://doi.org/10.1111/j.1083-6101.2007.00393.x. S2CID 52810295.

Brohan, E., Thornicroft, G., Rüsch, N., Lasalvia, A., Campbell, M. M., Yalçınkaya-Alkar, Ö., Lanfredi, M., Ochoa, S., Üçok, A., Tomás, C., Fadipe, B., Sebes, J., Fiorillo, A., Sampogna, G., Paula, C. S., Valverde, L., Schomerus, G., Klemm, P., Ouali, U., Castelein, S., Alexová, A., Oexle, N., Guimarães, P. N., Sportel, B. E., Chang, C. C., Li, J., Shanthi, C., Reneses, B., Bakolis, I., & Evans-Lacko, S. (2023). Measuring discrimination experienced by people with a mental illness: Replication of the short-form DISCUS in six world regions. *Psychological Medicine, 53*(9), 3963–3973. https://doi.org/10.1017/s0033291722000630

Brophy, L., Edan, V., Gooding, P., McSherry, B., Burkett, T., Carey, S., Carroll, A., Callaghan, S., Finch, A., Hansford, M., Hanson, S., Kisely, S., Lawn, S., Light, E., Maher, S., Patel, G., Ryan, C. J., Saltmarsh, K., Stratford, A., Tellez, J. J., Toko, M., & Weller, P. (2018). Community treatment orders: Towards a new research agenda. *Australasian Psychiatry, 26*(3), 299–302. https://doi.org/10.1177/1039856218758543

Caetano, D. F. (1974). Labeling theory and the presumption of mental illness in diagnosis: An experimental design. *Journal of Health and Social Behavior, 15*(3), 253–260. http://www.jstor.org/stable/pdfplus/2137025.pdf

Clement, S., Lassman, F., Barley, E., Evans-Lacko, S., Williams, P., Yamaguchi, S., Slade, M., Rüsch, N., & Thornicroft, G. (2013). Mass media interventions for reducing mental health-related stigma. *Cochrane Database of Systematic Reviews, 2013*(7), Cd009453. https://doi.org/10.1002/14651858.CD009453.pub2

Corrigan, P. W., & Penn, D. L. (1999). Lessons from social psychology on discrediting psychiatric stigma. *American Psychologist, 54*(9), 765–776. http://psycnet.apa.org/journals/amp/54/9/765/

Corrigan, P. W., & Watson, A. C. (2002). The paradox of self-stigma and mental illness. *Clinical Psychology: Science and Practice, 9*(1), 35–53. https://doi.org/10.1093/clipsy.9.1.35

Crawford, A. M. (1996). Stigma associated with AIDS: A meta-analysis. *Journal of Applied Social Psychology, 26*(5), 398–416. https://doi.org/10.1111/j.1559-1816.1996.tb01856.x

de Albuquerque, C. (2012, July 2). *Report of the Special Rapporteur on the human right to safe drinking water and sanitation, Catarina de Albuquerque: Stigma and the realization of the human rights to water and sanitation* [Report; A/HRC/21/42]. United Nations Human Rights Council. https://www.ohchr.org/sites/default/files/Documents/HRBodies/HRCouncil/RegularSession/Session21/A-HRC-21-42_en.pdf

Dubreucq, J., Plasse, J., & Franck, N. (2021). Self-stigma in serious mental illness: A systematic review of frequency, correlates, and consequences. *Schizophrenia Bulletin, 47*(5), 1261–1287. https://doi.org/10.1093/schbul/sbaa181

Ebuenyi, I. D., Regeer, B. J., Ndetei, D. M., Bunders-Aelen, J. F. G., & Guxens, M. (2019). Experienced and anticipated discrimination and social functioning in persons with mental disabilities in KIenya: Implications for employment. *Frontiers in Psychiatry, 10*, 181. https://doi.org/10.3389/fpsyt.2019.00181

Eisenberg, L. (1977). Psychiatry and society: A sociobiologic synthesis. *New England Journal of Medicine, 296*(16), 903–910. https://doi.org/10.1056/nejm197704212961604

European Parliament, Council, & Commission. (2012, Oct 26). *Charter of fundamental rights of the European Union* [2012/C 326/02](Official Journal of the European Union). https://eur-lex.europa.eu/legal-content/EN/TXT/?uri=CELEX:12012P/TXT

Evans-Lacko, S., Brohan, E., Mojtabai, R., & Thornicroft, G. (2012). Association between public views of mental illness and self-stigma among individuals with mental illness in 14 European countries. *Psychological Medicine, 42*(8), 1741–1752. https://doi.org/10.1017/s0033291711002558

Farrelly, S., Clement, S., Gabbidon, J., Jeffery, D., Dockery, L., Lassman, F., Brohan, E., Henderson, R. C., Williams, P., Howard, L. M., & Thornicroft, G. (2014). Anticipated and experienced discrimination amongst people with schizophrenia, bipolar disorder and major depressive disorder: A cross sectional study. *BMC Psychiatry, 14*, 157. https://doi.org/10.1186/1471-244x-14-157

Ge, X. (2020). Social media reduce users' moral sensitivity: Online shaming as a possible consequence. *Aggressive Behavior, 46*(5), 359–369. https://doi.org/10.1002/ab.21904

Goffman, E. (1961). *Asylums: Essays on the social situation of mental patients and other inmates.* Anchor Books.

Goffman, E. (1963). *Stigma: Notes on the management of spoiled identity.* Simon and Schuster.

Goldberg, S., Hemeida, H., Conyers-Tucker, L., & Brou, D. (2022). *Structural stigma in law: Implications and opportunities for health and health equity.* [Health Policy Brief]. Health Affairs. https://www.healthaffairs.org/do/10.1377/hpb20221104.659710/full/

Gove, W. R. (1970). Societal reaction as an explanation of mental illness: Evaluation. *American Sociological Review, 35*(5), 873–884. https://doi.org/10.2307/2093298

Gove, W. R. (1979). Labeling versus the psychiatric explanation of mental illness debate that has become substantively irrelevant. *Journal of Health and Social Behavior, 20*(3), 301–304. https://doi.org/10.2307/2136455

Gove, W. R. (1982). Labeling theory's explanation of mental-illness: An update of recent-evidence. *Deviant Behavior, 3*(4), 307–327. <Go to ISI>://WOS:A1982PT42600001.

Grunebaum, H., & Chasin, R. (1978). Relabeling and reframing reconsidered: The beneficial effects of a pathological label. *Family Process, 17*(4), 449–455.

Gupta, C., Jogdand, D. S., & Kumar, M. (2022). Reviewing the impact of social media on the mental health of adolescents and young adults. *Cureus, 14*(10), e30143. https://doi.org/10.7759/cureus.30143

Gwaikolo, W. S., Kohrt, B. A., & Cooper, J. L. (2017). Health system preparedness for integration of mental health services in rural Liberia. *BMC Health Services Research, 17*(1), 508. https://doi.org/10.1186/s12913-017-2447-1

Hanson, A. (2014). Illuminating the invisible voices in mental health policymaking. *Journal of Medicine and the Person, 12*(1), 13–18. https://doi.org/10.1007/s12682-014-0170-9

Hatzenbuehler, M. L., Phelan, J. C., & Link, B. G. (2013). Stigma as a fundamental cause of population health inequalities. *American Journal of Public Health, 103*(5), 813–821. https://doi.org/10.2105/ajph.2012.301069

Hogg, M. A., & Abrams, D. (1988). *Social identifications: A social psychology of intergroup relations and group processes.* Routledge.

Isaksson, A., Corker, E., Cotney, J., Hamilton, S., Pinfold, V., Rose, D., Rüsch, N., Henderson, C., Thornicroft, G., & Evans-Lacko, S. (2018). Coping with stigma and discrimination: Evidence from mental health service users in England. *Epidemiology & Psychiatric Sciences, 27*(6), 577–588. https://doi.org/10.1017/s204579601700021x

Jorm, A. F., & Oh, E. (2009). Desire for social distance from people with mental disorders. *Australian and New Zealand Journal of Psychiatry, 43*(3), 183–200. https://doi.org/10.1080/00048670802653349

Keusch, G. T., Wilentz, J., & Kleinman, A. (2006). Stigma and global health: Developing a research agenda. *Lancet, 367*(9509), 525–527. https://doi.org/10.1016/s0140-6736(06)68183-x

Kim, C., Teo, C., Nielsen, A., & Chum, A. (2022). Macro-level gender equality and women's depressive symptoms in South Korea: A longitudinal study. *Social Psychiatry and Psychiatric Epidemiology.* https://doi.org/10.1007/s00127-022-02335-6

Koschorke, M., Padmavati, R., Kumar, S., Cohen, A., Weiss, H. A., Chatterjee, S., Pereira, J., Naik, S., John, S., Dabholkar, H., Balaji, M., Chavan, A., Varghese, M., Thara, R., Patel, V., & Thornicroft, G. (2017). Experiences of stigma and discrimination faced by family caregivers of people with schizophrenia in India. *Social Science and Medicine, 178*, 66–77. https://doi.org/10.1016/j.socscimed.2017.01.061

Link, B. G., & Phelan, J. C. (2001). Conceptualizing stigma. *Annual Review of Sociology, 27*(1), 363–385. https://doi.org/10.1146/annurev.soc.27.1.363

Low, D. M., Rumker, L., Talkar, T., Torous, J., Cecchi, G., & Ghosh, S. S. (2020). Natural language processing reveals vulnerable mental health support groups and heightened health anxiety on reddit during COVID-19: Observational study. *Journal of Medical Internet Research, 22*(10), e22635. https://doi.org/10.2196/22635

Ludwig, K. A., Browne, J. W., Nagendra, A., Gleeson, J. F., D'Alfonso, S., Penn, D. L., & Alvarez-Jimenez, M. (2021). Horyzons USA: A moderated online social intervention for first episode psychosis. *Early Intervention in Psychiatry, 15*(2), 335–343. https://doi.org/10.1111/eip.12947

Lupton, D. (2003). *Medicine as culture illness, disease and the body in Western societies.* Sage. http://site.ebrary.com/id/10080891

Mahajan, A. P., Sayles, J. N., Patel, V. A., Remien, R. H., Sawires, S. R., Ortiz, D. J., Szekeres, G., & Coates, T. J. (2008). Stigma in the HIV/AIDS epidemic: A review of the literature and recommendations for the way forward. *AIDS, 22*(Suppl 2), S67–S79. https://doi.org/10.1097/01.aids.0000327438.13291.62

Manago, B., Pescosolido, B. A., & Olafsdottir, S. (2019). Icelandic inclusion, German hesitation and American fear: A cross-cultural comparison of mental-health stigma and the media. *Scandinavian Journal of Public Health, 47*(2), 90–98. https://doi.org/10.1177/1403494817750337

Meisenbach, R. J. (2010). Stigma management communication: A theory and agenda for applied research on how individuals manage moments of stigmatized identity. *Journal of Applied Communication Research, 38*(3), 268–292. https://doi.org/10.1080/00909882.2010.490841

Mental Health Million Project. (2021). *Mental health has bigger challenges than stigma: Rapid report* [Report]. Sapien Labs. https://mentalstateoftheworld.report/wp-content/uploads/2021/05/Rapid-Report-2021-Help-Seeking.pdf

Michels, K. M., Hofman, K. J., Keusch, G. T., & Hrynkow, S. H. (2006). Stigma and global health: Looking forward. *Lancet, 367*(9509), 538–539. https://doi.org/10.1016/s0140-6736(06)68190-7

Moore, D., Drey, N., & Ayers, S. (2017). Use of online forums for perinatal mental illness, stigma, and disclosure: An exploratory model. *JMIR Mental Health, 4*(1), e6. https://doi.org/10.2196/mental.5926

Morgiève, M., N'Diaye, K., Nguyen-Khac, A., Mallet, L., & Briffault, X. (2019). Crazy'App: A web survey on representations and attitudes toward mental disorders using video testimonies. *Encephale, 45*(4), 290–296. https://doi.org/10.1016/j.encep.2018.10.004

Murphy, J. M. (1977). Labeling theory. *Science, 196*(4289), 484–558. https://doi.org/10.1126/science.196.4289.484

Naslund, J. A., & Aschbrenner, K. A. (2019). Risks to privacy with use of social media: Understanding the views of social media users with serious mental illness. *Psychiatric Services, 70*(7), 561–568. https://doi.org/10.1176/appi.ps.201800520

Oakes, P. J., Haslam, S. A., & Turner, J. C. (1994). *Stereotyping and social reality.* Blackwell.

Olafsdottir, S., & Pescosolido, B. A. (2009). Drawing the line: The cultural cartography of utilization recommendations for mental health problems. *Journal of Health and Social Behavior, 50*(2), 228–244. https://doi.org/10.1177/002214650905000208

Olafsdottir, S., & Pescosolido, B. A. (2011). Constructing illness: How the public in eight Western nations respond to a clinical description of "schizophrenia". *Social Science and Medicine, 73*(6), 929–938. https://doi.org/10.1016/j.socscimed.2011.06.029

PAHO. (2023). *#DoYourShare to support mental health*. [Web page]. PAHO. https://www.paho.org/en/campaigns/do-your-share

Parker, R., & Aggleton, P. (2003). HIV and AIDS-related stigma and discrimination: A conceptual framework and implications for action. *Social Science and Medicine, 57*(1), 13–24. http://ac.els-cdn.com/S0277953602003040/1-s2.0-S0277953602003040-main.pdf?_tid=b946691a-b069-11e3-9cfd-00000aab0f6c&acdnat=1395345567_f577ba4f115b5df4b258a54c8e756d80

Pescosolido, B. A., Medina, T. R., Martin, J. K., & Long, J. S. (2013). The "backbone" of stigma: Identifying the global core of public prejudice associated with mental illness. *American Journal of Public Health, 103*(5), 853–860. https://doi.org/10.2105/ajph.2012.301147

Pescosolido, B. A., Martin, J. K., Olafsdottir, S., Long, J. S., Kafadar, K., & Medina, T. R. (2015). The theory of industrial society and cultural schemata: Does the "cultural myth of stigma" underlie the WHO schizophrenia paradox? *AJS. American Journal of Sociology, 121*(3), 783–825. https://doi.org/10.1086/683225

Pescosolido, B. A., Halpern-Manners, A., Luo, L., & Perry, B. (2021). Trends in public stigma of mental illness in the US, 1996-2018. *JAMA Network Open, 4*(12), e2140202. https://doi.org/10.1001/jamanetworkopen.2021.40202

Pokowitz, E. L., Stiles, B. J., Thomas, R., Bullard, K., Ludwig, K. A., Gleeson, J. F., Alvarez-Jimenez, M., Perkins, D. O., & Penn, D. L. (2023). User experiences of an American-adapted moderated online social media platform for first-episode psychosis: Qualitative analysis. *DIGITAL HEALTH, 9*, 20552076231176700. https://doi.org/10.1177/20552076231176700

President's New Freedom Commission on Mental Health. (2003). *Achieving the promise: Transforming mental health care in America*. Author. http://govinfo.library.unt.edu/mental-healthcommission/reports/FinalReport/downloads/FinalReport.pdf

Rai, S. S., Peters, R. M. H., Syurina, E. V., Irwanto, I., Naniche, D., & Zweekhorst, M. B. M. (2020). Intersectionality and health-related stigma: Insights from experiences of people living with stigmatized health conditions in Indonesia. *International Journal for Equity in Health, 19*(1), 206. https://doi.org/10.1186/s12939-020-01318-w

Read, J., Haslam, N., Sayce, L., & Davies, E. (2006). Prejudice and schizophrenia: A review of the 'mental illness is an illness like any other' approach. *Acta Psychiatrica Scandnavica, 114*(5), 303–318. https://doi.org/10.1111/j.1600-0447.2006.00824.x

Read, U. M., Sakyi, L., & Abbey, W. (2020). Exploring the potential of a rights-based approach to work and social inclusion for people with lived experience of mental illness in Ghana. *Health and Human Rights, 22*(1), 91–104. https://www.ncbi.nlm.nih.gov/pmc/articles/PMC7348440/pdf/hhr-22-01-091.pdf

Reece, A. G., & Danforth, C. M. (2017). Instagram photos reveal predictive markers of depression. *EPJ Data Science, 6*, Article 15. https://doi.org/10.1140/epjds/s13688-017-0110-z

Rideout, V., & Fox, S. (2018). *Digital health practices, social media use, and mental well-being among teens and young adults in the U.S.* [Report]. Hopelab and Well Being Trust. https://digitalcommons.providence.org/cgi/viewcontent.cgi?article=2092&context=publications

Rogers, H. -A. (2023, May 24). *Involuntary civil commitment: Fourteenth amendment due process protections*. [Report; R47571]. Authour (CRS). https://crsreports.congress.gov/product/pdf/R/R47571

Roman, P. M. (1971). Labeling theory and community psychiatry. The impact of psychiatric sociology on ideology and practice in American psychiatry. *Psychiatry, 34*(4), 378–390.

Rotenberg, M. (1974). Self-labelling: A missing link in the 'societal reaction' theory of deviance. *The Sociological Review, 22*(3), 335–354. https://doi.org/10.1111/j.1467-954X.1974.tb002

Rüsch, N., Lieb, K., Bohus, M., & Corrigan, P. W. (2006). Self-stigma, empowerment, and perceived legitimacy of discrimination among women with mental illness. *Psychiatric Services, 57*(3), 399–402. https://doi.org/10.1176/appi.ps.57.3.399

Rüsch, N., Corrigan, P. W., Powell, K., Rajah, A., Olschewski, M., Wilkniss, S., & Batia, K. (2009a). A stress-coping model of mental illness stigma: II. Emotional stress responses, coping behavior and outcome. *Schizophrenia Research, 110*(1–3), 65–71. https://doi.org/10.1016/j.schres.2009.01.005

Rüsch, N., Corrigan, P. W., Wassel, A., Michaels, P., Olschewski, M., Wilkniss, S., & Batia, K. (2009b). A stress-coping model of mental illness stigma: I. Predictors of cognitive stress appraisal. *Schizophrenia Research, 110*(1–3), 59–64. https://doi.org/10.1016/j.schres.2009.01.006

Rüsch, N., Müller, M., Lay, B., Corrigan, P. W., Zahn, R., Schönenberger, T., Bleiker, M., Lengler, S., Blank, C., & Rössler, W. (2014). Emotional reactions to involuntary psychiatric hospitalization and stigma-related stress among people with mental illness. *European Archives of Psychiatry and Clinical Neuroscience, 264*(1), 35–43. https://doi.org/10.1007/s00406-013-0412-5

Sarker, A., Lakamana, S., Hogg-Bremer, W., Xie, A., Al-Garadi, M. A., & Yang, Y. C. (2020). Self-reported COVID-19 symptoms on Twitter: An analysis and a research resource. *Journal of the American Medical Informatics Association, 27*(8), 1310–1315. https://doi.org/10.1093/jamia/ocaa116

Scheff, T. J. (1966). *Being mentally ill: A sociological theory*. Aldine.

Scheff, T. J. (1974). The labelling theory of mental illness. *American Sociological Review, 39*(3), 444–452. https://doi.org/10.2307/2094300

Schlosser, D., Campellone, T., Kim, D., Truong, B., Vergani, S., Ward, C., & Vinogradov, S. (2016). Feasibility of PRIME: A cognitive neuroscience-informed mobile app intervention to enhance motivated behavior and improve quality of life in recent onset schizophrenia. *JMIR Research Protocols, 5*(2), e77. https://doi.org/10.2196/resprot.5450

Schroeder, S., Tan, C. M., Urlacher, B., & Heitkamp, T. (2021). The role of rural and urban geography and gender in community stigma around mental illness. *Health Education & Behavior, 48*(1), 63–73. https://doi.org/10.1177/1090198120974963

Schwanberg, S. L. (1985). Changes in labeling homosexuality in health sciences literature: A preliminary investigation. *Journal of Homosexuality, 12*(1), 51–73.

Shahwan, S., Goh, C. M. J., Tan, G. T. H., Ong, W. J., Chong, S. A., & Subramaniam, M. (2022). Strategies to reduce mental illness stigma: Perspectives of people with lived experience and caregivers. *International Journal of Environmental Research and Public Health, 19*(3). https://doi.org/10.3390/ijerph19031632

Sharma, I., Tripathi, C. B., & Pathak, A. (2015). Social and legal aspects of marriage in women with mental illness in India. *Indian Journal of Psychiatry, 57*(Suppl 2), S324–S332. https://doi.org/10.4103/0019-5545.161499

Sharma, M. K., John, N., & Sahu, M. (2020). Influence of social media on mental health: A systematic review. *Current Opinion in Psychiatry, 33*(5), 467–475. https://doi.org/10.1097/yco.0000000000000631

Smith-Merry, J., Goggin, G., Campbell, A., McKenzie, K., Ridout, B., & Baylosis, C. (2019). Social connection and online engagement: Insights from interviews with users of a mental health online forum. *JMIR Mental Health, 6*(3), e11084. https://doi.org/10.2196/11084

Stickney, S., Yanosky, D., Black, D. R., & Stickney, N. L. (2012). Socio-demographic variables and perceptual moderators related to mental health stigma. *Journal of Mental Health, 21*(3), 244–256. https://doi.org/10.3109/09638237.2012.670878

Sugiura, K., Pertega, E., & Holmberg, C. (2020). Experiences of involuntary psychiatric admission decision-making: A systematic review and meta-synthesis of the perspectives of service users, informal carers, and professionals. *International Journal of Law and Psychiatry, 73*, 101645. https://doi.org/10.1016/j.ijlp.2020.101645

Thornicroft, G., Chatterji, S., Evans-Lacko, S., Gruber, M., Sampson, N., Aguilar-Gaxiola, S., Al-Hamzawi, A., Alonso, J., Andrade, L., Borges, G., Bruffaerts, R., Bunting, B., de Almeida,

J. M., Florescu, S., de Girolamo, G., Gureje, O., Haro, J. M., He, Y., Hinkov, H., Karam, E., Kawakami, N., Lee, S., Navarro-Mateu, F., Piazza, M., Posada-Villa, J., de Galvis, Y. T., & Kessler, R. C. (2017). Undertreatment of people with major depressive disorder in 21 countries. *British Journal of Psychiatry, 210*(2), 119–124. https://doi.org/10.1192/bjp.bp.116.188078

Trice, H. M., & Roman, P. M. (1968). The sick role, labelling theory, and the deviant drinker. *International Journal of Social Psychiatry, 14*(4), 245–251. http://isp.sagepub.com/content/14/4/245.full.pdf

Turner, J. C. (1987). *Rediscovering the social group: Self-categorization theory.* Blackwell.

Uçok, A., Brohan, E., Rose, D., Sartorius, N., Leese, M., Yoon, C. K., Plooy, A., Ertekin, B. A., Milev, R., & Thornicroft, G. (2012). Anticipated discrimination among people with schizophrenia. *Acta Psychiatrica Scandinavica, 125*(1), 77–83. https://doi.org/10.1111/j.1600-0447.2011.01772.x

U. S. Office of the Surgeon General. (1999). *Mental health: A report of the Surgeon General* [Report]. U.S. Department of Health and Human Services, Substance Abuse and Mental Health Services Administration, Center for Mental Health Services, National Institutes of Health, National Institute of Mental Health. https://profiles.nlm.nih.gov/spotlight/nn/catalog/nlm:nlm uid-101584932X120-doc

U. S. Office of the Surgeon General, Office of Disability. (2005). *The Surgeon General's call to action to improve the health and wellness of persons with disabilities.* [Report]. U.S. Department of Health and Human Services; Office of the Surgeon General. https://www.govinfo.gov/content/pkg/GOVPUB-HE20-PURL-LPS107697/pdf/GOVPUB-HE20-PURL-LPS107697.pdf.

van Brakel, W. H., Cataldo, J., Grover, S., Kohrt, B. A., Nyblade, L., Stockton, M., Wouters, E., & Yang, L. H. (2019). Out of the silos: Identifying cross-cutting features of health-related stigma to advance measurement and intervention. *BMC Medicine, 17*(1), 13. https://doi.org/10.1186/s12916-018-1245-x

van Doorn, M., Popma, A., van Amelsvoort, T., McEnery, C., Gleeson, J. F., Ory, F. G. M. W. M. J., Alvarez-Jimenez, M., & Nieman, D. H. (2021). ENgage YOung people earlY (ENYOY): A mixed-method study design for a digital transdiagnostic clinical - and peer- moderated treatment platform for youth with beginning mental health complaints in The Netherlands. *BMC Psychiatry, 21*(1), 368. https://doi.org/10.1186/s12888-021-03315-x

van Doorn, M., Monsanto, A., Boeschoten, C. M., van Amelsvoort, T., Popma, A., Öry, F. G., Alvarez-Jimenez, M., Gleeson, J., Jaspers, M. W. M., & Nieman, D. H. (2022). Moderated digital social therapy for young people with emerging mental health problems: A user-centered mixed-method design and usability study. *Frontiers in Digital Health, 4*, 1020753. https://doi.org/10.3389/fdgth.2022.1020753

Webb, P., Falls, D., Keenan, F., Norris, B., Owens, A., Davidson, G., Edge, R., Kelly, B., McLaughlin, A., Montgomery, L., Mulvenna, C., & Irvine, R. S. (2022). Peer researchers' experiences of a co-produced research project on supported decision-making. *Research Involvement and Engagement, 8*(1), 70. https://doi.org/10.1186/s40900-022-00406-1

Welch, V., Petkovic, J., Pardo, J., Rader, T., & Tugwell, P. (2016). Interactive social media interventions to promote health equity: An overview of reviews. *Health Promotion and Chronic Disease Prevention in Canada: Research, Policy and Practice, 36*(4), 63–75.

Wergeland, N. C., Fause, Å., Weber, A. K., Fause, A. B. O., & Riley, H. (2022). Health professionals' experience of treatment of patients whose community treatment order was revoked under new capacity-based mental health legislation in Norway: Qualitative study. *BJPsych Open, 8*(6), e183. https://doi.org/10.1192/bjo.2022.592

World Health Organization. (2001). *Mental health: New understanding, new hope: The World Health Report.* WHO. http://www.who.int/whr/2001/en/

World Health Organization. (2017). *International classification of functioning, disability and health.* [Interactive Online Web Site]. Author. http://apps.who.int/classifications/icfbrowser/Default.aspx

World Health Organization. (2022, June 16). *World mental health report: Transforming mental health for all* [Report]. Author [WHO]. https://apps.who.int/iris/rest/bitstreams/1433523/retrieve

Wormdahl, I., Husum, T. L., Kjus, S. H. H., Rugkåsa, J., Hatling, T., & Rise, M. B. (2021). Between no help and coercion: Toward referral to involuntary psychiatric admission. A qualitative interview study of stakeholders' perspectives. *Frontiers in Psychiatry, 12*, 708175. https://doi.org/10.3389/fpsyt.2021.708175

Xu, Z., Lay, B., Oexle, N., Drack, T., Bleiker, M., Lengler, S., Blank, C., Müller, M., Mayer, B., Rössler, W., & Rüsch, N. (2019). Involuntary psychiatric hospitalisation, stigma stress and recovery: A 2-year study. *Epidemiology & Psychiatric Sciences, 28*(4), 458–465. https://doi.org/10.1017/s2045796018000021

Yeung, D. (2018). Social media as a catalyst for policy action and social change for health and well-being: Viewpoint. *Journal of Medical Internet Research, 20*(3), e94. https://doi.org/10.2196/jmir.8508

Part III
Services Delivery

Chapter 9
Integration of Behavioral Health and Primary Care Services for Women

Amanda Koire, Elizabeth Richards, Juan Aparicio, Koriann Cox, and Amritha Bhat

Introduction

Women with behavioral health concerns, including mood and substance use disorders, often present to primary or prenatal care settings before presenting to specialty mental health care. This first point of contact is an opportunity to improve behavioral health outcomes for individuals who may not have the desire or ability to access specialty care. The goal of integrated behavioral health is to identify these patients through screening, facilitate patient access to mental health services, and support primary care providers in delivering these services. Care may be integrated into clinical or community settings, and the unifying premise of differing models is to take the care to the patient and minimize barriers to receiving behavioral health interventions. Women in particular may benefit from integrated behavioral health models not only because of higher rates of depressive and anxiety disorders compared to men but also due to unique mental health needs and frequent health-care interventions during pregnancy and postpartum.

Here we describe the rationale for and various implementations of integrated models that have been designed to address women's behavioral health concerns. By the end of the chapter, readers should be able to compare and contrast common integrated behavioral health models that can be implemented in a primary care or prenatal setting, describe how integrated behavioral health models address barriers

A. Koire
Department of Psychiatry, Brigham and Women's Hospital, Harvard Medical School, Boston, MA, USA
e-mail: akoire@bwh.harvard.edu

E. Richards · J. Aparicio · K. Cox · A. Bhat (✉)
Department of Psychiatry and Behavioral Sciences, University of Washington, Seattle, WA, USA
e-mail: esricha@uw.edu; Japaric1@uw.edu; broussea@uw.edu; amritha@uw.edu

© The Author(s), under exclusive license to Springer Nature Switzerland AG 2024
A. Hanson, B. L. Levin (eds.), *Women's Behavioral Health*,
https://doi.org/10.1007/978-3-031-58293-6_9

to accessing mental health services and align with patient needs, and be able to describe factors that facilitate the successful implementation of an integrated behavioral health program for women.

Definition of Integrated Behavioral Health

Integrated behavioral health (IBH) is a model of health-care delivery that aims to provide comprehensive care to address physical and behavioral health concerns in a single setting. Though this concept has taken shape over the last 50 years, the term was first introduced in the late twentieth century (Blount & Bayona, 1994) to describe an approach that acknowledges the interconnected nature of physical and behavioral health and the need to create a holistic care team for patients. There are several models of integrated behavioral health care (American Psychological Association, 2022). In the collaborative care model (CoCM), a care manager, primary care physician, and a psychiatric consultant develop a coordinated treatment plan and discuss patient progress as a team, using principles of measurement-based treatment to target, population-based patient-centered team care, evidence-based treatments, and accountable care. In the Primary Care Behavioral Health model, a co-located behavioral health specialist provides time-limited (usually six or fewer sessions) behavioral treatments designed for primary care. There are also programs that allow primary care physicians to consult mental health specialists directly to inform their clinical decision-making and decrease need for referral out of the primary clinic, and community-based programs that bring mental health care directly to the patient.

While the nature and degree of the integration may vary between models, fundamentally all seek to decrease barriers to mental health-care access and improve patient outcomes, satisfaction, and health-care savings (Prom et al., 2021). There is a recognition inherent to these approaches that mental health and substance use concerns often present first within a primary care setting, that receiving behavioral health-care treatment in this setting may be more accessible and socially acceptable to patients, and that primary care providers find it feasible to treat common mental disorders, such as depression and anxiety. In these programs, patients presenting with chronic physical health conditions may have access to treatment to address comorbid behavioral health concerns. Gynecologic conditions encountered by obstetricians and gynecologists (OB-GYNs) and primary care doctors, for example, endometriosis, infertility, recurrent pregnancy loss, polycystic ovarian syndrome, and premature ovarian insufficiency, are associated with depressive symptoms (Bhat et al., 2017). Health-care encounters with OB-GYNs and primary care doctors in their practices can therefore be an ideal setting for integration of mental health treatment for women.

Services to screen for and treat mental health conditions can be expanded by integrating mental health professionals into primary care and other health settings. This, in turn, allows providers to treat mental health conditions more confidently within their own clinic, providing brief therapeutic interventions and facilitating referral to more intensive mental health care when needed.

Screening for Women's Mental Health and Substance Use Disorders

Screening is a critical part of preventive care and allows health-care providers to identify individuals who may be at risk of developing mental or substance use disorders and to provide early interventions to prevent these conditions from becoming more severe or chronic. Screening is often the first step in integrated mental health care. Researchers have examined and compared the presentation of symptoms for various mental health disorders, such as autism spectrum disorder, attention-deficit hyperactivity disorder (ADHD), substance use disorders, eating disorders, depression, and anxiety, across different developmental stages and considering gender differences. Moreover, research is ongoing to investigate the potential influence of estrogen and other hormonal variations between women and men on the prevalence and manifestation of mental health disorders (Ma et al., 2019). Additional research in this field is necessary to evaluate and adjust current screening practices accordingly. By incorporating validated screening tools into routine care, health-care providers can effectively identify at-risk individuals and provide timely interventions, improving outcomes, and promoting overall well-being for women.

The lifetime prevalence of depressive disorders is 14.4% for men and 22% for women, and prevalence of anxiety disorders is 26.4% for men and 40.4% for women, highlighting the higher burden of common mental disorders among women (Kessler et al., 2012). The U. S. Preventive Services Task force (USPSTF) recommends screening for depressive (Siu, 2016) and anxiety disorders (Barry et al., 2023) in adults (ages 64 and younger), including pregnant and postpartum women. The Women's Preventive Services Initiative recommends all female patients 13 years or older not currently diagnosed with an anxiety disorder should be screened for anxiety disorder (Gregory et al., 2020). Commonly used tools include the Patient Health Questionnaire (PHQ-9) (Kroenke & Spitzer, 2002) and the Generalized Anxiety Disorder scale (GAD-7) (Spitzer et al., 2006).

Within an integrated care setting, other life events warrant screening in women, such as intimate partner violence (IPV). Numerous studies consistently demonstrate a significant link between IPV and substance use disorders, suicidal ideation, depression, and anxiety among women. Equipping clinicians with the necessary training to recognize and address the consequences of violence can alleviate the severity of mental and substance use disorders in women experiencing such situations. The American College of Obstetricians and Gynecologists (ACOG) recommends screening all perinatal women for a history of sexual assault, with particular attention paid to women who report relevant symptoms. The recommendations also recommend annual screening for all women of childbearing age and all perinatal women for IPV at periodic intervals, including the first prenatal visit, at least once per trimester, and at the postpartum checkup (Randel, 2019). The USPSTF recommends the following tools when screening for IPV in perinatal women: Humiliation, Afraid, Rape, Kick (HARK), Hurt/Insult/Threaten/Scream (HITS), Extended Hurt/Insult/Threaten/Scream (E-HITS), Partner Violence Screen (PVS), and Woman Abuse Screening Tool (WAST) (Moyer & US Preventive Services Task Force*, 2013).

The perinatal period is a time of increased contact with the health-care system for many women and an opportunity to screen for mental health conditions. Since mental and substance use disorders are the most common complication of pregnancy (Byatt et al., 2020), several organizations recommend screening for these conditions in pregnancy and postpartum (American College of Obstetricians and Gynecologists, 2015; Siu, 2016). Despite recommendations, universal screening is variably implemented, with reported rates of screening for depression during the perinatal periods, ranging from 50% to 98% (Byatt et al., 2020). Common tools include the Edinburgh Postnatal Depression Scale (EPDS) and the Patient Health Questionnaire-9 (PHQ-9). Both screening tools can be completed in under 5 minutes and have been translated to many languages and validated in diverse cultural settings. Anxiety is frequently comorbid with depression, and anxiety screening is often administered with depression screening. As in general adult populations, the General Anxiety Disorder-7 (GAD-7) is commonly used to screen for perinatal anxiety. Other perinatal anxiety screening tools include the Edinburgh Postnatal Depression Scale-3A (EPDS 3A) and pregnancy-specific anxiety scales (Brunton et al., 2015). Compared to screening for depression in the perinatal period, the rate of screening for anxiety is lower in obstetric settings (Toler et al., 2018). This may be partly attributed to a lack of perceived preparedness among obstetric providers to successfully manage symptoms of anxiety. Despite the progress made in screening in both primary care settings and obstetric practices, there remain few formal structures and systems in place to ensure proper referral, treatment, and follow-up for those individuals with positive depression and anxiety screens.

When someone screens positive for depression in the perinatal period, it is critical to rule out a bipolar spectrum disorder, as up to 20% of women who screen positive for perinatal depression may have bipolar disorder (Clark et al., 2015). This becomes clinically relevant, as misdiagnosis in this scenario can lead to treatment with an unopposed antidepressant, which can result in hypomania, mania, or poor treatment response. Validated tools for bipolar disorder screening include the Mood Disorder Questionnaire (MDQ) and the Composite International Diagnostic Interview (CIDI). Both tools have high sensitivity and specificity and take 5–10 minutes to complete.

Many women are at increased risk for substance use during the perinatal period, particularly those who are experiencing anxiety or mood disorders. Several professional organizations recommend universal screening for perinatal substance use disorders. This screening is typically performed during the initial obstetric visit, with ongoing screening at subsequent appointments in perinatal care if the initial screening is positive. Validated screening tools in the perinatal period include 4Ps Plus (Chasnoff et al., 2007), NIDA Quick Screen (Coleman-Cowger et al., 2019),

Substance Use Risk Profile-Pregnancy (SURP-P) (Yonkers et al., 2010), and the CRAFFT (CAR, RELAX, ALONE, FORGET, FRIENDS, TROUBLE) (Knight et al., 2002), which is recommended in adolescent populations. It is important to note that using blood or urine testing is not recommended for screening purposes for several reasons, including possible legal ramifications of a positive test, the inability of a positive test to indicate use patterns or severity, and the risk of false positive tests. There must be ongoing efforts to provide appropriate education regarding reporting requirements and psychoeducation to address the stigma associated with perinatal substance use disorder. These efforts ensure a transparent screening process that results in therapeutic outcomes. Providers are also encouraged to screen for behavioral addictions, as these may also have impacts during the perinatal period (Cox, 2023).

Barriers and Facilitators to Access of Mental Health and Substance Use Care

Mental health is an essential part of overall well-being. When an individual is experiencing symptoms of mental illnesses and/or using substances, receiving care to support their needs may be critical to their functioning. However, not everyone is able to access care when needed, and women report experiencing barriers to care at higher rates than their male counterparts (Agterberg et al., 2020), especially barriers related to family responsibilities, relationship factors, and mental health concerns.

From a systems perspective, general availability (Goel et al., 2023; Jackson & Shannon, 2012; Priester et al., 2016) is a commonly and frequently identified barrier. Elements may include a lack of providers or appointments (Espinoza-Kulick & Cerdeña, 2022; Tyokighir et al., 2022), a lack of access to the level of care needed (e.g., inpatient beds, residential treatment, or intensive outpatient care) (Priester et al., 2016), or a lack of available specialty care, such as gender-specific treatment or services including perinatal mental health providers (Jackson & Shannon, 2012; Owens et al., 2007; Priester et al., 2016; Solway et al., 2010; Webb et al., 2021). Another common systemic barrier is transportation when the actual location of services is cited as being inaccessible or difficult to access via public transportation (Espinoza-Kulick & Cerdeña, 2022; Miranda & Green, 1999; Priester et al., 2016). However, the nature of this barrier has evolved since the onset of telemedicine services during the COVID-19 pandemic. Lack of childcare is also frequently cited as something that prevents women from accessing care (Agterberg et al., 2020; Espinoza-Kulick & Cerdeña, 2022; Priester et al., 2016; Tyokighir et al., 2022).

A major systemic barrier to accessing needed mental and/or substance use services is cost, exacerbated by a lack of insurance or being underinsured (Miranda & Green, 1999; Owens et al., 2007; Roll et al., 2013; Tyokighir et al., 2022), especially for those individuals who have Medicaid insurance (Barnett & Huskamp, 2020). An analysis of reports from the National Center for Health Statistics found the rates of unmet mental health-care needs, prior to the implementation of the Affordable Care Act, rose from 4.3 million individuals in 1997 to 7.2 million individuals in 2011, primarily among 18–64-year-olds. The rates of unmet need were five times higher in those individuals who did not have insurance compared to those individuals who held private insurance. Women also reported more unmet needs than men (Roll et al., 2013).

Staff-related concerns are another systemic barrier to accessing care. These include rude or disinterested staff (including perceived stigma of a provider towards a patient) or previous bad experiences with care (DeSa et al., 2022; Owens et al., 2007; Webb et al., 2021). An added layer of difficulty is racial/cultural/ethnic discrimination which can also include a lack of knowledge from providers about the impact of immigration, cultural experiences, and systemic racism on mental health symptoms and/or symptom presentation. Additionally, a lack of providers with a similar cultural, ethnic, or other "like me" identities (Goel et al., 2023) or general cultural competence (DeSa et al., 2022; Owens et al., 2007) can be a barrier.

A nationally representative survey (Williams et al., 2022) found sexual minority women (defined as bisexual and gay-lesbian women) reported poorer self-rated behavioral health care, the largest number of barriers in accessing care, and a greater need for this type of care. When comparing heterosexual women to heterosexual men, women reported poorer self-rated behavioral health care and greater barriers. The researchers hypothesized that sexism may be a factor in access and quality of care in both heterosexual and LGBTQIA+ women. They noted that identifying the discrepancies in quality and access barriers in sexual minority groups may be further hindered by this sexism, as most research within this community tends to focus on gay men (Williams et al., 2022). Older LGBTQIA+ adults reported they waited longer or not sought care because they would not be able to see a provider with a similar identity to their own (Solway et al., 2010).

In addition to cultural competence, lack of services in languages other than English are identified as a barrier to care. This could include not only a lack of services in one's preferred spoken language but also a lack of services that matches a linguistic or cultural understanding of terminology versus a direct word-for-word translation. Other staffing-related barriers include a lack of collaboration between providers, lack of resources, a lack of confidence or training in providing services, or a lack of knowledge needed to recognize specific symptoms and related disorders (Solway et al., 2010; Tyokighir et al., 2022; Webb et al., 2021). Many individuals first access mental health care with their primary care providers (Goel et al., 2023); these providers may not have enough knowledge to accurately diagnose a mental health concern and/or to recommend appropriate treatment.

Other systemic barriers include societal stigma and the involvement with multiple systems (e.g., criminal justice system or Child Protective Services agencies) where a woman might be punished for experiencing a mental disorder or using substances (Agterberg et al., 2020; Priester et al., 2016; Stone, 2015).

Given all the potential barriers to access, what then helps women to access much needed care? According to Webb et al. (2021), "to understand fully what women need in terms of appropriate care, flexibility, and choice, care should be designed with women at the center and co-produced with women with lived experience..." (p. 531). In a comprehensive review of treatment for women with substance use disorders, several factors were found to facilitate treatment completion and better outcomes. Outcomes were defined as decreased use, reduced mental health symptoms, improved birth outcomes in women who were pregnant, higher employment rates, and improved general health status. Facilitators included access to childcare, engagement in prenatal care, women-only programming, psychoeducation about supplemental topics of interest and/or focus for women, concurrent mental health treatment, and overall comprehensive treatment options (e.g., therapeutic communities) (Ashley et al., 2003).

Staff can act as either as systemic barriers or facilitators. This includes having clear referral pathways, dedicated staff to complete outreach or assessment, supportive management and/or good supervision of staff (Webb et al., 2021), strong relationships between staff and patients, and culturally sensitive and competent staff, including those who have the knowledge of potential cultural differences in symptom presentation (Goel et al., 2023). Specifically, having the ability to see a provider with a similar background might increase access, recognition, and understanding of mental health concerns in historically underrepresented communities (Goel et al., 2023).

Facilitators for access include increased availability, accessibility, and flexibility of treatment, such as a wider range of scheduled times, including "after hours" appointments (Webb et al., 2021), and flexibility in how interventions are applied such as in person, via telehealth, or in home. When appointments shifted to telehealth during the COVID-19 pandemic, women accessed mental health appointments at higher rates than they had during pre-pandemic (Egan et al., 2022). Offering services (both specialty and gender-specific) within underserved communities (Ashley et al., 2003; DeSa et al., 2022) and in locations that are connected to good public transit options (Webb et al., 2021) with accessible buildings (e.g., ramps for wheelchairs or strollers) or offering transportation facilitated access to care. Childcare services also allowed women to access care at higher rates (Ashley et al., 2003; Miranda & Green, 1999). Social support and education can facilitate access, especially when women were able to engage in open intergenerational conversations (DeSa et al., 2022). Education for patients and providers should include information on specific disorders and symptoms, available services, and supplemental or gender-specific topics (Ashley et al., 2003). Integrated mental health-care models offer many of the facilitators described above.

Barriers and Facilitators to Integrating Mental Health Care

In general, integrated mental health care is considered feasible and acceptable by patients, providers, and health-care systems. Barriers reported pertain mainly to implementation challenges, such as underutilization, team dynamics, and financial and interdepartmental issues (Prom et al., 2021). Facilitators of successful implementation of integrated care models, such as CoCM, include strong inter-professional communication through standardized workflows and care managers with clear role definitions and personal qualities such as being adaptable, motivated, and organized (Wood et al., 2017). Factors associated with improved patient outcomes in CoCM include strong leadership support, a strong primary care physician who champions patients, an accessible on-site care manager, psychiatrists who are engaged with patients, and warm handoffs (face-to-face communication) between the care manager and the primary care physician for new patients (Whitebird et al., 2014).

Unique Barriers and Facilitators to Integration in Perinatal Care Settings

The perinatal period provides unique opportunities and challenges for the integration of collaborative care. These may be best understood by dividing them into system factors, provider factors, and patient factors.

Systemwide challenges to the development and running of an integrated care model in perinatal care settings include complexities in reimbursement. For example, while there have been new developments in how collaborative care services may be coded to receive reimbursement, prenatal and postnatal care is often covered via bundled payments (Miller et al., 2020). This bundling may make justifying additional costs of operating the collaborative care program difficult. Additionally, another challenge for initiating care in the prenatal period is that this period is both time sensitive and time limited. While being able to quickly access mental health services is always the goal, the quickly changing nature of the prenatal period increases the urgency to access these services. Women's bodies, social circumstances, economic opportunities, and medical conditions change rapidly over the course of weeks in this setting, while they may be more stable or slow to change when an individual is not pregnant or postpartum (Sakowicz et al., 2022).

Facilitators to the implementation of collaborative care programs in the peripartum period are multiple validated screening and monitoring scales that already exist for this population. These tools include the PHQ-9 (depression), EPDS (depression), GAD-7 (anxiety), and WHIPLASHED (bipolar disorder) (Miller et al., 2020). These tools are necessary for population and measurement-based care, essential elements of collaborative care. Additionally, the peripartum period is often a time in which women may have access to health insurance when they otherwise would not.

Provider-associated challenges to the success of an integrated care program in the perinatal period include discomfort, insufficient training, and concerns about scope of practice for OB-GYNs in the treatment of psychiatric illness (Byatt et al., 2012b). Most research on collaborative care has been in primary care settings. The difference in expertise and comfort between obstetric providers and primary care providers may necessitate distinct types of training and levels of support. A unique element of the postnatal period revolves around which providers patients see most frequently. During prenatal care, patients will have higher-frequency contact with obstetric providers which then shifts to pediatricians in the postpartum period. The need to include pediatric providers to adequately maintain ease of contact with patients in the postpartum period increases the complexity of optimized interventions (Cox et al., 2016).

The largest facilitator to the implementation of a collaborative care model for this population is the frequency with which women will interact with their OB-GYNs. One-third of all visits for reproductive age women and many non-illness-related visits for women under age 65 are provided by OB-GYNs (Scholle et al., 2002). Routine prenatal care for an uncomplicated pregnancy includes approximately 15 encounters over the course of 40 weeks, which would provide numerous time points for screening, treatment, and monitoring of psychiatric illness (Committee on Obstetric Practice, 2015; Earls et al., 2019).

The prenatal period may provide a window of opportunity during which pregnant patients may be more willing or motivated to effect change in their life. The substance use and nicotine use disorder treatment literature indicates that pregnancy is a time of heightened motivation and willingness for a patient to engage in life changes, including engaging with mental health issues (Orleans et al., 2001). However, pregnancy may also be a period of heightened vulnerability for many patients. Patients report concerns about discussing depressive symptoms with their providers. Patients worry that providers will negatively judge their ability to mother their children or are fearful that they will lose custody of their children due to being depressed (Byatt et al., 2012b). Patients also may minimize, normalize, or confuse depressive symptoms as signs of normal pregnancy. Additionally, patients express increased hesitancy about pharmacotherapy in pregnancy due to concerns (founded or not) for what effects it may have on their pregnancy or child (Byatt et al., 2012b). The postpartum period also brings changes which may increase barriers to patients receiving care. Physical demands and changing priorities of childcare, breastfeeding, or physical recovery may limit a patient's time and capacity to engage in mental health care (Miller et al., 2020).

Approaches to Integration of Women's Evidence-Based Mental and Substance Use Treatment

Integrated behavioral health models are most frequently designed for the treatment of common mental disorders, such as depression and anxiety. However, collaborative care for substance use disorder and indirect psychiatric consultation for bipolar disorder have emerging evidence for successful treatment (Wendt et al., 2020). Approaches to integration of women's behavioral health care are summarized below.

Perinatal Psychiatry Access Programs

Perinatal psychiatry access programs (referred to as access programs) are population-level programs that improve perinatal mental health. Modeled after child psychiatry access programs, these state-specific programs increase access to pediatric mental health services by supporting pediatric primary care providers through telephone consultation, care coordination, and in-person clinical consultations (Straus & Sarvet, 2014). The aim of access programs is to increase access to perinatal mental health and substance use disorder treatments. These programs increase the capacity of frontline providers (such as obstetric and primary care providers) to identify and manage common mental disorders within the obstetric or primary care setting.

Access programs are based on the observation that mental health issues are common during the perinatal period and can be identified in prenatal and primary care settings using standardized screening tools. However, referral to specialty mental health care may not be effective, as only 22% of women with depression obtain mental health care when referred out after a positive screening (Byatt et al., 2015). Mental health treatment provided as part of regular prenatal care is more easily accessed. Additionally, the perinatal period (pregnancy through 1 year postpartum), with its frequent health-care encounters, is an ideal setting for identification and follow-up within the framework of a longitudinal trusting relationship between the patient and prenatal provider. Access programs were therefore developed as a scalable solution to perinatal mental health treatment gaps, by building the capacity of frontline providers to screen for and to manage common mental disorders in pregnancy and postpartum. Although access programs began with a focus on depression and anxiety, many programs have since expanded to provide consultation on perinatal bipolar disorder and substance use disorders as well.

The Massachusetts Child Psychiatry Access Program (MCPAP) for Moms, established in 2014, was the first access program in the United States (Massachusetts Child Psychiatry Access Program for Moms (Boston), 2017), followed by the Washington State's Perinatal Psychiatry Consultation Line (PPCL) in 2016 (Cowley et al., 2022) and Wisconsin's Periscope Project in 2017 (Wichman et al., 2019). There are currently 14 programs in the United States, and Postpartum Support International's Perinatal Psychiatry Consultation Line can answer calls nationally.

The three most common components of access programs are (1) real-time provider-to-provider teleconsultation, (2) community resource information, and (3) provider education. Additional services include one-time provider to patient clinical consultation.

Provider-to-Provider Teleconsultation

Typically, a perinatal or reproductive psychiatrist is available to provide real-time psychiatric telephone consultation to frontline providers. Depending on the caller's question, many issues, such as diagnosis, treatment planning, choice or dose of medication and considerations during pregnancy and lactation, and type of evidence-based therapy, can be addressed. The psychiatrist provides recommendations and case-based education for each caller, tailored to the caller's skills and comfort level (Byatt et al., 2012a). This real-time consultation supports the frontline provider who may not have confidence managing perinatal mental health disorders and improves patient care since recommendations can be received and implemented during the patients' prenatal or postpartum visit.

Programs also differ in the type of provider who is eligible to call (prescriber or not) and whether organizations or clinics are "enrolled" into the access programs before the providers can call for consultation. Access programs serve a diverse set of providers who care for perinatal individuals such as obstetric, pediatric, primary care, therapists, and community health workers. Approximately 15–16% of consultations are from psychiatric providers, perhaps reflecting the lack of standardized training in perinatal mental health during psychiatry residency training.

Community Resource Information

Access programs may have a resource and referral specialist or team who helps to connect the patient to outpatient mental health and substance use treatment including individual and group therapy or prescribers. Programs vary in whether this resource information is provided to the caller or directly to the patient.

Provider Education

Programs provide education to frontline providers through webinars, trainings, and toolkits. Education is provided on topics, such as screening for perinatal mental health and substance use disorders, how to discuss the results of screening with patients, treatment planning, and risks and benefits of medication during pregnancy and postpartum. Interestingly, there is emerging evidence that the process of providing telephone consultation itself may serve an educational purpose. The complexity of calls to access programs has increased over time, reflecting the fact that frontline providers are caring for perinatal patients who have increasingly complex psychiatric presentations. This could be due to the increased availability of perinatal mental health training and consultation which improves the callers' knowledge level, confidence, and motivation to treat perinatal mental health conditions because of consultation.

Patient Consultation

Access programs may provide a one-time patient evaluation and consultation with recommendations to the obstetric and primary care providers. This is often offered when the complexity of a case makes it challenging to provide adequate recommendations by telephone consultation alone. The advent of telepsychiatry has made this component more accessible.

Access program evaluations have mostly been descriptive and focused on utilization and caller satisfaction. All programs, which have reported metrics, have found high rates of utilization and caller satisfaction. Utilization of call lines has increased over time. Medication management and diagnostic questions were most common in all programs reporting this metric, indicative of the topic areas in which perinatal clinicians require the most support. There is a need to improve evaluation of access programs and include evaluation of patient outcomes when possible.

The total costs of these programs (after start up) range from $5.60 (Wichman et al., 2019) to $8.38 per pregnant and postpartum individual per year (Byatt et al., 2018). Funding comes from a variety of sources. In the first ever federal funding specifically to address perinatal mental health in the United States, the "Bringing Postpartum Depression out of the Shadows Act" awarded seven states five-year grants to create perinatal psychiatry access programs (Maternal Mental Health Leadership Alliance, 2020, November 23). Funding for other perinatal psychiatry access programs is from state and philanthropic grants.

Collaborative Care Model

Using a registry and a multidisciplinary team, the CoCM approach uses systematic screening and tracking of patient mental health outcomes (e.g., depression and/or anxiety). An on-site behavioral care manager provides brief psychological interventions (behavioral activation, brief interpersonal therapy, or problem-solving treatment). Cases are reviewed regularly with a psychiatrist who provides recommendations to the primary care team, modifying recommendations in response to measurement of symptoms. Collaborative care models have well established effectiveness in primary care populations and more recently in women's mental health and in prenatal care (Bhat et al., 2018; Grote et al., 2016; Huang et al., 2017; Miller et al., 2020). Implementation of a perinatal CoCM program leads to an increase in the rates of antenatal screening for depression, and women with a positive antenatal screen for depression are more likely to receive a treatment recommendation (Miller et al., 2021).

Women who engage in CoCM are more likely to initiate and continue breastfeeding compared to those who do not engage in CoCM (Allen et al., 2022). CoCM, with or without cultural/linguistic tailoring, can improve depression for racial/ethnic minorities, as well as women from low socioeconomic backgrounds (Hu et al., 2020). This is particularly relevant to women's mental health given the well-documented racial and ethnic disparities in depression care and outcomes (Huang et al., 2012; Kozhimannil et al., 2011). Specifically, in the perinatal population, an evaluation of racial disparities found that before implementation of CoCM, Black individuals were more likely to receive screening but less likely to have a treatment recommended when a positive screen was identified. After implementation of CoCM, there were no significant differences by race in screening or treatment recommendations (Snowber et al., 2022). Also, there is emerging evidence of the cost effectiveness of CoCM; the highest costs per depression-free day were $24 US (van Steenbergen-Weijenburg et al., 2010). For women with probable major depression and post-traumatic stress disorder, CoCM has significant clinical benefit with only a moderate increase in health services cost (Grote et al., 2017).

Co-located Integrated Care

Primary Care Behavioral Health (PCBH) is an approach which shares some of the features of the CoCM but is distinct in several regards (Reiter et al., 2018). In this model, the behavioral health specialist (also known as the "primary care behaviorist") is on the team, typically a psychologist, clinical social worker, or counselor, and is physically co-located within the primary care clinic and available to all patients within the practice rather than exclusively those with mental health diagnoses. The specialist often assists in addressing issues that can affect patient treatment and health, including stress management for episodic stressors and behavioral strategies for smoking cessation, exercise, and diet. The behaviorist may offer services, including evidence-based screenings and time-limited therapeutic interventions. Their presence within the clinic allows primary care physicians to communicate directly with the behaviorist about the patient and their needs and for patients to have coordinated behavioral health access with their visits to the primary care physician for convenience, decreased stigma, and lessened barrier to engagement in care.

The PCBH model has been demonstrated in research studies to improve patient outcomes. One randomized controlled trial found that PCBH approaches for depression management led to greater use of coping strategies, improved adherence to treatment regimens recommended by the primary care physician, and increased patient satisfaction (Robinson et al., 2020). A second study indicated that implementation of the PCBH model was associated with fewer "all-cause" emergency room visits and hospital admissions (Maeng et al., 2022). When integrated into a women's health clinic, the PCBH model was well received by patients, with attendance and engagement rates for referred patients similar to other PCBH settings (Carroll et al., 2020). While to date the model has been primarily used in the women's health setting for managing depressive symptoms (Lomonaco-Haycraft et al., 2019), it has also been proposed as a way to improve care after miscarriage (Hiefner & Villareal, 2021) and to provide care in a resident OB-GYN clinic (Dang & Salcedo, 2023).

The OB-GYN PCBH model has been found to be feasible and acceptable. Patients want to receive education on pregnancy-related topics, such as exercise, healthy eating, and mood disorders. They also appreciated the support of the collocated behavioral health counselor in managing pregnancy-related stress, depression, and anxiety. Despite overall acceptability, there was also stigma among patients about seeking mental health support within the PCBH. In general, the PCBH model is best suited for behavioral and lifestyle interventions and more mild mental health issues given its short-term nature and the absence of a psychiatrist on the team to address more complex mental health needs.

Peer Mentored Care Models

In addition to perinatal access programs, other models, under the umbrella of Peer Mentored Care Models, have been introduced to increase access to expert specialty care and knowledge by educating providers. One such approach is that of eConsults within a given hospital system. In 2014, the American Association of Medical Colleges (AAMC) launched "Project CORE" to improve efficiency of communication between primary care physicians and specialist clinicians in academic medical center settings in cases. A primary care physician may have a question that may not require in-person evaluation of the patient (AAMC, 2023). Primary care physicians place an order for an "eConsult" where they can provide information about the case and their question for the specialist electronically. The physician then receives an asynchronous text-based response within 3 days with guidance for next steps in clinical management.

As of 2023, Project CORE has expanded to over 50 academic medical centers and estimates that 2000 eConsults are placed every month. Evaluations of the model have suggested that patients have been receptive to this framework, especially when they report a positive relationship with their primary care physician. Patients note benefits such as fewer referral appointments with associated costs as well as accelerated workups when referral appointments were considered indicated by the specialist (Ackerman et al., 2020). The eConsults model was also considered acceptable by 89% of primary health-care providers and met key indicators of clinical safety while decreasing patient care costs (Thompson et al., 2021). Optimizing design features that improve usability, and protecting clinical time for the additional administrative burden posed to primary care providers further improves the sustainability of such models (Gleason et al., 2018).

The Extension for Community Healthcare Outcomes (ECHO) model, first launched in 2003 by the University of New Mexico (UNM) (Arora et al., 2007), similarly seeks to educate providers and increase access to feedback from specialists but does so in a virtual group setting. Primary care providers present anonymized cases to a specialist and receive feedback in real time. Sometimes referred to as "tele-mentoring" and "tele-education," these sessions are intended to mimic academic case conferences. Typically, the ECHO model entails a team of specialists at a regional academic center hosting a weekly teleconsultation hour for affiliated remote primary care sites, typically in underserved locations. Primary care providers learn from both their peers and the specialist and, due to the interactive format, can communicate in detail about nuances of the case that may influence management. In the field of psychiatry, ECHO models have been used to improve evidence-based suboxone prescribing in rural areas (Anderson et al., 2022) and are supported by the American Psychiatric Association (2023) to expand access to child and adolescent psychiatry specialists. Attendance at these case conferences has expanded beyond the academic institution to better serve local needs. UNM currently hosts ECHO programs for reproductive health and perinatal health that each meet twice monthly and encompass mental health intersections with these topics. The target audience for these sessions includes not only clinicians at UNM but also midwives, community health workers, and peer support specialists from across the state (New Mexico Perinatal ECHO, 2023).

Similarly, the Georgia Maternal Health ECHO (2023, January 25) meets monthly to address cases involving maternal morbidity and mortality, including perinatal substance use, and the Washington State Mom's Access Project ECHO (Ramaraj et al., 2023) and the Colorado Perinatal Mental Health ECHO program (2023) focus on perinatal mental health and substance use. All ECHOs are open to clinicians and community advocates from across the state. Other clinicians within the field have recreated the spirit of the ECHO model tele-mentoring model while eliminating the hub-and-spoke framework that connects specific sites within the community. One example of this adjusted model is the weekly "virtual rounds" hosted by the Massachusetts General Hospital's Center for Women's Mental Health (MGH Center for Women's Mental Health, 2023), which provides similar case-based discussion with peers and experts but accepts participation from behavioral health specialists of all role descriptions in addition to primary care providers across the nation.

Community-Based Programs and Providers

Community-based programs can support mental health indirectly or directly. Given the well-established connection between the social determinants of health and mental health, it follows that addressing an individual's social determinants of health can indirectly have a beneficial effect on their mental health. For example, people with severe mental illnesses face significant marginalization and vulnerability in society, underscoring the importance of interventions to enhance their social and economic participation. A recent systematic review by Killaspy et al. (2022) examined various interventions targeting either the service level or individuals directly. Encouraging evidence was found for the Housing First model (team assisting persons to find, move into, and sustain a tenancy), Individual Placement and Support model (supported employment), and family psychoeducation. However, diverse models are necessary to address the diverse needs of individuals. It was emphasized that contextual factors and local adaptations are crucial when implementing interventions from different settings. Peer-led/supported interventions, recovery colleges, and community participation support also displayed emerging evidence. Overall, social interventions offer significant benefits but are complex to implement, needing commitment and investment from multiple stakeholders to be successful.

In the perinatal period, community-based programs, such as home visiting and doula services, are vital for promoting women's mental health during pregnancy, childbirth, and the postpartum period. These programs provide support, resources, and guidance, leading to improved maternal mental health outcomes. Home visiting programs involve professionals visiting homes, offering education, support, and mental health screening, resulting in reduced perinatal depression rates and better parenting skills. Doulas provide continuous emotional and physical support, leading to lower intervention rates, higher satisfaction, and reduced postpartum depression (Quiray et al., 2024). Both interventions alleviate stress, anxiety, and isolation, contributing to the prevention and early detection of mood disorders. By prioritizing the utilization of social support, home visiting programs show significant potential to add structural support and achieve health equity at the system level (Bhat et al., 2021). They empower women, enhance their well-being and resilience, and should be integrated into health care systems for widespread accessibility and improved overall family well-being. Further, there is emerging evidence on the success of directly providing mental health services within community settings. Integrating mental health screening and treatment into community settings has the added advantage of addressing mental health and substance use concerns in the context of other needs and social determinants of health.

The mental health workforce faces challenges in reaching the growing population of individuals with mental illnesses, particularly among disadvantaged groups. Task sharing, an approach used commonly in global mental health, is one way to address mental health workforce challenges in low-resource settings. In this approach, tasks are shifted from individuals with more specialized training to individuals with less specialized training (Hoeft et al., 2016). Peers or community health workers (CHWs) are trained to provide screening and brief behavioral interventions. Recent reviews suggest that mental health CHWs have the potential to improve mental health outcomes, especially for underserved communities, by providing culturally competent care, reducing stigma and improving access to referrals and treatment (Weaver & Lapidos, 2018).

Although the feasibility of screening for perinatal depression in community-based settings is well established, there is a need to evaluate feasibility of screening for perinatal anxiety. Importantly, there are no studies examining the feasibility of integrating mental health care into community settings or social services (Webb et al., 2021). A recent project that included community-based organizations within a CoCM team for the treatment of late life depression found adaptability, opportunities for multi-level partnerships within and across organizations, and fostering a commitment to partnership can support the work of partnering across health care and community-based organizations (Henderson et al., 2020). Factors that contribute to program success include actively bridging nonmedical and medical service delivery systems, addressing the unique needs of specific local populations, building on community strengths and resources, and participating in strategic collaborative partnerships with local community organizations (Sherry et al., 2016).

Most importantly, as women with more severe symptoms cannot be managed in community-based settings and need to be referred to the health-care system, any program that aims to integrate mental health screening and treatment into community-based settings will need to have a strong and secure care and communication pathway. This aspect of bidirectional connection between traditionally siloed health care and community-based services needs further attention. While developing such models is a complex challenge (Henderson et al., 2020), ideal patient-centered service delivery models will seamlessly integrate medical, social, and other services.

Integration of Women's Mental Health Treatment: A Global Perspective

Globally, mental health accounts for the highest number of disability-adjusted life years (DALYs) (Ferrari et al., 2013) . Efforts to integrate mental health care have focused on doing so within existing priority platforms, such as HIV care and maternal and child health care (Collins et al., 2011; Patel et al., 2013; Prince et al., 2007). However, social determinants of mental health (poverty, discrimination, and interpersonal violence) are disproportionately higher among women. In addition to increasing access to mental health treatments, effective promotion of women's mental health will need to include attention to eliminating discrimination and involve women in decision-making, not only in treatment planning but also in decisions which affect their lives more broadly. Women have lower income relative to men, and more women live in absolute poverty than men; women account for approximately 70% of the world's poor (Action Steps for Improving Women's Mental Health, U. S. Department of Health and Human Services Department, Office on Women's Health [2009]). In low-income and middle-income countries, mental illness and poverty perpetuate negative cycles. Economic programs (conditional cash transfer and asset promotion programs) have been shown to have some mental health benefits, and conversely, some mental health interventions are associated with improved economic outcomes (Lund et al., 2011).

Women's autonomy or "control over their lives" includes freedom from violence, participation in family decisions (both noneconomic and economic), and community involvement (Agarwala & Lynch, 2006). Autonomy is directly associated with the ability to access health care. In many countries, ratings of autonomy and empowerment among women are disproportionately low. It is therefore critically important to strengthen social networks for additional support to women and reduce income inequality. Self-help groups (SHGs) are one such example of broader social and economic support to women, which can be used to provide health education and connect women to treatment. Ubiquitous in low- and middle-income countries, such as India and Bangladesh, especially in rural areas, these SHGs include groups of 10–15 women from the same community, who meet every week to build skills, such as sewing, and to participate in microfinancing. Recently, SHGs have been used as a platform for health education, as one study found prenatal education delivered in SHGs led to improved birth outcomes (Tripathy et al., 2010). There is a move to similarly include mental health education in SHGs, which could serve the dual role of education and destigmatization.

Implications for Women's Behavioral Health

Ensuring high-quality integrated behavioral health treatment for women requires coordination and collaboration between women's health, prenatal, primary care, pediatric, public health and allied health providers, payors, and policymakers. Evidence-based models of integrated behavioral health treatment can be success-fully applied to women's health care with some modifications. For example, in the case of perinatal mental health treatments, extending the duration of the postpartum period beyond the traditionally defined 6 weeks can expand mental health treatment access to more women in need, through 1 year postpartum. Policy changes to the definition of the postpartum period for the purposes of insurance can support this modification. This may indirectly decrease racial-ethnic disparities, as Hispanic, Black, and indigenous women who are disproportionally enrolled in pregnancy Medicaid experience higher rates of loss of insurance in the postpartum period. Integrated approaches can also be enriched by close collaboration with other health-care and community-based providers who interact frequently with women, such as pediatric providers and home visiting nurses. There is a need for reimbursement for the non-encounter-based case management and navigation that is often required to support coordination across multiple systems of care. Other policies that may sup-port integrated behavioral health treatments for women include adding quality met-rics such as rates of depression screening and follow-up and rates of mental health treatment completion.

Further research is needed to evaluate the effectiveness of access programs and of peer mentor models in the treatment of women's behavioral health treatments. Given the critical importance of community-based providers and programs in improving access to women's behavioral health treatments, it is essential to include the perspectives of community-based providers in designing and implementing integrated models of care.

References

Ackerman, S. L., Dowdell, K., Clebak, K. T., Quinn, M., & Shipman, S. A. (2020). Patients assess an eConsult Model's acceptability at 5 US academic medical centers. *Annals of Family Medicine, 18*(1), 35–41. https://doi.org/10.1370/afm.2487

Agarwala, R., & Lynch, S. M. (2006). Refining the measurement of women's autonomy: An inter-national application of a multi-dimensional construct. *Social Forces, 84*(4), 2077–2098. https://doi.org/10.1353/sof.2006.0079

Agterberg, S., Schubert, N., Overington, L., & Corace, K. (2020). Treatment barriers among individuals with co-occurring substance use and mental health problems: Examining gender differences. *Journal of Substance Abuse Treatment, 112,* 29–35. https://doi.org/10.1016/j. jsat.2020.01.005

Allen, E. C., Sakowicz, A., Parzyszek, C. L., McDonald, A., & Miller, E. S. (2022). The association between engagement in a perinatal collaborative care program and breastfeeding among people with identified mental health conditions. *American Journal of Obstetrics & Gynecology MFM, 4*(3), 100591. https://doi.org/10.1016/j.ajogmf.2022.100591

American College of Obstetricians and Gynecologists. (2015). Committee Opinion No. 630. Screening for perinatal depression. *Obstetrics and Gynecology, 125*(5), 1268–1271. https:// doi.org/10.1097/01.AOG.0000465192.34779.dc

American Psychiatric Association. (2023). *Child & adolescent telepsychiatry.* [Web page]. APA. https://www.psychiatry.org/psychiatrists/practice/telepsychiatry/toolkit/ child-adolescent/project-echo

American Psychological Association. (2022). *Behavioral Health Integration* [Fact sheet]. https:// www.apa.org/health/behavioral-health-factsheet.pdf

Anderson, J. B., Martin, S. A., Gadomski, A., Krupa, N., Mullin, D., Cahill, A., & Jenkins, P. (2022). Project ECHO and primary care buprenorphine treatment for opioid use disorder: Implementation and clinical outcomes. *Substance Abuse, 43*(1), 222–230. https://doi.org/1 0.1080/08897077.2021.1931633

Arora, S., Geppert, C. M., Kalishman, S., Dion, D., Pullara, F., Bjeletich, M. B., Simpson, G., Alverson, D. C., Moore, L. B., & Kuhl, D. (2007). Academic health center management of chronic diseases through knowledge networks: Project ECHO. *Academic Medicine: Journal of the Association of American Medical Colleges, 82*(2), 154–160. https://doi.org/10.1097/ ACM.0b013e31802d8f68

Ashley, O. S., Marsden, M. E., & Brady, T. M. (2003). Effectiveness of substance abuse treatment programming for women: A review. *The American Journal of Drug and Alcohol Abuse, 29*(1), 19–53. https://doi.org/10.1081/ada-120018838

Association of American Medical Colleges. (2023). *Project CORE: Coordinating Optimal Referral Experiences.* [Web page]. AAMC. https://www.aamc.org/what-we-do/mission-areas/ health-care/project-core

Barnett, M. L., & Huskamp, H. A. (2020). Telemedicine for mental health in the United States: Making progress, still a long way to go. *Psychiatric Services, 71*(2), 197–198. https://doi. org/10.1176/appi.ps.201900555

Barry, M. J., Nicholson, W. K., Silverstein, M., Coker, T. R., Davidson, K. W., Davis, E. M., Donahue, K. E., Jaén, C. R., Li, L., & Ogedegbe, G. (2023). Screening for anxiety disorders in adults: US Preventive Services Task Force Recommendation Statement. *JAMA, 329*(24), 2163–2170. https://doi.org/10.1001/jama.2023.9301

Bhat, A., Reed, S. D., & Unützer, J. (2017). The obstetrician–gynecologist's role in detecting, preventing, and treating depression. *Obstetrics & Gynecology, 129(1), 157–163.*

Bhat, A., Reed, S., Mao, J., Vredevoogd, M., Russo, J., Unger, J., Rowles, R., & Unützer, J. (2018). Delivering perinatal depression care in a rural obstetric setting: A mixed methods study of feasibility, acceptability and effectiveness. *Journal of Psychosomatic Obstetrics & Gynecology, 39*(4), 273–280. https://doi.org/10.1080/0167482X.2017.1367381

Bhat, A., Nanda, A., Murphy, L., Ball, A. L., Fortney, J., & Katon, J. (2021). A systematic review of screening for perinatal depression and anxiety in community-based settings. *Archives of Women's Mental Health, 25*(1), 1–17. https://doi.org/10.1007/s00737-021-01151-2

Blount, A., & Bayona, J. (1994). Toward a system of integrated primary care. *Family Systems Medicine, 12*(2), 171–182. https://doi.org/10.1037/h0089151

Brunton, R. J., Dryer, R., Saliba, A., & Kohlhoff, J. (2015). Pregnancy anxiety: A systematic review of current scales. *Journal of Affective Disorders, 176,* 24–34. https://doi.org/10.1016/j. jad.2015.01.039

Byatt, N., Biebel, K., Lundquist, R. S., Moore Simas, T. A., Debordes-Jackson, G., Allison, J., & Ziedonis, D. (2012a). Patient, provider, and system-level barriers and facilitators to addressing perinatal depression. *Journal of Reproductive and Infant Psychology, 30*(5), 436–449. https://doi.org/10.1080/02646838.2012.743000

Byatt, N., Simas, T. A. M., Lundquist, R. S., Johnson, J. V., & Ziedonis, D. M. (2012b). Strategies for improving perinatal depression treatment in North American outpatient obstetric settings. *Journal of Psychosomatic Obstetrics & Gynecology, 33*(4), 143–161. https://doi.org/10.3109/0167482X.2012.728649

Byatt, N., Levin, L. L., Ziedonis, D., Moore Simas, T. A., & Allison, J. (2015). Enhancing participation in depression care in outpatient perinatal care settings: A systematic review. *Obstetrics and Gynecology, 126*(5), 1048–1058. https://doi.org/10.1097/aog.0000000000001067

Byatt, N., Straus, J., Stopa, A., Biebel, K., Mittal, L., & Simas, T. A. M. (2018). Massachusetts Child Psychiatry Access Program for Moms: Utilization and quality assessment. *Obstetrics and Gynecology, 132*(2), 345. https://doi.org/10.1097/AOG.0000000000002688

Byatt, N., Masters, G. A., Bergman, A. L., & Moore Simas, T. A. (2020). Screening for mental health and substance use disorders in obstetric settings. *Current Psychiatry Reports, 22*(11), 1–13. https://doi.org/10.1007/s11920-020-01182-z

Carroll, A. J., Jaffe, A. E., Stanton, K., Guille, C., Lazenby, G. B., Soper, D. E., Gilmore, A. K., & Holland-Carter, L. (2020). Program evaluation of an integrated behavioral health clinic in an outpatient women's health clinic: Challenges and considerations. *Journal of Clinical Psychology in Medical Settings, 27*(2), 207–216. https://doi.org/10.1007/s10880-019-09684-6

Chasnoff, I., Wells, A., McGourty, R., & Bailey, L. (2007). Validation of the 4P's Plus© screen for substance use in pregnancy validation of the 4P's Plus. *Journal of Perinatology, 27*(12), 744–748. https://doi.org/10.1038/sj.jp.7211823

Clark, C. T., Sit, D. K., Driscoll, K., Eng, H. F., Confer, A. L., Luther, J. F., Wisniewski, S. R., & Wisner, K. L. (2015). Does screening with the MDQ and EPDS improve identification of bipolar disorder in an obstetrical sample? *Depression and Anxiety, 32*(7), 518–526. https://doi.org/10.1002/da.22373

Coleman-Cowger, V. H., Oga, E. A., Peters, E. N., Trocin, K. E., Koszowski, B., & Mark, K. (2019). Accuracy of three screening tools for prenatal substance use. *Obstetrics and Gynecology, 133*(5), 952–961. https://doi.org/10.1097/AOG.0000000000003230

Collins, P. Y., Patel, V., Joestl, S. S., March, D., Insel, T. R., Daar, A. S., Bordin, I. A., Costello, E. J., Durkin, M., & Fairburn, C. (2011). Grand challenges in global mental health. *Nature, 475*(7354), 27–30. https://doi.org/10.1038/475027a

Committee on Obstetric Practice. (2015). The American College of Obstetricians and Gynecologists Committee Opinion no. 630. Screening for perinatal depression. *Obstetrics and Gynecology, 125*(5), 1268–1271. https://doi.org/10.1097/01.AOG.0000465192.34779.dc

Cowley, D. S., Yadama, A., Adachi, J., Kerlee, A., Forrester, M., & Bhat, A. (2022). Training and professional development needs of consultation line perinatal psychiatrists. *General Hospital Psychiatry, 78*, 130–132. https://doi.org/10.1016/j.genhosppsych.2022.04.008

Cox, K. (2023). Clinical considerations of behavioural addiction in pregnancy. In F. Prever, G. Blycker, & L. Brandt (Eds.), *Behavioural addiction in women* (pp. 47–52). Routledge.

Cox, E. Q., Sowa, N. A., Meltzer-Brody, S. E., & Gaynes, B. N. (2016). The perinatal depression treatment cascade: Baby steps toward improving outcomes. *The Journal of Clinical Psychiatry, 77*(9), 1189–1200. https://doi.org/10.4088/JCP.15r10174

Dang, D., & Salcedo, J. (2023). Patient acceptance of primary care behavioral health in a resident obstetrics and gynecology clinic. *Southern Medical Journal, 116*(9), 733–738. https://doi.org/10.14423/smj.0000000000001596

DeSa, S., Gebremeskel, A. T., Omonaiye, O., & Yaya, S. (2022). Barriers and facilitators to access mental health services among refugee women in high-income countries: A systematic review. *Systematic Reviews, 11*(1), Article 62. https://doi.org/10.1186/s13643-022-01936-1

Earls, M. F., Mattson, G., Rafferty, J., Yogman, M. W., & Committee on Psychosocial Aspects of Child Family Health. (2019). Incorporating recognition and management of perinatal depression into pediatric practice. *Pediatrics, 143*(1), Article e20183260. https://doi.org/10.1542/peds.2018-3260

ECHO Colorado. (2023). *Perinatal mental health: An interdisciplinary approach.* [Web page]. https://echocolorado.org/echo/perinatal-mental-health/

Egan, R. P., Hurley, D. B., Goetz, M. C., Smith, C. S., Palmer, B. A., & St Hill, C. A. (2022). Disparities in mental health access before and after transitioning to telehealth. *Journal of Rural Mental Health, 46*(4), 271–276. https://doi.org/10.1037/rmh0000214

Espinoza-Kulick, M. A. V., & Cerdeña, J. P. (2022). "We need health for all": Mental health and barriers to care among Latinxs in California and Connecticut. *International Journal of Environmental Research and Public Health, 19*(19), Article 12817. https://doi.org/10.3390/ijerph191912817

Ferrari, A. J., Charlson, F. J., Norman, R. E., Patten, S. B., Freedman, G., Murray, C. J., Vos, T., & Whiteford, H. A. (2013). Burden of depressive disorders by country, sex, age, and year: Findings from the Global Burden of Disease Study 2010. *PLoS Medicine, 10*(11), e1001547. https://doi.org/10.1371/journal.pmed.1001547

Georgia Maternal Health ECHO. (2023, Jan 25). *Maternal Health ECHO.* [Web page]. Georgia Department of Mental Health. https://dph.georgia.gov/maternal-health-echo

Gleason, N., Ackerman, S., & Shipman, S. A. (2018). eConsult: Transforming primary care or exacerbating clinician burnout? *JAMA Internal Medicine, 178*(6), 790–791. https://doi.org/10.1001/jamainternmed.2018.0762

Goel, N. J., Thomas, B., Boutté, R. L., Kaur, B., & Mazzeo, S. E. (2023). "What will people say?": Mental health stigmatization as a barrier to eating disorder treatment-seeking for South Asian American women. *Asian American Journal of Psychology, 14*(1), 96. https://doi.org/10.1037/aap0000271

Gregory, K. D., Chelmow, D., Nelson, H. D., Van Niel, M. S., Conry, J. A., Garcia, F., Kendig, S. M., O'Reilly, N., Qaseem, A., Ramos, D., Salganicoff, A., Son, S., Wood, J. K., Zahn, C., & Women's Preventive Services, I. (2020). Screening for anxiety in adolescent and adult women: A recommendation from the Women's Preventive Services Initiative. *Annals of Internal Medicine, 173*(1), 48–56. https://doi.org/10.7326/M20-0580

Grote, N. K., Katon, W. J., Russo, J. E., Lohr, M. J., Curran, M., Galvin, E., & Carson, K. (2016). A randomized trial of collaborative care for perinatal depression in socioeconomically disadvantaged women: The impact of comorbid posttraumatic stress disorder. *The Journal of Clinical Psychiatry, 77*(11), 1527–1537. https://doi.org/10.4088/JCP.15m10477

Grote, N. K., Simon, G. E., Russo, J., Lohr, M. J., Carson, K., & Katon, W. (2017). Incremental benefit-cost of MOMCare: Collaborative care for perinatal depression among economically disadvantaged women. *Psychiatric Services, 68*(11), 1164–1171. https://doi.org/10.1176/appi.ps.201600411

Henderson, S., Wagner, J. L., Gosdin, M. M., Hoeft, T. J., Unützer, J., Rath, L., & Hinton, L. (2020). Complexity in partnerships: A qualitative examination of collaborative depression care in primary care clinics and community-based organisations in California, United States. *Health & Social Care in the Community, 28*(4), 1199–1208. https://doi.org/10.1111/hsc.12953

Hiefner, A. R., & Villareal, A. (2021). A multidisciplinary, family-oriented approach to caring for parents after miscarriage: The integrated behavioral health model of care. *Frontiers in Public Health, 9*, 725762. https://doi.org/10.3389/fpubh.2021.725762

Hoeft, T. J., Fortney, J. C., Patel, V., & Unützer, J. (2016). Task-sharing approaches to improve mental health care in rural and other low-resource settings: A systematic review. *Journal of Rural Health, 34*(1), 48–62. https://doi.org/10.1111/jrh.12229

Hu, J., Wu, T., Damodaran, S., Tabb, K. M., Bauer, A., & Huang, H. (2020). The effectiveness of collaborative care on depression outcomes for racial/ethnic minority populations in primary care: A systematic review. *Psychosomatics, 61*(6), 632–644. https://doi.org/10.1016/j.psym.2020.03.007

Huang, H., Chan, Y. F., Katon, W., Tabb, K., Sieu, N., Bauer, A. M., Wasse, J. K., & Unutzer, J. (2012). Variations in depression care and outcomes among high-risk mothers from different racial/ethnic groups. *Family Practice, 29*(4), 394–400. https://doi.org/10.1093/fampra/cmr108

Huang, H. M., Tabb, K. M., Cerimele, J., Ahmed, N., Bhat, A., & Kester, R. (2017). Collaborative care for women with depression: A systematic review. *Psychosomatics, 58*(1), 11–18. https://doi.org/10.1016/j.psym.2016.09.002

Jackson, A., & Shannon, L. (2012). Barriers to receiving substance abuse treatment among rural pregnant women in Kentucky. *Maternal and Child Health Journal, 16*(9), 1762–1770. https://doi.org/10.1007/s10995-011-0923-5

Kessler, R. C., Petukhova, M., Sampson, N. A., Zaslavsky, A. M., & Wittchen, H. U. (2012). Twelve-month and lifetime prevalence and lifetime morbid risk of anxiety and mood disorders in the United States. *International Journal of Methods in Psychiatric Research, 21*(3), 169–184. https://doi.org/10.1002/mpr.1359

Killaspy, H., Harvey, C., Brasier, C., Brophy, L., Ennals, P., Fletcher, J., & Hamilton, B. (2022). Community-based social interventions for people with severe mental illness: A systematic review and narrative synthesis of recent evidence. *World Psychiatry, 21*(1), 96–123. https://doi.org/10.1002/wps.20940

Knight, J. R., Sherritt, L., Shrier, L. A., Harris, S. K., & Chang, G. (2002). Validity of the CRAFFT substance abuse screening test among adolescent clinic patients. *Archives of Pediatrics & Adolescent Medicine, 156*(6), 607–614. https://doi.org/10.1001/archpedi.156.6.607

Kozhimannil, K. B., Trinacty, C. M., Busch, A. B., Huskamp, H. A., & Adams, A. S. (2011). Racial and ethnic disparities in postpartum depression care among low-income women. *Psychiatric Services, 62*(6), 619–625. https://doi.org/10.1176/appi.ps.62.6.619

Kroenke, K., & Spitzer, R. L. (2002). The PHQ-9: A new depression diagnostic and severity measure. *Psychiatric Annals, 32*(9), 509–515. https://doi.org/10.3928/0048-5713-20020901-06

Lomonaco-Haycraft, K. C., Hyer, J., Tibbits, B., Grote, J., Stainback-Tracy, K., Ulrickson, C., Lieberman, A., van Bekkum, L., & Hoffman, M. C. (2019). Integrated perinatal mental health care: A national model of perinatal primary care in vulnerable populations. *Primary Health Care Research & Development, 20*, e77. ARTN e77. https://doi.org/10.1017/S1463423618000348

Lund, C., De Silva, M., Plagerson, S., Cooper, S., Chisholm, D., Das, J., Knapp, M., & Patel, V. (2011). Poverty and mental disorders: Breaking the cycle in low-income and middle-income countries. *The Lancet, 378*(9801), 1502–1514. https://doi.org/10.1016/S0140-6736(11)60754-X

Ma, L., Xu, Y., Wang, G., & Li, R. (2019). What do we know about sex differences in depression: A review of animal models and potential mechanisms. *Progress in Neuro-Psychopharmacology and Biological Psychiatry, 89*, 48–56. https://doi.org/10.1016/j.pnpbp.2018.08.026

Maeng, D. D., Poleshuck, E., Rosenberg, T., Kulak, A., Mahoney, T., Nasra, G., Lee, H. B., & Li, Y. (2022). Primary care behavioral health integration and care utilization: Implications for patient outcome and healthcare resource use. *Journal of General Internal Medicine, 37*(11), 2691–2697. https://doi.org/10.1007/s11606-021-07372-6

Massachusetts Child Psychiatry Access Program for Moms (Boston). (2017). Gold award: Building the capacity of frontline providers to treat mental and substance use disorders among pregnant and postpartum women. *Psychiatric Services, 68*(10), e1–e3. https://doi.org/10.1176/appi.ps.681001

Maternal Mental Health Leadership Alliance. (2020, Nov 23). *Fact sheet: Perinatal psychiatry access programs* [Fact sheet]. MMHLA. https://web.archive.org/web/20220628000001/https://www.mmhla.org/wp-content/uploads/2020/07/MMHLA-Psychiatry-Fact-Sheet-2.pdf

MGH Center for Women's Mental Health. (2023). *Virtual rounds at the CWMH*. Massachusetts General Hospital; Harvard Medical School. https://womensmentalhealth.org/educational-programs/virtual-rounds-at-the-cwmh/

Miller, E. S., Jensen, R., Hoffman, M. C., Osborne, L. M., McEvoy, K., Grote, N., & Moses-Kolko, E. L. (2020). Implementation of perinatal collaborative care: A health services approach to perinatal depression care. *Primary Health Care Research & Development, 21*, e30. https://doi.org/10.1017/S1463423620000110

Miller, E. S., Grobman, W. A., Ciolino, J. D., Zumpf, K., Sakowicz, A., Gollan, J., & Wisner, K. L. (2021). Increased depression screening and treatment recommendations after implementation of a perinatal collaborative care program. *Psychiatric Services, 72*(11), 1268–1275. https://doi.org/10.1176/appi.ps.202000563

Miranda, J., & Green, B. L. (1999). The need for mental health services research focusing on poor young women. *The Journal of Mental Health Policy and Economics, 2*(2), 73–80. https://doi.org/10.1002/(sici)1099-176x(199906)2:2<73::aid-mhp40>3.0.co;2-3

Moyer, V. A., & US Preventive Services Task Force*. (2013). Screening for intimate partner violence and abuse of elderly and vulnerable adults: US Preventive Services Task Force Recommendation Statement. *Annals of Internal Medicine, 158*(6), 478–486. https://doi.org/10.7326/0003-4819-158-6-201303190-00588

New Mexico Perinatal ECHO. (2023). *Improving Perinatal Health ECHO Program.* [Web page]. University of New Mexico. https://hsc.unm.edu/echo/partner-portal/programs/new-mexico/perinatal/

Orleans, C. T., Johnson, R. W., Barker, D. C., Kaufman, N. J., & Marx, J. F. (2001). Helping pregnant smokers quit: Meeting the challenge in the next decade. *Western Journal of Medicine, 174*(4), 276. https://doi.org/10.1136/ewjm.174.4.276

Owens, G. P., Riggle, E. D., & Rostosky, S. S. (2007). Mental health services access for sexual minority individuals. *Sexuality Research & Social Policy, 4*, 92–99. https://doi.org/10.1525/srsp.2007.4.3.92

Patel, V., Belkin, G. S., Chockalingam, A., Cooper, J., Saxena, S., & Unützer, J. (2013). Grand challenges: Integrating mental health services into priority health care platforms. *PLoS Medicine, 10*(5), ARTICLE e1001448. https://doi.org/10.1371/journal.pmed.1001448

Perinatal Mental Health & Substance Use Education, Research, & Clinical Consultation (PERC) Center. (2023). *Mom's Access Project ECHO: Perinatal Psychiatry Case Conference Series.* [Web page]. University of Washington, Department of Psychiatry and Behavioral Sciences. https://www.mcmh.uw.edu/echo

Priester, M. A., Browne, T., Iachini, A., Clone, S., DeHart, D., & Seay, K. D. (2016). Treatment access barriers and disparities among individuals with co-occurring mental health and substance use disorders: An integrative literature review. *Journal of Substance Abuse Treatment, 61*, 47–59. https://doi.org/10.1016/j.jsat.2015.09.006

Prince, M., Patel, V., Saxena, S., Maj, M., Maselko, J., Phillips, M. R., & Rahman, A. (2007). No health without mental health. *The Lancet, 370*(9590), 859–877. https://doi.org/10.1016/S0140-6736(07)61238-0

Prom, M. C., Canelos, V., Fernandez, P. J., Gergen Barnett, K., Gordon, C. M., Pace, C. A., & Ng, L. C. (2021). Implementation of integrated behavioral health care in a large medical center: Benefits, challenges, and recommendations. *The Journal of Behavioral Health Services & Research, 48*(3), 346–362. https://doi.org/10.1007/s11414-020-09742-0

Quiray, J., Richards, E., Navarro-Aguirre, Y., Glazer, D., Adachi, J., Trujillo, E., ... & Bhat, A. (2024). The role of doulas in supporting perinatal mental health–a qualitative study. *Frontiers in Psychiatry, 15, 1272513*.

Ramaraj, A. B., Franz, N. A., Bhat, A., Adachi, J., Quiray, J. A., Bespalova, N., ... & Cowley, D. S. (2023). Project ECHO in psychiatric workforce development: The example of a perinatal mental health ECHO. *Academic Psychiatry, 1–5*.

Randel, A. (2019). Interpregnancy care: Guidelines from ACOG and SMFM. *American Family Physician, 100*(2), 121–123. https://www.aafp.org/pubs/afp/issues/2019/0715/p121.html

Reiter, J. T., Dobmeyer, A. C., & Hunter, C. L. (2018). The primary care behavioral health (PCBH) model: An overview and operational definition. *Journal of Clinical Psychology in Medical Settings, 25*(2), 109–126. https://doi.org/10.1007/s10880-017-9531-x

Robinson, P., Von Korff, M., Bush, T., Lin, E. H., & Ludman, E. J. (2020). The impact of primary care behavioral health services on patient behaviors: A randomized controlled trial. *Families, Systems & Health, 38*(1), 6. https://doi.org/10.1037/fsh0000474

Roll, J. M., Kennedy, J., Tran, M., & Howell, D. (2013). Disparities in unmet need for mental health services in the United States, 1997–2010. *Psychiatric Services, 64*(1), 80–82. https://doi.org/10.1176/appi.ps.201200071

Sakowicz, A., Allen, E. C., Nugooru, A., Grobman, W. A., & Miller, E. S. (2022). Timing of perinatal mental health needs: Data to inform policy. *American Journal of Obstetrics & Gynecology MFM, 4*(2), 100482. https://doi.org/10.1016/j.ajogmf.2021.100482

Scholle, S. H., Chang, J. C., Harman, J., & McNeil, M. (2002). Trends in women's health services by type of physician seen: Data from the 1985 and 1997–98 NAMCS. *Women's Health Issues, 12*(4), 165–177. https://doi.org/10.1016/S1049-3867(02)00139-1

Sherry, M., Wolff, J. L., Ballreich, J., DuGoff, E., Davis, K., & Anderson, G. (2016). Bridging the silos of service delivery for high-need, high-cost individuals. *Population Health Management, 19*(6), 421–428. https://doi.org/10.1089/pop.2015.0147

Siu, A. L., & U. S. Preventive Services Task Force. (2016). Screening for depression in adults: US Preventive Services Task Force Recommendation Statement. *JAMA, 315*(4), 380–387. https://doi.org/10.1001/jama.2015.18392

Snowber, K., Ciolino, J. D., Clark, C. T., Grobman, W. A., & Miller, E. S. (2022). Associations between implementation of the collaborative care model and disparities in perinatal depression care. *Obstetrics and Gynecology, 140*(2), 204–211. https://doi.org/10.1097/Aog.0000000000004859

Solway, E., Estes, C. L., Goldberg, S., & Berry, J. (2010). Access barriers to mental health services for older adults from diverse populations: Perspectives of leaders in mental health and aging. *Journal of Aging & Social Policy, 22*(4), 360–378. https://doi.org/10.1080/08959420.2010.507650

Spitzer, R. L., Kroenke, K., Williams, J. B., & Löwe, B. (2006). A brief measure for assessing generalized anxiety disorder: The GAD-7. *Archives of Internal Medicine, 166*(10), 1092–1097. https://doi.org/10.1001/archinte.166.10.1092

Stone, R. (2015). Pregnant women and substance use: Fear, stigma, and barriers to care. *Health & Justice, 3*(1), 1–15. https://doi.org/10.1186/s40352-015-0015-5

Straus, J. H., & Sarvet, B. (2014). Behavioral health care for children: The Massachusetts child psychiatry access project. *Health Affairs, 33*(12), 2153–2161. https://doi.org/10.1377/hlthaff.2014.0896

Thompson, M. A., Fuhlbrigge, A. L., Pearson, D. W., Saxon, D. R., Oberst-Walsh, L. A., & Thomas, J. F. (2021). Building eConsult (electronic consults) capability at an academic medical center to improve efficiencies in delivering specialty care. *Journal of Primary Care & Community Health, 12*, 21501327211005303. https://doi.org/Artn21501327211005303 10.1177/21501327211005303

Toler, S., Stapleton, S., Kertsburg, K., Callahan, T. J., & Hastings-Tolsma, M. (2018). Screening for postpartum anxiety: A quality improvement project to promote the screening of women suffering in silence. *Midwifery, 62*, 161–170. https://doi.org/10.1016/j.midw.2018.03.016

Tripathy, P., Nair, N., Barnett, S., Mahapatra, R., Borghi, J., Rath, S., Rath, S., Gope, R., Mahto, D., & Sinha, R. (2010). Effect of a participatory intervention with women's groups on birth outcomes and maternal depression in Jharkhand and Orissa, India: A cluster-randomised controlled trial. *The Lancet, 375*(9721), 1182–1192. https://doi.org/10.1016/S0140-6736(09)62042-0

Tyokighir, D., Hervey, A. M., Schunn, C., Clifford, D., & Ahlers-Schmidt, C. R. (2022). Qualitative assessment of access to perinatal mental health care: A social-ecological framework of barriers. *Kansas. Journal of Medicine, 15*, 48–54. https://doi.org/10.17161/kjm.vol15.15853

van Steenbergen-Weijenburg, K. M., van der Feltz-Cornelis, C. M., Horn, E. K., van Marwijk, H. W., Beekman, A. T., Rutten, F. F., & Hakkaart-van Roijen, L. (2010). Cost-effectiveness of collaborative care for the treatment of major depressive disorder in primary care. A systematic review. *BMC Health Services Research, 10*(1), 1–10. https://doi.org/10.1186/1472-6963-10-19

Weaver, A., & Lapidos, A. (2018). Mental health interventions with community health workers in the United States: A systematic review. *Journal of Health Care for the Poor and Underserved, 29*(1), 159–180. https://doi.org/10.1353/hpu.2018.0011

Webb, R., Uddin, N., Ford, E., Easter, A., Shakespeare, J., Roberts, N., Alderdice, F., Coates, R., Hogg, S., & Cheyne, H. (2021). Barriers and facilitators to implementing perinatal mental health care in health and social care settings: A systematic review. *The Lancet Psychiatry, 8*(6), 521–534. https://doi.org/10.1016/S2215-0366(20)30467-3

Wendt, A. C., Stamper, G., Howland, M., Cerimele, J. M., & Bhat, A. (2020). Indirect psychiatric consultation for perinatal bipolar disorder: A scoping review. *General Hospital Psychiatry, 68*, 19–24. https://doi.org/10.1016/j.genhosppsych.2020.11.011

Whitebird, R. R., Solberg, L. I., Jaeckels, N. A., Pietruszewski, P. B., Hadzic, S., Unützer, J., Ohnsorg, K. A., Rossom, R. C., Beck, A., Joslyn, K. E., & Rubenstein, L. V. (2014). Effective implementation of collaborative care for depression: What is needed? *American Journal of Managed Care, 20*(9), 699–707. https://www.ajmc.com/view/effective-implementation-of-collaborative-care-for-depression-what-is-needed

Wichman, C. L., Laszewski, A., Doering, J. J., & Borchardt, S. (2019). Feasibility of model adaptations and implementation of a perinatal psychiatric teleconsultation program. *General Hospital Psychiatry, 59*, 51–57. https://doi.org/10.1016/j.genhosppsych.2019.05.007

Williams, N. D., Turpin, R. E., Akré, E.-R. L., Boekeloo, B. O., & Fish, J. N. (2022). Disparities in mental health care access among persons differing in sexual identity: Nationally representative findings. *Psychiatric Services, 73*(4), 456–459. https://doi.org/10.1176/appi.ps.202100045

Wood, E., Ohlsen, S., & Ricketts, T. (2017). What are the barriers and facilitators to implementing collaborative care for depression? A systematic review. *Journal of Affective Disorders, 214*, 26–43. https://doi.org/10.1016/j.jad.2017.02.028

Yonkers, K. A., Gotman, N., Kershaw, T., Forray, A., Howell, H. B., & Rounsaville, B. J. (2010). Screening for prenatal substance use: Development of the substance use risk profile-pregnancy scale. *Obstetrics and Gynecology, 116*(4), 827. https://doi.org/10.1097/AOG.0b013e3181ed8290

Chapter 10
Financing Behavioral Health Services: Influence on Access to and Quality of Behavioral Health Care

Maureen T. Stewart, Thuong Nong, and Anika Kumar

Introduction

Mental health and substance use disorders (SUD) are common (Substance Abuse and Mental Health Service Administration, SAMHSA, 2022), and there is a concern that these behavioral health conditions have worsened since the start of the COVID-19 pandemic (Panchal et al., 2023). Depression and anxiety are more common among women than men, and alcohol use among women is increasing at a faster rate than among men; thus, attention to women's behavioral health services is needed (Jalnapurkar et al., 2018; Kuehner, 2017; White, 2020).

Financing and payment for behavioral health services influence the organization of services, access, and quality of care and, therefore, are essential to the delivery of behavioral health services for women. This chapter provides an overview of the financing and payment for behavioral health services and examines how these factors influence women's access to and quality of behavioral health care. The chapter begins with a brief description of the financing of behavioral health services historically in the USA. Then, it describes the impact of federal policy changes, including the Patient Protection and Affordable Care Act of 2010 (ACA) and the Paul Wellstone and Pete Domenici Mental Health Parity and Addiction Equity Act of 2008 (referred to here as the federal parity law) on financing for behavioral health services for women. The chapter then covers how payment models may influence access to and quality of care. The chapter concludes with behavioral health payment and financing implications for research, practice, and policy.

M. T. Stewart (✉) · T. Nong · A. Kumar
Institute for Behavioral Health, The Heller School for Social Policy and Management, Brandeis University, Waltham, MA, USA
e-mail: mstewart@brandeis.edu

A. Hanson, B. L. Levin (eds.), *Women's Behavioral Health*,
https://doi.org/10.1007/978-3-031-58293-6_10

Background

The USA has historically had a fragmented approach to financing and delivering behavioral health services (McGinty & Daumit, 2020). The fragmentation partly exists because behavioral health conditions were historically viewed differently from physical health conditions (Glied & Frank, 2006). As a result, behavioral health financing and delivery systems developed and evolved separately from medical care (Druss, 2002). The stigmatized and slow adoption of mental illness and addiction as primary concerns of medicine is partly responsible for what many still experience as two parallel and unequal systems with behavioral health services separated from physical health services. Behavioral health care was delivered in settings separate from medical care and financed primarily through state and local governments, with some funding from federal block grants. The block grants provide lump sums to each state to support mental health and substance use prevention and treatment services.

With the development of Medicare and Medicaid in the 1960s, followed by the approval of antidepressant medications, financing for physical and mental health treatment services shifted to an insurance-based system. Between 1986 and 2014, mental health treatment spending shifted from primarily publicly financed by state and local governments, outside the insurance-based system, to being insurance-financed (Glied & Frank, 2006; Mark et al., 2016). Over the same period, substance use treatment services continued to be financed primarily by state and local governments (Mark et al., 2016). This historic separation of behavioral health from physical health continues to affect the current financing and delivery of behavioral health services. Further, the stigma around mental health and substance use disorders still persists today, affecting access to and quality of care (Thornicroft et al., 2022; Wakeman & Rich, 2018).

Despite the health consequences, behavioral health conditions are often untreated. For example, fewer than 10% of individuals with alcohol use disorders receive evidence-based treatment (e.g., behavioral interventions, three FDA-approved medications), and women and racial and ethnic minorities are less likely to receive alcohol treatment services than male and White counterparts (Cook & Alegría, 2011; Mulia, 2020; Mulvaney-Day et al., 2012; Williams et al., 2017). In 2021, over half of all individuals with serious mental illnesses (SMI) resulting in substantial impairment in the USA did not receive evidence-based treatment for behavioral health (e.g., medication treatment, counseling, and inpatient/outpatient programs). Of the approximately 14 million adults (ages 18+) in the USA with SMI, approximately 52% perceived an unmet need for behavioral health treatment in the previous 12 months (SAMHSA, 2022).

Reasons for low rates of behavioral health treatment are varied. According to the National Survey on Drug Use and Health (NSDUH), the most common barrier to behavioral health treatment was the cost of care (SAMHSA, 2022). Financial barriers may disproportionately affect some populations, including non-Hispanic American Indian and Alaskan Native (AIAN), non-Hispanic Black, and Hispanic individuals, who are more likely to be uninsured than their counterparts (Artiga et al., 2022). Additional barriers to behavioral health-care access and treatment include stigma, treatment setting appeal, childcare difficulties, and concerns about losing custody of children, all of which may prevent women from seeking care (Alvarez et al., 2022; Copeland & Snyder, 2011; Knaak et al., 2017). System barriers to care include health insurance benefit design, lack of integration between behavioral and physical health, payment policies that limit flexibility and prevent billing for multiple services on the same day, and provider availability (Andrilla et al., 2018; McGinty & Daumit, 2020; Roby & Jones, 2016; Roman et al., 2011). Further, providers' attitudes and assumptions may also represent barriers (e.g., providers' beliefs regarding the effectiveness and risks of pharmacotherapy for SUD) (Oliva et al., 2011; Priester et al., 2016).

The milieu of barriers that prevent access to comprehensive behavioral health care harms populations with substantial behavioral health needs and those least represented in the US health-care financing structure. Although prevalence rates of mental illness (MI) and substance use disorders (SUDs) are typically higher among White individuals, rates of MI and SUDs are still consistently high among AIAN individuals and those who report two or more races (SAMHSA, 2022). Importantly, non-White individuals experience higher rates of negative consequences from behavioral health conditions including delayed care, comorbidities, poor quality of life, higher mortality, and lower overall wellness (Karaye et al., 2023). Prevalence of behavioral health needs among non-White racial and ethnic groups became especially apparent during the pandemic, when mortality by suicide and drug overdose was found to be increasing more rapidly among people of color compared to their White counterparts (Panchal et al., 2022). Specifically, Black and AIAN people saw the greatest increases in rates of death by suicide between 2010 and 2020 (Panchal et al., 2022).

Despite evident need for services, research demonstrates that Black, Hispanic, and Asian individuals are less likely to access behavioral health services compared to non-Hispanic White individuals (Cook et al., 2017; Thomeer et al., 2023). Reasons for low utilization are complex and numerous. Structural inequities (e.g., lack of health insurance coverage, financial, logistical barriers) contribute to the disparity in behavioral health-care utilization, as does a lack of culturally informed screening tools and treatment options (Rice & Harris, 2021), discrimination (Gabbidon et al., 2014), and harmful racial/ethnic stereotypes (Eylem et al., 2020).

Literature suggests that the impacts of lockdown restrictions, isolation, and distancing have resulted in increased anxiety, loneliness, and depression (Jia et al., 2021). Drug overdose deaths increased 31% between 2019 and 2021 (Hedegaard et al., 2021; SAMHSA, 2022). Three years after the onset of the COVID-19 pandemic, mental health professionals are still struggling to accommodate the increased need and demand for mental health services. In the American Psychological Association's, 2022 COVID-19 Practitioner Impact Survey, 79% of psychologists reported an increased number of patients with anxiety disorders, and 66% reported an increased number of patients with depression since the pandemic's beginning (American Psychological Association, 2022). Low rates of behavioral health treatment are concerning, especially with the increasing need for services due to the COVID-19 pandemic.

Financing for Behavioral Health Care

Today, behavioral health care is financed through public and private insurance, out-of-pocket payments, and direct public funding. Changes in social policies and cultural perspectives that recognize behavioral health conditions as diseases have shifted financing for mental health and substance use treatment services. Factors contributing to changing the delivery of behavioral health services in the USA include a shift in health-care financing toward managed care, state and federal mental health parity laws that regulate managed care, the ACA, efforts to reduce the stigma associated with behavioral health conditions, and therapeutic developments including new medications and telehealth approaches.

Financing Behavioral Health Services by Payer

In 2016, the United States (U. S.) spent an estimated $181 billion on mental health and SUD treatment services (Dieleman et al., 2020). This amount represents nearly 7% of all health spending, a relatively small portion of all health spending. An estimated 57% of the almost $181 billion in behavioral health spending is financed through public insurance (Medicare and Medicaid), 34% through private (i.e., employer-based) insurance, and 8% through out-of-pocket expenditures (Dieleman et al., 2020). Public insurance's share of behavioral health spending is higher than the public insurance share of any other type of health spending. In 2021, approximately18% of the US population had Medicare, approximately 19% had Medicaid, 66% had employer-sponsored or other private insurance, and approximately 8% were uninsured (United States Census Bureau, 2022). Public insurance disproportionately finances behavioral health care because public insurance programs disproportionately cover people with behavioral health conditions. Insurance coverage for behavioral health services has traditionally been more limited than coverage for physical health care (Barry et al., 2003; McLellan & Woodworth, 2014).

Medicare Spending and Coverage for Behavioral Health Services

Medicare is a federal insurance program available to Americans aged 65 years and older. The program covers over 62 million beneficiaries (KFF State Health Facts, 2021). In 2019, over 49% of Americans 65 years or older had at least one form of Medicare (Medicare only, Medicare Advantage, or dual-eligible covered by Medicare and Medicaid) (Cohen et al., 2021). Approximately 30% of Medicare enrollees have a mental health disorder (Figueroa et al., 2020), a rate higher than the general population rate of 20%. Almost two million Medicare beneficiaries, or approximately 3% of Medicare beneficiaries, have substance use disorders (Parish et al., 2022). Alcohol use disorder is the most common, affecting 77% of those with a substance use disorder (Parish et al., 2022). Medicare spends an estimated $3 billion on behavioral health treatment services annually, representing 4% of total Medicare spending (Figueroa et al., 2020). Medicare pays an additional $5.5 billion on medical expenditures associated with mental illness; almost 13% of Medicare spending is related to behavioral health conditions (Figueroa et al., 2020).

When the Medicare program was adopted in the 1960s, Medicare coverage for behavioral health services was limited (Lave & Goldman, 1990). The program imposed a lifetime limit on the number of days covered in freestanding psychiatric hospitals and limited inpatient care to 90 days per benefit period to ensure the federal government was not responsible for services for people with chronic mental illnesses, leaving that responsibility to states (Lave & Goldman, 1990). However, changes made over time have expanded behavioral health coverage and benefits for Medicare beneficiaries.

Traditional (fee-for-service [FFS]) Medicare and Medicare Advantage plans cover inpatient and outpatient behavioral health care and medications for behavioral health conditions. Inpatient services are subject to a lifetime limit of 190 days of coverage for services delivered in a psychiatric hospital. Medicare covers outpatient services provided by clinical nurse specialists, clinical psychologists, clinical social workers, nurse practitioners, physician assistants, and psychiatrists or other physicians. Coverage for services and medications to treat individuals with behavioral health conditions can vary by Medicare Advantage plan policies.

Beginning January 1, 2024, Medicare will reimburse for services delivered by licensed professional counselors, a new policy included in the 2023 federal appropriations bill (Consolidated Appropriations Act, 2023). However, Medicare does not cover licensed and certified substance use disorder counselors (Weber & Steinberg, 2021). The 2008 Medicare Improvements for Patients and Providers Act required cost-sharing for mental health services should not be higher than cost-sharing for physical health coverage (Medicare Improvements for Patients and Providers Act, 2008). This law helped to decrease out-of-pocket expenses for Medicare enrollees when accessing mental health services. It was associated with an increase in the use of psychotropic medications among Medicare enrollees (Cook et al., 2020).

Medicare coverage for SUD treatment has additional gaps. Medicare covers the most intense level of care (inpatient care) and the least intense level of care (outpatient care) but does not cover mid-level treatment for SUD, including intensive outpatient, partial hospital, specialty addiction treatment, residential treatment, or many of the providers who work in these programs (Weber & Steinberg, 2021). Medicare also does not cover substance use services delivered in community-based, specialty substance use treatment facilities (Weber & Steinberg, 2021). In 2020, Medicare started covering opioid treatment programs with the passage of the SUPPORT for Patients and Communities Act of 2018 (2018). These programs provide methadone and other medication treatments for opioid use disorder.

Furthermore, unlike most employer-sponsored insurance and Medicaid managed care plans, Medicare is not subject to the federal parity law, which requires coverage of and access to mental health and SUD benefits equal to medical and surgical benefits. Adding these benefits to the Medicare program would total close to $2 billion annually, covering SUD residential ($935 million), intensive outpatient ($928 million), and counseling ($66 million) services (Parish & Mark, 2022). Analyses of the cost offsets from reduced incidence of comorbid conditions and reduced SUD-related hospitalizations and emergency department (ED) visits are $1.5 million annually (Parish & Mark, 2022). Thus, the net impact of expanding Medicare coverage for SUD residential, intensive outpatient, and counseling exceeds $360 million annually (Parish & Mark, 2022).

Medicaid Spending and Coverage for Behavioral Health Services

Medicaid is an insurance program for low-income and disabled Americans funded jointly by federal and state governments. Each state determines its own Medicaid eligibility requirements within federal regulations. Medicaid programs provide health insurance for more than 92 million people in the USA, including 18% of women and approximately 36% of children (Centers for Medicare & Medicaid Services, 2023; KFF, 2022a; Mykyta et al., 2022). Medicaid covers a large and disproportionate share of women, individuals from racial and ethnic minority groups, and rural Americans (Foutz et al., 2017; KFF, 2012, 2020).

Medicaid is a critical payer for women. In 2021, Medicaid covered 18% of all non-elderly women and 14% of all non-elderly men in the USA, ages 19–64 (KFF, 2022a). Before the ACA, women typically were required to have very low incomes and be pregnant, parenting, or disabled to qualify for Medicaid benefits. Through the ACA, 39 states and Washington D.C. have expanded Medicaid access to non-elderly, low-income women and men with incomes below 138% of the federal poverty line (FPL) regardless of pregnancy, parenting, or disability status (KFF, 2022a). Women are less likely to be uninsured when compared to men in the USA (11% and 14% uninsured, respectively, in 2021). Women are now more apt to qualify for Medicaid benefits due to income and meeting Medicaid's other stringent enrollment requirements (KFF, 2022a).

Rates of mental health and SUD in the Medicaid population are exceptionally high (Saunders & Rudowitz, 2022). In 2020, an estimated 29% of Medicaid enrollees had a mental health condition, and 21% had a SUD, rates that are higher than among privately insured enrollees. Nearly 40% of Medicaid enrollees have either a mental illness or SUD (Saunders & Rudowitz, 2022). Thus, Medicaid programs are among the most essential payers for behavioral health services. In the most recent data, Medicaid is the second largest payer for SUD services, covering 21% of all treatment services, second to only state and local spending (Mark et al., 2016).

States have discretion in how their Medicaid program is managed and how care is delivered, but states must comply with federal requirements regarding eligibility, coverage, and administration, including the federal parity law. Medicaid services may be delivered and managed by states (traditional state fee-for-service [FFS]), or states may contract with health plans that manage care. Most state Medicaid FFS programs cover a range of behavioral health services, including inpatient care, outpatient care, and medication services (Guth, 2021b). Almost all state Medicaid programs contract with managed care organizations (MCOs) to deliver and manage health-care services (Hinton & Raphael, 2023). In 2021, 72% of Medicaid enrollees were in managed care, with the balance treated in Medicaid FFS programs (KFF, 2023). Clearly, there is a lack of comprehensive information about managed care plan behavioral health benefits and policies.

Publicly Financed Direct Care Spending

In addition to public insurance programs, the federal and state governments directly finance behavioral health prevention and treatment services. The federal government provides lump sum payments to states through the Substance Abuse Prevention and Treatment (SAPT) Block Grant program, which provides funding and technical assistance to US states and territories. Funding is used to support substance use prevention and treatment services. Similarly, the Community Mental Health Services Block Grant (MHBG) provides funding to US states and territories to support community-based mental health services for adults with SMI and children with serious emotional disturbances as well as to support the community-based mental health system. Block grant funding is used for prevention, treatment, recovery support, and other services to supplement insurance-based services. Block grant dollars can be used for people without health insurance, for services not covered by insurance, and for primary prevention services, to collect performance and outcomes data needed to assess the effectiveness of block grant-funded services.

SAMHSA administers the federal block grants, and funding is allocated to each state based on an algorithm that considers population size and cost of care. Under the block grant, there is little accountability, quality measurement, monitoring, or oversight, and therefore, it is difficult to ensure evidence-based services are provided. In each fiscal year from 2016 to 2021, the federal government provided $1.86 billion to states through the SAPT block grant. An additional $1.65 billion in supplemental funds were delivered in 2021 for COVID-19 relief funding (National Association of State Alcohol and Drug Abuse Directors, 2021). The Mental Health Block Grant totaled $715 million in FY 2022 and over $1 billion in FY 2023 (Tracking Accountability in Government Grants System [TAGGS], 2023).

In addition to federal block grant funding, states finance behavioral health services through state budgets and allocate those funds to state agencies. On average, from 2010 to 2019, states allocated $48 million per year from state budgets for substance use agencies (Andrews et al., 2023). State funding per capita varied substantially by state from \$0.61 per capita in Arizona to \$51.11 in Wyoming (Andrews et al., 2023). State funding allocations to state substance use agencies have declined by nearly an estimated \$10 million in expansion states relative to states that did not expand Medicaid, indicating states are substituting Medicaid funding for state funding (Andrews et al., 2023).

Private Insurance Financing and Coverage

An estimated 66% of Americans have private insurance, which includes employer-sponsored insurance (approximately 54%) which covers many working adults and their families (Keisler-Starkey & Bunch, 2022). Individuals may also purchase insurance on their own, either in the individual market or through the Marketplace Plans established by the ACA. Private insurance generally covers detoxification, inpatient hospital, partial hospitalization, intensive outpatient, and outpatient counseling services for both mental illnesses and SUDs (Horgan et al., 2016). Residential treatment for mental health is also usually covered, but residential treatment for SUDs is covered by fewer plans (Horgan et al., 2016). Medications for SUDs are commonly covered by private health plans, but utilization management strategies are also common (Reif et al., 2016). The federal parity law substantially strengthened behavioral health coverage offered by private insurance plans (Hodgkin et al., 2018). Changes due to the federal parity law are described in more detail below.

Out-of-Pocket Financing

Despite insurance coverage, individuals also pay out-of-pocket for behavioral health treatment services. This includes cost sharing associated with insurance (i.e., deductible, co-payments, co-insurance) and out-of-pocket expenditures where insurance is not used. People with behavioral health conditions have higher out-of-pocket expenditures than people with physical health conditions (Xu et al., 2019). High out-of-pocket expenditures are one of the reasons people do not seek behavioral health care. In an analysis of people with mental health conditions who perceived a need for treatment but did not receive treatment, 51% reported the inability to afford the cost of treatment as a barrier, and 12% reported insurance not covering enough of the cost as a barrier (Walker et al., 2015).

Financing by Type of Care

Analyses of behavioral health spending by type of care show 46% of behavioral health spending is for ambulatory care, 19% for inpatient care, 20% for prescribed pharmaceuticals, 3% for nursing facilities, 2% for emergency department care, and nearly 10% for government administration and cost of insurance programs (Dieleman et al., 2020). The proportion of behavioral health spending for ambulatory care is higher than ambulatory care for many other conditions, reflecting that most behavioral health care takes place in ambulatory settings (Dieleman et al., 2020).

Financing by Condition

Estimates of behavioral health spending by condition show health-care costs for depressive disorders represent the largest share of behavioral health spending and are estimated at approximately $68 billion, the 13th most expensive health condition (Dieleman et al., 2020). Health expenditures for anxiety disorders are an estimated in excess of $42 billion, attention-deficit/hyperactive disorder $17 billion, bipolar disorder approximately $14 billion, schizophrenia approximately $14 billion, drug use disorders approximately $13 billion, and alcohol use disorders in excess of $8 billion (Dieleman et al., 2020). Importantly, these are underestimates of the true health-care costs of behavioral health conditions because these estimates include only direct health-care expenditures for each condition and not expenditures for other conditions resulting from mental illnesses or SUDs (e.g., cirrhosis of the liver from alcohol use or endocarditis from drug use).

Federal Policy Changes Affecting Behavioral Health Financing

The Paul Wellstone and Pete Domenici Mental Health Parity and Addiction Equity Act (2008), combined with the Patient Protection and Affordable Care Act (ACA, 2010), dramatically changed financing for SUD treatment in the USA. The federal parity law greatly expanded behavioral health service coverage in the USA by requiring insurance coverage for mental health and SUD treatment be no more restrictive than coverage for medical services (Beronio et al., 2014). As a result, annual and lifetime limits on behavioral health services and differential cost-sharing for behavioral health services were eliminated, and procedures for determining behavioral health coverage must be substantially similar to procedures used for physical health conditions (Beronio et al., 2014).

There were concerns behavioral health treatment spending might increase following coverage expansion with the federal parity law. While behavioral health services use increased following the parity law, and there were moderate increases in insurance-financed spending (Mark et al., 2016), large increases in spending did not materialize and the law provided financial protections for enrollees (Busch et al., 2014; Huskamp et al., 2017; Stuart et al., 2017b). States that expanded Medicaid also reduced state support for substance use treatment services, and this may have prevented some of the anticipated large spending increases (Andrews et al., 2023).

The ACA included mental health and SUD treatment in the essential benefits package, thereby requiring SUD services must be covered by small group and individual plans (Beronio et al., 2014). The ACA also mandated Medicaid MCOs comply with the federal parity law requirements. Together these laws resulted in coverage expansion by making more people eligible for insurance coverage and by making behavioral health coverage more generous because it had to be at parity with medical care (Beronio et al., 2014). The number of uninsured individuals in the USA declined from 48 million in 2010, prior to the ACA, to 28 million in 2016 (Finegold et al., 2021). Today, an estimated 8.4% of Americans are not covered by health insurance, reflecting an expansion of health insurance coverage (Cohen & Cha, 2022). However, there are differences in insurance coverage by demographic characteristics and state. For example, people who are Hispanic are more likely to be uninsured than people who are White, and those living in non-expansion states are more likely to be uninsured than people living in states which expanded Medicaid eligibility (Cohen & Cha, 2022) (for more about policy and financing, see Chap. 15 in this volume).

Health Insurance: Function and Challenges

Over time, health insurance, both publicly and privately financed, has become a more important payer for behavioral health services (Mark et al., 2016). The purpose of health insurance is to shield the recipient from financial risk for health-care expenditures. Insurance markets work effectively when they can spread risk for expenditures among many people. However, individual decision-making based on personal health information distorts insurance markets and undermines the ability of markets to spread risk.

Adverse selection occurs in health insurance markets in two scenarios. The first scenario occurs when individuals with acute, chronic, or recurring illnesses, who are more likely to need services, buy insurance and those who are healthier do not. The second scenario occurs when individuals who are more frequently ill buy more generous insurance than healthier individuals. When an individual's health information is taken into account when deciding which health insurance, provider, or policy to purchase, adverse selection may occur, often resulting in higher health-care expenditures for insurers. In countries with universal health insurance (e.g., France, UK), issues related to information asymmetry and how knowledge of one's health influences demand for insurance are irrelevant. In the USA, however, there is substantial variation in how one purchases insurance, as insurance markets are complicated by the potential for adverse selection.

Requiring people to purchase insurance, regardless of their perceived need for health-care services, is one strategy to ensure well-functioning health insurance markets include healthy people. The 2006 Massachusetts health reform law requires all its residents to have health insurance (Long et al., 2012). This mandate ensures health expenditures are spread among healthy and sick individuals because everyone must buy insurance. Employer-sponsored insurance is another solution to adverse selection. Since the insurance policy is selected for large groups of employees, adverse selection is limited because the people in the group do not have any influence over specific insurance benefits/plan purchased.

Adverse selection may be more detrimental for people with behavioral health needs because behavioral health services have been shown to be more sensitive to price (Keeler et al., 1988). Risk adjustment is a strategy developed to ensure that both high-risk and low-risk enrollees are attractive to health plans (Frank et al., 1997). Under risk adjustment, plans receive a higher rate for people who are not healthy. However, the risk adjustment methods for behavioral health conditions often have limited accuracy, leaving plans with strong incentives to avoid high-cost enrollees (McGuire & Sinaiko, 2010). To try to discourage people with behavioral health conditions, who are expected to have higher health expenditures from purchasing a specific insurance product, the insurer may offer less generous behavioral health coverage. Preventing insurers from selecting only healthier members or those without behavioral health conditions is a key role for public policy to improve insurance coverage for behavioral health services.

The Role of Managed Care in Financing Behavioral Health Services in the USA

Most health insurance in the USA is offered by MCOs on behalf of financing entities (e.g., federal Medicare programs, state Medicaid programs, or employers). An estimated 48% of Medicare enrollees, 72% of Medicaid enrollees, and 99% of those with employer-sponsored insurance are in managed care plans (KFF, 2022b; KFF, 2023; Ochieng et al., 2023).

Under this arrangement, the financing entity pays a fixed rate per member per month to MCOs. The MCO is responsible for all aspects of coverage, including determining covered services and utilization management policies, establishing provider networks, conducting quality monitoring and measurement, and paying providers. MCOs follow federal, state, and employer contracting requirements and have substantial leeway to establish their own policies.

Features of Managed Care

Important features of managed care plans include coverage design, cost sharing requirements, utilization management policies, quality measurement, provider payment models, and reimbursement rates. Differences in MCO coverage policies may influence enrollees' access to and quality of care. For example, some Medicaid MCOs do not cover the same treatment services in the state FFS programs, and many limit access to residential treatment (Andrews et al., 2018). In a study reviewing coverage handbooks, the authors found 100% of state FFS programs covered buprenorphine, but only 80% of Medicaid managed care plans indicated coverage (Andrews et al., 2018). Further, requiring co-payments for services may result in lower utilization (Lo Sasso & Lyons, 2002; Quinn et al., 2017b).

Utilization management policies (e.g., prior authorization, continuing review) are used to manage access to high-cost services and medications. When prior authorization is required, the provider must request permission and receive approval from the MCO for a medication or service to be covered under the policy (Quinn et al., 2017b). Step-therapy (or "fail-first") policies require members to try less expensive medications before starting another higher-cost medication (Hodgkin et al., 2014, 2015; Reif et al., 2016). Delays and denials resulting from utilization management present barriers to accessing services. Administrative burden introduced by these policies may discourage providers from offering services which will require time-intensive interactions with payers (Andrews et al., 2019).

Some insurers subcontract the risk and management of mental health and substance use care to specialized companies. These companies are called managed behavioral health organizations (MBHOs), and this arrangement is often called a "behavioral health carve-out." MBHOs specialize in managing and delivering behavioral health services and, therefore, may generate efficiencies and be able to better deliver high-quality care and control costs without limiting behavioral health coverage. The use of MBHOs has declined over time. In 2003, most commercial plans (72%) contracted with an MBHO to deliver and manage behavioral health services (Horgan et al., 2016). However, by 2010, less than 15% of commercial health plans used this arrangement. Instead, most commercial plans took on the management and risk of behavioral health services themselves (Horgan et al., 2016). Some Medicaid managed care plans also carve-out behavioral health services, but systematic information on how often this occurs is not available. Separately, the financing entity may also choose to contract out behavioral health services as one approach to limiting problems associated with adverse selection. In this case, the employer or the state Medicaid agency selects an MBHO to manage all behavioral health services.

Provider networks are a key tool for managed care plans to facilitate and manage access to care. Adequate network size is necessary to ensure provider availability and offer timely appointments. Provider networks are developed to include a range of provider expertise and to provide sufficient geographic coverage for enrollees. To maintain provider networks, health plans may use a combination of reduced administrative burden and higher reimbursement rates for select providers (Garnick et al., 2008). However, there is evidence managed care networks for behavioral health providers are too narrow and this is a consistent problem across all private insurance, Medicare, and Medicaid plans. In a survey of employer-sponsored insurance, only 44% of employers reported that behavioral health provider networks were sufficiently large to offer timely access to care, compared to 82% of primary care provider networks (Claxton et al., 2022). An analysis of psychiatrist networks in Medicare managed care plans found 65% of psychiatrist networks in Medicare

Advantage met the threshold for narrow (defined as a median network size of less than 25% of the area's providers), compared with 43% in Medicaid managed care. However, the analysis found 20% of primary care provider networks were narrow. Medicaid enrollees report difficulty finding primary and specialty providers that take their insurance (Kemmick Pintor et al., 2019). Medicaid MCOs do not offer out-of-network access, so enrollees have few options when encountering network barriers. The lack of providers may be due to the lack of available providers, low reimbursement rates, or high administrative burden.

Provider payment policies and reimbursement rates are key to ensuring the availability of quality behavioral health care. Managed care plans determine payment models and rates for network providers. Medicaid MCO payment rates are typically lower than Medicare or private insurance rates for the same services (Zuckerman et al., 2017). Low payment rates are often cited as a barrier in the Medicaid program and likely limit providers' willingness to accept Medicaid patients (Candon et al., 2018). Low Medicaid payment rates for buprenorphine prescribing in Medicaid may discourage physicians from offering buprenorphine treatment (Stein et al., 2015).

A 2018 analysis of Medicaid FFS payment rates showed reimbursement rates for psychiatrists are 81% of the Medicare rate and vary substantially by state (Zhu et al., 2023). There is evidence payment rates influence providers' willingness to accept Medicaid patients. When the ACA established a temporary increase in Medicaid payments to match the amount paid by Medicare, Medicaid patients' access to primary care providers increased (Polsky et al., 2015). While efforts to lower the cost of care are ongoing in general health care, there are some efforts in place to increase reimbursement rates for behavioral health providers. For example, Oregon increased its Medicaid FFS rates for behavioral health services an average of 30% in July 2022 (Oregon Health Authority, 2022).

MCOs are developing and implementing policies to better integrate medical and behavioral health care through health homes, programs to address social determinants of health, reimbursing for peer recovery services, and paying for care provided via telemedicine (Huskamp et al., 2018; Kushner & McConnell, 2019; SAMHSA, 2018). These policies may benefit individuals who experience more barriers to treatment and thus reduce disparities or inequities in care. Innovative policies often depend on more flexibility in payment models and are supported by a shift away from FFS to alternative payment models.

Payment Models

Health insurers generally pay providers for care using a FFS payment model or a per-member-per-month capitated payment model or some combination of the two. The models differ in how they distribute the risk of health-care expenses between payer and provider and, therefore, in the incentives providers face regarding quality and quantity of care delivered. Achieving the right balance between financial risk and incentives has been a focus of health policy for decades.

Payment for behavioral health care evolved differently from payment for physical health care because behavioral health services were historically separate from physical health care. As previously described, behavioral health systems were initially supported by state and local government funding and block grant funding rather than insurance. These financing mechanisms have less accountability and transparency. Under the block grant system, behavioral health organizations receive a fixed payment, regardless of the number of people they served or the quality of the care they delivered. The shift to insurance-based payment has some benefits for behavioral health organizations and providers because FFS payment facilitates reimbursement for more services and allows organizations maximize the services they are delivering.

Just as the delivery systems for physical and behavioral health services have developed differently over time, the problems with payment for behavioral health care and physical health care are different. Issues for behavioral health include lack of funding and accountability under block grant systems and low reimbursement rates in the insurance-based system. This is very different from the problems associated with payment models for physical health care which are driven by high rate of cost growth. The behavioral health service systems need improved access to care and increased use of evidence-based treatment services, while challenges in the health care systems more broadly are focused on reducing health-care cost growth and improving quality of care. Below we describe several common payment models followed by specific considerations for behavioral health care, given the different ways the systems have developed.

Traditionally, health-care services were paid for using a FFS system in which health insurers either paid medical providers directly or reimbursed beneficiaries for each covered medical expense. FFS payment reward providers based on volume rather than patient health outcomes and quality of care (Robinson, 2001). Providers have an incentive to offer more services, can only be paid for services with payment codes, and do not have an incentive to control costs or focus on quality. Often, care coordination is not paid for under FFS, and innovative approaches to managing behavioral health care, such as peer-based care, may be difficult to pay for under a FFS model.

To lower the overall cost of care and add incentives for quality, MCOs and the Centers for Medicare and Medicaid Services (CMS) are moving away from FFS and using a range of 'alternative' payment models. Alternative payment models that move beyond FFS offer the potential to lend needed flexibility to substance use treatment programs to provide services in a more innovative way and incentivize delivery of high quality of care. These payment models align payer and provider interests in improved performance while preventing payers from becoming too directive and allowing providers flexibility in achieving improved performance. Despite arguments that alternative payment models are needed, they are not widely used for behavioral health services. Alternative payment models have potential implications for care delivery, cost, and quality. Several payment approaches have been implemented and tested in the USA to reduce spending and improve the quality of care. These models are often referred to as value-based payments and include pay-for-performance (P4P), accountable care organizations (ACOs), and bundled payments.

P4P is an alternative payment model designed to address the shortcomings (inefficiency and high cost) of the FFS payment model (Abrams et al., 2015). P4P utilizes the FFS system but adds a focus on quality by offering financial incentives to providers for meeting pre-defined performance measures (NEJM Catalyst, 2018). Measures commonly included in P4P programs for behavioral health care include number of visits per month or per episode, length of time in treatment, or proportion of patients who receive appropriate follow-up care after hospitalization or ED visit (National Committee for Quality Assurance, 2023). P4P models also may promote transparency and accountability by using publicly reported metrics. Providers concerned about their public reputation may strive to improve performance in order to maintain their reputation. Thus, providers have both financial and nonfinancial incentives to improve quality and lower costs, resulting in increased efficiency and value in the health-care system (Sinaiko et al., 2021).

However, P4P models may create barriers for low-income or less healthy patients to access health-care services. Providers are incentivized to avoid treating people whose services are less likely to meet the quality metrics and focus on healthier patients who are more likely to achieve clinical targets necessary for rewards (Casalino, 1999; Shen, 2003; Stewart et al., 2017). In addition, medical providers must deal with a higher burden of administrative complexity, requiring a costly system to acquire and verify metrics data (Quinn et al., 2017a). This approach often focuses on clinical process measures which may not be associated with improved health outcomes (Mathes et al., 2019; Mendelson et al., 2017).

Evidence of the effectiveness of P4P programs in behavioral health care is limited. A P4P program implemented in Delaware outpatient substance use treatment programs was associated with longer retention in treatment and shorter waiting times for care (Brucker & Stewart, 2011). However, several other studies of P4P in Maine, Delaware, and Maryland did not identify strong relationships between P4P and improved patient outcomes (Stewart et al., 2017, 2018). Providers face challenges in defining and measuring behavioral outcomes because many disorders are co-occurring; hence, desirable outcomes must include clinical and nonclinical changes (Hodgkin et al., 2020).

ACOs are an alternative payment model designed to shift the focus to rewarding providers for providing high-quality care and improving health instead of offering more services. ACOs are comprised of groups of health-care providers who coordinate and ensure high-quality care to lower the total cost of care for a population of patients. Participating ACOs receive a fixed amount per member per month. Total spending for the ACO population is tracked and savings or losses may be shared depending on the ACO contract (Abrams et al., 2015). Participating providers are motivated to provide comprehensive care and preventive care earlier. The ACO model offers flexibility so providers can use innovative approaches that are not billable under FFS models (e.g., peer navigators or consultations between primary care and specialty behavioral health providers) to support behavioral health in primary care (Fullerton et al., 2016).

Research shows ACOs are associated with cost reduction for physician groups and hospitals (McWilliams et al., 2018). ACO implementation is associated with reduced inpatient use, improved measures of preventive care, reduced ED visits, and chronic disease management (McWilliams et al., 2018). However, the impact of this model on patient outcomes and people with behavioral health conditions needs further study (Kaufman et al., 2019). A study of ACOs' implementation in Massachusetts found the model did not increase SUD service use during its first 3 years of implementation (Stuart et al., 2017a).

Bundled payment (BP) is another value-based alternative payment method. Under this model, payers reimburse one or more providers a set amount for services provided during a defined episode of care (Quinn et al., 2017a). BPs are commonly used for discrete episodes of care, for example, joint replacement surgery or labor and delivery, which begin with a specific diagnosis and continue for a discrete period. This differs from an ACO model, which begins with a patient population. In BPs, savings and risks are shared by physicians and hospitals in the form of bonuses or penalties based on P4P structures (Berenson et al., 2016; Ginsburg, 2012). This arrangement encourages providers to coordinate care across settings to reduce costs and redundant services and better manage patient care (Freeman et al., 2020; Ginsburg, 2012). Similar to ACO models, under BP, providers have more flexibility regarding service delivery (Steenhuis et al., 2020). Although the main strength of the BP model is to drive providers toward higher-value care and more efficient use of resources, it may also lead to increased admissions, limits on beneficial services, or avoiding patients with complicated health issues (Mechanic & Altman, 2017).

Although people with behavioral health conditions are among the highest users of health-care services, payment reform has not focused on behavioral health. The shift to accountable care models and the associated emphasis on care coordination has the potential to benefit people with behavioral health conditions. However, attention to equity and selection issues is needed. In addition to using performance benchmarks that include behavioral health conditions, equity-focused measures are equally important to support providers caring for underserved populations (Crook et al., 2021).

To effectively respond to incentives in alternative payment models, programs need resources to make changes. As alternative payment models expand, ensuring enough resources are available to respond is essential. Historically, behavioral health treatment has been underfunded, and shifting the same amount to a new payment model will not likely result in improvements in care and outcomes. The approach and underlying data used to design alternative payment models is particularly important for behavioral health. Ensuring the payment rate is adequate for delivering quality care under the alternative payment model and not based on retrospective data of episodes which do not meet quality metrics is key (Quinn et al., 2017a). Programs face structural barriers in responding to incentive models (Davis et al., 2021). Successful alternative payment models for behavioral health providers will offer both flexibility for providers to innovate and provide additional funding necessary to deliver high-quality, patient-centered, and evidence-based treatment services.

Payment Considerations for Quality Improvement

Implementing quality improvements often requires flexibility from financing and payment systems. Innovations are not always aligned with standard payment models. In fact, many novel interventions include components not covered by insurance. Implementing these models requires subsidizing nonreimbursable activities with revenue from reimbursed activities (Hodgkin et al., 2021). For example, offering office-based opioid treatment in primary care typically uses care coordination services delivered by a nurse care manager or other professional, and in many settings, those services are not covered by insurers. Therefore, financing the full office-based opioid treatment model through FFS billing has been impractical for many clinics and physician practices. Instead, office-based opioid treatment programs continue to be financed through federal substance use or opioid response grants. Efforts to implement accountable care offer more flexibility for innovative programs because providers do not have to worry about which aspects of innovations are billable through FFS.

Today, there are efforts toward integrating behavioral and physical health together and toward integrating behavioral health services in social service settings. For example, EDs increasingly help to initiate patients on medication for opioid use disorder and connect them to outpatient care, rather than simply offering information or a referral to outpatient care as they may have done previously. In addition, primary care practices are employing therapists to facilitate 'warm handoffs' to outpatient mental health care, and medical care is offered in some specialty behavioral health clinics. These and additional efforts are needed to improve access to behavioral health services and to facilitate a 'no-wrong-door' approach to entering care. As these innovations are implemented and tested, it will be important to ensure payment models are not barriers to innovation.

Financing Behavioral Health Services Outside the USA

Many of the features of the organization, financing, and delivery of behavioral health services described here is unique to the US health-care delivery systems. In other countries with national health insurance programs, the issues faced by providers and policymakers may be different. However, the need for strong behavioral health-care systems is consistent around the world. Globally, spending on mental health care in low- and middle-income countries is low. We describe here the financing system in South Africa as one example.

Low- and middle-income countries have identified behavioral health as a high priority and critical component to global development (Docrat et al., 2019a). South Africa has declared a national commitment to the development and upscaling of their mental health system as demonstrated in the South African National Mental Health Policy Framework and Strategic Plan 2013–2020 (MHPF). Behavioral health disorders are one of the leading causes of disease burden in South Africa with nearly one in three people experiencing mental illness but only one in four receiving treatment among those with behavioral health needs (Craig et al., 2022; Herman et al., 2009; Petersen et al., 2016). With an explicit need for robust behavioral health treatment pathways, South Africa's health-care system is examining strategies to integrate behavioral health into the existing, disease-centric model of care and to develop a financial structure that sustains these efforts (Docrat et al., 2019b). However, there have been minimal policy changes to execute the proposed plans. These initiatives are stunted by poor infrastructure and a lack of data-driven methods to communicate the importance and long-term vision of a transformed behavioral health-care systems, as well as inadequate technical support for policy implementation (Docrat et al., 2019a).

Currently, South Africa spends 5% of the national public health budget on mental health care (USD 615.3 million), with 86% of expenditures concentrated in inpatient, specialized care (AxessHealth, 2023; Docrat et al., 2019b). Few financial resources are allocated toward disease prevention and behavioral health promotion in outpatient or community-based settings despite a lower prevalence of SMI. There are also inequitable expenditures and distribution of resources, such as mental health clinicians between provinces, which contributes to widespread disparities (Freeman, 2022). With an overextended and under-resourced public health-care system serving nearly 80% of the population, there is a growing interest in establishing universal health care to distribute health-care resources more equitably, increase coverage, and decrease the treatment gap (Freeman, 2022).

To implement South Africa's commitment to behavioral health care, scholars recommend a redistribution of resources and investment in key initiatives. First, the development of data infrastructure technologies to inform evidence-based decision-making and transparency will demonstrate the benefits of an integrated behavioral health system and address associated stigmas (Freeman, 2022). Second, increased investment in disease prevention and promotion programming is also a critical driver to achieve long-term public health and mental wellness. Finally, to address province-wide disparities, behavioral health resources must target underserved localities. The nation's initiative to establish universal health care may also reduce barriers to quality treatment. South Africa's goal to achieve an equitable and efficient behavioral health-care system relies upon structural changes to the public health financing system and an intentional investment in the population's health needs.

Implications for Women's Behavioral Health

Although more than one-third of Americans have behavioral health conditions, behavioral health services are underutilized, exacerbated by the low total expenditures for behavioral health care. Research is needed on how payment and financing approaches can be used to improve the utilization and quality of behavioral health care. Medicaid programs pay a substantial portion of behavioral health-care costs, yet there is almost no information on Medicaid managed care plan policies related to behavioral health services. Research that systematically examines policies of managed care plans is needed. At the delivery system level, studies are needed to determine the effectiveness and optimal implementation approaches for delivery system changes to improve the availability and appeal of behavioral health services. The use of peer recovery specialists in EDs and telehealth expansion for behavioral health services are two approaches which may improve the accessibility and availability of services.

Policies at multiple levels, from the federal government to payers and providers, influence access to and outcomes of behavioral health treatment services. State policy plays an active role in influencing which managed care plans are offered, as well as regulating the plans in terms of enrollment, premiums, benefits, and other policies. In turn, managed care plans set their policies for both provider networks and patients in response to their own goals and state policies. Providers make decisions about whether to participate in managed care networks and the types of care they deliver in response to managed care policies. A more rigorous understanding of how policies and decisions made by states, plans, and providers influence patient access to care, quality, and outcomes of behavioral health care will help to identify policy levers to improve care.

Policy changes, including the federal parity law, the ACA, and telehealth expansion, have transformed behavioral health services. New grants and policies which support innovations to improve service delivery must consider financing and payment from the outset to ensure changes are sustainable going forward. Due to the systematic underuse of behavioral health services, payment models that incentivize and support improved access and use of evidence-based treatment services are needed. The COVID-19 pandemic affected both the availability and delivery of behavioral health treatment. In the wake of the COVID-19 pandemic in the USA, the need to expand the availability of quality behavioral health treatment for both mental illnesses and SUDs is even more urgent.

Acknowledgments The authors thank Sage Feltus, MS, for very capable research assistance, and Kurt D. Lebeck, MSW, for contributing to a first draft of the chapter.

References

Abrams, M. K., Nuzum, R., Zezza, M. A., Ryan, J., Kiszla, J., & Guterman, S. (2015). *The Affordable Care Act's payment and delivery system reforms: A progress report at five years.* [Report]. The Commonwealth Fund. https://doi.org/10.26099/fx69-kq34

Alvarez, K. S., Bhavan, K., Mathew, S., Johnson, C., McCarthy, A., Garcia, B., Callies, M., Stovall, K., Harms, M., & Kho, K. A. (2022). Addressing childcare as a barrier to healthcare access through community partnerships in a large public health system. *BMJ Open Quality, 11*(4), e001964. https://doi.org/10.1136/bmjoq-2022-001964

American Psychological Association. (2022). *Psychologists struggle to meet demand amid mental health crisis.* [Report]. https://www.apa.org/pubs/reports/practitioner/2022-covid-psychologist-workload.pdf

Andrews, C. M., Grogan, C. M., Westlake, M. A., Abraham, A. J., Pollack, H. A., D'Aunno, T. A., & Friedmann, P. D. (2018). Do benefits restrictions limit Medicaid acceptance in addiction treatment? Results from a national study. *Journal of Substance Abuse Treatment, 87*, 50–55.

Andrews, C. M., Abraham, A. J., Grogan, C. M., Westlake, M. A., Pollack, H. A., & Friedmann, P. D. (2019). Impact of Medicaid restrictions on availability of buprenorphine in addiction treatment programs. *American Journal of Public Health, 109*(3), 434–436. https://doi.org/10.2105/AJPH.2018.304856

Andrews, C. M., Hinds, O. M., Lozano-Rojas, F., Besmann, W. L., Abraham, A. J., Grogan, C. M., & Silverman, A. F. (2023). State funding for substance use disorder treatment declined in the wake of Medicaid expansion. *Health Affairs, 42*(7), 981–990. https://doi.org/10.1377/hlthaff.2022.01568

Andrilla, C. H. A., Patterson, D. G., Garberson, L. A., Coulthard, C., & Larson, E. H. (2018). Geographic variation in the supply of selected behavioral health providers. *American Journal of Preventive Medicine, 54*(6), S199–S207. https://doi.org/10.1016/j.amepre.2018.01.004

Artiga, S., Hill, L., & Damico, A. (2022). *Health coverage by race and ethnicity, 2010-201.* [Report]. KFF.

AxessHealth. (2023). *Mental health in SA in dire need of better funding: Society of South African Society of Psychiatrists.* [Report]. https://www.axesshealth.org/blog/mental-health-in-sa-in-dire-need-of-better-funding-sasop

Barry, C. L., Gabel, J., Frank, R. G., Hawkins, S., Whitmore, H., & Pickreign, J. (2003). Design of mental health benefits: Still unequal after all these years. *Health Affairs, 22*(5), 127–137. https://doi.org/10.1377/hlthaff.22.5.127

Berenson, R. A., Upadhyay, D. K., Delbanco, S. F., & Murray, R. (2016, May 3). *Payment methods: How they work.* [Research report]. Urban Institute. https://www.urban.org/research/publication/payment-methods-how-they-work

Beronio, K., Glied, S., & Frank, R. (2014). How the Affordable Care Act and Mental Health Parity and Addiction Equity Act greatly expand coverage of behavioral health care. *The Journal of Behavioral Health Services & Research, 41*(4), 410–428. https://doi.org/10.1007/s11414-014-9412-0

Brucker, D. L., & Stewart, M. (2011). Performance-based contracting within a state substance abuse treatment system: A preliminary exploration of differences in client access and client outcomes. *The Journal of Behavioral Health Services & Research, 38*(3), 383–397. https://doi.org/10.1007/s11414-010-9228-5

Busch, S. H., Epstein, A. J., Harhay, M. O., Fiellin, D. A., Un, H., Leader, D., & Barry, C. L. (2014). The effects of federal parity on substance use disorder treatment. *The American Journal of Managed Care, 20*(1), 76–82. https://www.ajmc.com/view/the-effects-of-federal-parity-on-substance-use-disorder-treatment

Candon, M., Zuckerman, S., Wissoker, D., Saloner, B., Kenney, G. M., Rhodes, K., & Polsky, D. (2018). Declining Medicaid fees and primary care appointment availability for new Medicaid patients. *JAMA Internal Medicine, 178*(1), 145–146. https://doi.org/10.1001/jamainternmed.2017.6302

Casalino, L. P. (1999). The unintended consequences of measuring quality on the quality of medical care. *New England Journal of Medicine, 341*(15), 1147–1150. https://doi.org/10.1056/NEJM199910073411511

Centers for Medicare & Medicaid Services. (2023). *December 2022 Medicaid & CHIP enrollment data highlights.* [Web page]. https://www.medicaid.gov/sites/default/files/2023-03/December-2022-medicaid-chip-enrollment-trend-snapshot.pdf

Claxton, G., Rae, M., Damico, A., Wager, E., Young, G., & Whitmore, H. (2022). Health benefits in 2022: Premiums remain steady, many employers report limited provider networks for behavioral health. *Health Affairs, 41*(11), 1670–1680. https://doi.org/10.1377/hlthaff.2022.01139

Cohen, R. A., & Cha, A. E. (2022). *Health insurance coverage: Early release of estimates from the National Health Interview Survey, 2022.* https://www.cdc.gov/nchs/data/nhis/earlyrelease/insur202305_1.pdf

Cohen, R. A., Cha, A. E., Terlizzi, E. P., & Martinez, M. E. (2021). *Demographic variation in health insurance coverage: United States, 2019.* National Health Statistics Reports, no. 159, 1–15. Number 159. https://www.cdc.gov/nchs/data/nhsr/nhsr159-508.pdf

Consolidated Appropriations Act, 2023, Pub. L. 117–328. (2023). https://www.govinfo.gov/content/pkg/PLAW-117publ328/pdf/PLAW-117publ328.pdf

Cook, B. L., & Alegría, M. (2011). Racial-ethnic disparities in substance abuse treatment: The role of criminal history and socioeconomic status. *Psychiatric Services, 62*(11), 1273–1281. https://doi.org/10.1176/ps.62.11.pss6211_1273

Cook, B. L., Trinh, N., Li, Z., Hou, S. S., & Progovac, A. M. (2017). Trends in racial-ethnic disparities in access to mental health care 2004–2012. *Psychiatric Services 68*(1), 9–16. https://doi.org/10.1176/appi.ps.201500453

Cook, B. L., Flores, M., Zuvekas, S. H., Newhouse, J. P., Hsu, J., Sonik, R., Lee, E., & Fung, V. (2020). The impact of Medicare's mental health cost-sharing parity on use of mental health care services. *Health Affairs, 39*(5), 819–827. https://doi.org/10.1377/hlthaff.2019.01008

Copeland, V. C., & Snyder, K. (2011). Barriers to mental health treatment services for low-income African American women whose children receive behavioral health services: An ethnographic investigation. *Social Work in Public Health, 26*(1), 78–95. https://doi.org/10.1080/10911350903341036

Craig, A., Rochat, T., Naicker, S. N., Mapanga, W., Mtintsilana, A., Dlamini, S. N., Ware, L. J., Du Toit, J., Draper, C. E., Richter, L., & Norris, S. A. (2022). The prevalence of probable depression and probable anxiety, and associations with adverse childhood experiences and socio-demographics: A national survey in South Africa. *Frontiers in Public Health, 10*, 1–13. https://www.frontiersin.org/articles/10.3389/fpubh.2022.986531

Crook, H. L., Saunders, R. S., Roiland, R., Higgins, A., & McClellan, M. B. (2021). A decade of value-based payment: Lessons learned and implications for the Center for Medicare and Medicaid Innovation, Part 2. *Health Affairs Forefront.* https://www.healthaffairs.org/do/10.1377/forefront.20210607.656313/

Davis, M. T., Torres, M., Nguyen, A., Stewart, M., & Reif, S. (2021). Improving quality and performance in substance use treatment programs: What is being done and why is it so hard? *Journal of Social Work (London, England), 21*(2), 141–161. https://doi.org/10.1177/1468017319867834

Dieleman, J. L., Cao, J., Chapin, A., Chen, C., Li, Z., Liu, A., Horst, C., Kaldjian, A., Matyasz, T., Scott, K. W., Bui, A. L., Campbell, M., Duber, H. C., Dunn, A. C., Flaxman, A. D., Fitzmaurice, C., Naghavi, M., Sadat, N., Shieh, P., et al. (2020). US health care spending by payer and health condition, 1996–2016. *JAMA, 323*(9), 863–884. https://doi.org/10.1001/jama.2020.0734

Docrat, S., Besada, D., Cleary, S., Daviaud, E., & Lund, C. (2019a). Mental health system costs, resources and constraints in South Africa: A national survey. *Health Policy and Planning, 34*(9), 706–719. https://doi.org/10.1093/heapol/czz085

Docrat, S., Lund, C., & Chisholm, D. (2019b). Sustainable financing options for mental health care in South Africa: Findings from a situation analysis and key informant interviews. *International Journal of Mental Health Systems, 13*(1), 4. https://doi.org/10.1186/s13033-019-0260-4

Druss, B. G. (2002). The mental health/primary care interface in the United States: History, structure, and context. *General Hospital Psychiatry, 24*(4), 197–202. https://doi.org/10.1016/S0163-8343(02)00170-6

Eylem, O., de Wit, L., van Straten, A., Steubl, L., Melissaourgaki, Z., Danisman, G. T., de Vries, R., Kerhof, A. J. F. M., Bhui, K., & Cuijpers, P. (2020). Stigma for common mental disorders in racial minorities and majorities a systematic review and meta-analysis. *BMC Public Health, 20*, 879. https://doi.org/10.1186/s12889-020-08964-3

Figueroa, J. F., Phelan, J., Orav, E. J., Patel, V., & Jha, A. K. (2020). Association of mental health disorders with health care spending in the Medicare population. *JAMA Network Open, 3*(3), e201210. https://doi.org/10.1001/jamanetworkopen.2020.1210

Finegold, K., Conmy, A., Chu, R. C., Bosworth, A., & Sommers, B. D. (2021). *Trends in the U.S. Uninsured Population, 2010-2020 (Issue Brief No. HP-2021-02)*. Office of the Assistant Secretary for Planning and Evaluation, U.S. Department of Health and Human Services. https://aspe.hhs.gov/sites/default/files/private/pdf/265041/trends-in-the-us-uninsured.pdf

Foutz, J., Artiga, S., & Garfield, R. (2017). *The role of Medicaid in rural America*. [Medicaid Issue Brief]. KFF. https://www.kff.org/medicaid/issue-brief/the-role-of-medicaid-in-rural-america/

Frank, R. G., McGuire, T. G., Bae, J. P., & Rupp, A. (1997). Solutions for adverse selection in behavioral health care. *Health Care Financing Review, 18*(3), 109–122. https://www.ncbi.nlm.nih.gov/pmc/articles/PMC4194506/

Freeman, M. (2022). Investing for population mental health in low and middle income countries: Where and why? *International Journal of Mental Health Systems, 16*, 38. https://doi.org/10.1186/s13033-022-00547-6

Freeman, R., Coyne, J., & Kingsdale, J. (2020). Successes and failures with bundled payments in the commercial market. *The American Journal of Managed Care, 26*, e300–e304. https://doi.org/10.37765/ajmc.2020.88503

Fullerton, C. A., Henke, R. M., Crable, E. L., Hohlbauch, A., & Cummings, N. (2016). The Impact of Medicare ACOs on improving integration and coordination of physical and behavioral health care. *Health Affairs, 35*(7), 1257–1265. https://doi.org/10.1377/hlthaff.2016.0019

Gabbidon, J., Farrelly, S., Hatch, S. L., Henderson, C., Williams, P., Bhugra, D., Dockery, L., Lassman, F., Thornicroft, G., & Clement, S. (2014). Discrimination attributed to mental illness or race-ethnicity by users of community psychiatric services. *Psychiatric Services, 65*(11), 1360–1366. https://doi.org/10.1176/appi.ps.201300302

Garnick, D. W., Horgan, C. M., Reif, S., Merrick, E. L., & Hodgkin, D. (2008). Management of behavioral health provider networks in private health plans. *The Journal of Ambulatory Care Management, 31*(4), 330. https://doi.org/10.1097/01.JAC.0000336552.62084.3b

Ginsburg, P. B. (2012). Fee-for-service will remain a feature of major payment reforms, requiring more changes in Medicare physician payment. *Health Affairs, 31*(9), 1977–1983. https://doi.org/10.1377/hlthaff.2012.0350

Glied, S. A., & Frank, R. G. (2006). *Better but not well: Mental health policy in the United States since 1950*. Johns Hopkins University Press. https://doi.org/10.1353/book.3252

Guth, M. (2021b, December 9). *State policies expanding access to behavioral health care in Medicaid*. [Issue brief]. KFF. https://www.kff.org/medicaid/issue-brief/state-policies-expanding-access-to-behavioral-health-care-in-medicaid/

Hedegaard, H., Miniño, A., Spencer, M. R., & Warner, M. (2021). *Drug overdose deaths in the United States, 1999–2020*. NCHS Data Brief, no. 428, 1–8. https://doi.org/10.15620/cdc:112340

Herman, A. A., Stein, D. J., Seedat, S., Heeringa, S. G., Moomal, H., & Williams, D. R. (2009). The South African Stress and Health (SASH) study: 12-month and lifetime prevalence of common mental disorders. *South African Medical Journal = Suid-Afrikaanse Tydskrif Vir Geneeskunde, 99*(5 Pt 2), 339–344. https://www.ncbi.nlm.nih.gov/pmc/articles/PMC3191537/

Hinton, E., & Raphael, J. (2023). *10 Things to know about Medicaid managed care*. [Report]. KFF. https://www.kff.org/medicaid/issue-brief/10-things-to-know-about-medicaid-managed-care/

Hodgkin, D., Horgan, C. M., Quinn, A. E., Merrick, E. L., Stewart, M. T., & Leslie, L. K. (2014). Management of newer medications for attention-deficit/hyperactivity disorder in commercial health plans. *Clinical Therapeutics, 36*(12), 2034–2046. https://doi.org/10.1016/j.clinthera.2014.09.019

Hodgkin, D., Horgan, C. M., Creedon, T. B., Merrick, E. L., & Stewart, M. T. (2015). Management of newer antidepressant medications in U.S. commercial health plans. *The Journal of Mental Health Policy and Economics, 18*(4), 165–173. https://www.ncbi.nlm.nih.gov/pmc/articles/PMC4812668/

Hodgkin, D., Horgan, C. M., Stewart, M. T., Quinn, A. E., Creedon, T. B., Reif, S., & Garnick, D. W. (2018). Federal parity and access to behavioral health care in private health plans. *Psychiatric Services, 69*(4), 396–402. https://doi.org/10.1176/appi.ps.201700203

Hodgkin, D., Garnick, D. W., Horgan, C. M., Busch, A. B., Stewart, M. T., & Reif, S. (2020). Is it feasible to pay specialty substance use disorder treatment programs based on patient outcomes? *Drug and Alcohol Dependence, 206*, 107735. https://doi.org/10.1016/j.drugalcdep.2019.107735

Hodgkin, D., Horgan, C. M., Stewart, M., & Brown, S. J. (2021). New interventions io address substance use disorder must take financial sustainability into account. *Health Affairs Forefront.* https://doi.org/10.1377/forefront.20210129.865724

Horgan, C. M., Stewart, M. T., Reif, S., Garnick, D. W., Hodgkin, D., Merrick, E. L., & Quinn, A. E. (2016). Behavioral health services in the changing landscape of private health plans. *Psychiatric Services, 67*(6), 622–629. https://doi.org/10.1176/appi.ps.201500235

Huskamp, H. A., Samples, H., Hadland, S. E., McGinty, E. E., Gibson, T. B., Goldman, H. H., Busch, S. H., Stuart, E. A., & Barry, C. L. (2017). Mental health spending and intensity of service use among individuals with diagnoses of eating disorders following federal parity. *Psychiatric Services, 69*(2), 217–223. https://doi.org/10.1176/appi.ps.201600516

Huskamp, H. A., Busch, A. B., Souza, J., Uscher-Pines, L., Rose, S., Wilcock, A., Landon, B. E., & Mehrotra, A. (2018). How is telemedicine being used in opioid and other substance use disorder treatment? *Health Affairs, 37*(12), 1940–1947. https://doi.org/10.1377/hlthaff.2018.05134

Jalnapurkar, I., Allen, M., & Pigott, T. (2018). Sex differences in anxiety disorders: A review. *Journal of Psychiatry Depression & Anxiety, 4*, 012. https://doi.org/10.24966/PDA-0150/100012

Jia, H., Guerin, R. J., Barile, J. P., Okun, A. H., McKnight-Eily, L., Blumberg, S. J., Njai, R., & Thompson, W. W. (2021). National and state trends in anxiety and depression severity scores among adults during the COVID-19 pandemic: United States, 2020–2021. *MMWR. Morbidity and Mortality Weekly Report, 70*(40), 1427–1432. https://doi.org/10.15585/mmwr.mm7040e3

Karaye, I. M., Maleki, N., Hassan, N., & Yunusa, I. (2023). Trends in alcohol-related deaths by sex in the US, 1999–2020. *JAMA Network Open, 6*(7), e2326346. https://doi.org/10.1001/jamanetworkopen.2023.26346

Kaufman, B. G., Spivack, B. S., Stearns, S. C., Song, P. H., & O'Brien, E. C. (2019). Impact of accountable care organizations on utilization, care, and outcomes: A systematic review. *Medical Care Research and Review: MCRR, 76*(3), 255–290. https://doi.org/10.1177/1077558717745916

Keeler, E. B., Manning, W. G., & Wells, K. B. (1988). The demand for episodes of mental health services. *Journal of Health Economics, 7*(4), 369–392. https://doi.org/10.1016/0167-6296(88)90021-5

Keisler-Starkey, K. & Bunch, L. N. (2022, September 13). *Health insurance coverage in the United States: 2021.* [Report; P60–278]. U. S. Census Bureau. https://www.census.gov/library/publications/2022/demo/p60-278.html

Kemmick Pintor, J., Alcalá, H. E., Roby, D. H., Grande, D. T., Alberto, C. K., McKenna, R. M., & Ortega, A. N. (2019). Disparities in pediatric provider availability by insurance type after the ACA in California. *Academic Pediatrics, 19*(3), 325–332. https://doi.org/10.1016/j.acap.2018.09.003

KFF. (2012). *Medicaid's role for women across the lifespan: Current issues and the impact of the Affordable Care Act.* [Fact sheet], Henry J. Kaiser Family Foundation. https://files.kff.org/attachment/medicaid-role-for-women-across-the-lifespan-issue-brief

KFF. (2021). *Total number of Medicare beneficiaries by type of coverage* (State Health Facts). https://www.kff.org/medicare/state-indicator/total-medicare-beneficiaries/

KFF. (2022a). *Women's health insurance coverage.* [Fact sheet]. https://www.kff.org/womens-health-policy/fact-sheet/womens-health-insurance-coverage/

KFF. (2022b). *2022 employer health benefits survey: Summary of findings.* [Report]. https://www.kff.org/report-section/ehbs-2022-summary-of-findings/

KFF. (2023). *Total Medicaid MCO enrollment.* [Medicaid Managed Care Tracker; Timeframe: 2021]. https://www.kff.org/other/state-indicator/total-medicaid-mco-enrollment/

Knaak, S., Mantler, E., & Szeto, A. (2017). Mental illness-related stigma in healthcare. *Healthcare Management Forum, 30*(2), 111–116. https://doi.org/10.1177/0840470416679413

Kuehner, C. (2017). Why is depression more common among women than among men? *The Lancet Psychiatry, 4*(2), 146–158. https://doi.org/10.1016/S2215-0366(16)30263-2

Kushner, J., & McConnell, K. J. (2019). Addressing social determinants of health through Medicaid: Lessons from Oregon. *Journal of Health Politics, Policy and Law, 44*(6), 919–935. https://doi.org/10.1215/03616878-7785823

Lave, J. R., & Goldman, H. H. (1990). Medicare financing for mental health care. *Health Affairs, 9*(1), 19–30. https://doi.org/10.1377/hlthaff.9.1.19

Lo Sasso, A. T., & Lyons, J. S. (2002). The effects of copayments on substance abuse treatment expenditures and treatment reoccurrence. *Psychiatric Services, 53*(12), 1605–1611. https://ps.psychiatryonline.org/doi/10.1176/appi.ps.53.12.1605

Long, S. K., Stockley, K., & Dahlen, H. (2012). Massachusetts health reforms: Uninsurance remains low, self-reported health status improves as state prepares to tackle costs. *Health Affairs, 31*(2), 444–451. https://doi.org/10.1377/hlthaff.2011.0653

Mark, T. L., Yee, T., Levit, K. R., Camacho-Cook, J., Cutler, E., & Carroll, C. D. (2016). Insurance financing increased for mental health conditions but not for substance use disorders, 1986–2014. *Health Affairs, 35*(6), 958–965. https://www.healthaffairs.org/doi/10.1377/hlthaff.2016.0002

Mathes, T., Pieper, D., Morche, J., Polus, S., Jaschinski, T., & Eikermann, M. (2019). Pay for performance for hospitals. *The Cochrane Database of Systematic Reviews, 2019*(7), CD011156. https://doi.org/10.1002/14651858.CD011156.pub2

McGinty, E. E., & Daumit, G. L. (2020). Integrating mental health and addiction treatment into general medical care: The role of policy. *Psychiatric Services, 71*(11), 1163–1169. https://doi.org/10.1176/appi.ps.202000183

McGuire, T. G., & Sinaiko, A. D. (2010). Regulating a health insurance exchange: Implications for individuals with mental illness. *Psychiatric Services, 61*(11), 1074–1080. https://doi.org/10.1176/ps.2010.61.11.1074

McLellan, A. T., & Woodworth, A. M. (2014). The Affordable Care Act and treatment for "substance use disorders": Implications of ending segregated behavioral healthcare. *Journal of Substance Abuse Treatment, 46*(5), 541–545. https://doi.org/10.1016/j.jsat.2014.02.001

McWilliams, J. M., Hatfield, L. A., Landon, B. E., Hamed, P., & Chernew, M. E. (2018). Medicare spending after 3 years of the Medicare Shared Savings Program. *New England Journal of Medicine, 379*(12), 1139–1149. https://doi.org/10.1056/NEJMsa1803388

Mechanic, R. E., & Altman, S. H. (2017). Payment reform options: Episode payment is a good place to start. *Health Affairs, 28*(Supplement 2), w262–w271. https://doi.org/10.1377/hlthaff.28.2.w262

Medicare Improvements for Patients and Providers Act, 2008, Pub. L. 110–275. (2008). https://www.congress.gov/bill/110th-congress/house-bill/6331?overview=closed

Mendelson, A., Kondo, K., Damberg, C., Low, A., Motúapuaka, M., Freeman, M., O'Neil, M., Relevo, R., & Kansagara, D. (2017). The effects of pay-for-performance programs on health, health care use, and processes of care: A systematic review. *Annals of Internal Medicine, 166*(5), 341. https://doi.org/10.7326/M16-1881

Mulia, N. (2020). Alcohol-related disparities among women: Evidence and potential explanations. *Alcohol Research: Current Reviews, 40*(2), arcr.v40.2.09. https://doi.org/10.35946/arcr.v40.2.09

Mulvaney-Day, N., DeAngelo, D., Chen, C., Cook, B. L., & Alegría, M. (2012). Unmet need for treatment for substance use disorders across race and ethnicity. *Drug & Alcohol Dependence, 125*(Suppl 1), S44–S50. https://doi.org/10.1016/j.drugalcdep.2012.05.005

Mykyta, L., Keisler-Starkey, K. & Bunch, L. (2022). *More children were covered by Medicaid and CHIP in 2021.* [Report]. United States Census Bureau. https://www.census.gov/library/stories/2022/09/uninsured-rate-of-children-declines.html

National Association of State Alcohol and Drug Abuse Directors. (2021). *Substance abuse prevention and treatment (SAPT) block grant.* [Fact Sheet]. https://nasadad.org/wp-content/uploads/2019/03/SAPT-Block-Grant-Fact-Sheet-Feb.-2021-FINAL.pdf

National Committee for Quality Assurance. (2023). *HEDIS measures and technical resources.* NCQA. https://www.ncqa.org/hedis/measures/

NEJM Catalyst. (2018). What is pay for performance in healthcare? *NEJM Catalyst, 4*(2). https://doi.org/10.1056/CAT.18.0245

Ochieng, N., Fuglesten Biniek, J., Freed, M., Damico, A., & Neuman, T. (2023). *Medicare Advantage in 2023: Enrollment update and key trends.* [Issue brief]. https://www.kff.org/medicare/issue-brief/medicare-advantage-in-2023-enrollment-update-and-key-trends/

Oliva, E. M., Maisel, N. C., Gordon, A. J., & Harris, A. H. S. (2011). Barriers to use of pharmacotherapy for addiction disorders and how to overcome them. *Current Psychiatry Reports, 13*(5), 374–381. https://doi.org/10.1007/s11920-011-0222-2

Oregon Health Authority. (2022). *Fee-for-service rate increase for Medicaid behavioral health services, effective July 1, 2022.* [Announcement]. https://www.oregon.gov/oha/HSD/OHP/Announcements/BH-Rate-Increase1222.pdf

Panchal, N., Saunders, H., & Ndugga, N. (2022). *Five key findings on mental health and substance use disorders by race/ethnicity.* [Report]. https://www.kff.org/mental-health/issue-brief/five-key-findings-on-mental-health-and-substance-use-disorders-by-race-ethnicity/

Panchal, N., Saunders, H., Rudowitz, R., & Cox, C. (2023, March 20). *The implications of COVID-19 for mental health and substance use.* [Issue brief]. KFF. https://www.kff.org/coronavirus-covid-19/issue-brief/the-implications-of-covid-19-for-mental-health-and-substance-use/

Parish, W., & Mark, T. L. (2022). *The cost of adding substance use disorder services and professionals to Medicare* (p. 13) [Report]. The Legal Action Center. https://www.lac.org/assets/files/LAC_Medicare_Budget_Impact_Report_08_08_2022-submitted.pdf

Parish, W. J., Mark, T. L., Weber, E. M., & Steinberg, D. G. (2022). Substance use disorders among Medicare beneficiaries: Prevalence, mental and physical comorbidities, and treatment barriers. *American Journal of Preventive Medicine, 63*(2), 225–232. https://doi.org/10.1016/j.amepre.2022.01.021

Patient Protection and Affordable Care Act, Pub. L. No. 111–148, 42 U.S.C. §18001. (2010). https://www.govinfo.gov/content/pkg/PLAW-111publ148/pdf/PLAW-111publ148.pdf

Paul Wellstone and Pete Domenici Mental Health Parity and Addiction Equity Act, Pub. L. 110–343. (2008). https://www.govinfo.gov/content/pkg/PLAW-110publ343/pdf/PLAW-110publ343.pdf

Petersen, I., Fairall, L., Bhana, A., Kathree, T., Selohilwe, O., Brooke-Sumner, C., Faris, G., Breuer, E., Sibanyoni, N., Lund, C., & Patel, V. (2016). Integrating mental health into chronic care in South Africa: The development of a district mental healthcare plan. *The British Journal of Psychiatry, 208*(Suppl 56), s29–s39. https://doi.org/10.1192/bjp.bp.114.153726

Polsky, D., Richards, M., Basseyn, S., Wissoker, D., Kenney, G. M., Zuckerman, S., & Rhodes, K. V. (2015). Appointment availability after increases in Medicaid payments for primary care. *New England Journal of Medicine, 372*(6), 537–545. https://doi.org/10.1056/NEJMsa1413299

Priester, M. A., Browne, T., Iachini, A., Clone, S., DeHart, D., & Seay, K. D. (2016). Treatment access barriers and disparities among individuals with co-occurring mental health and substance use disorders: An integrative literature review. *Journal of Substance Abuse Treatment, 61,* 47–59. https://doi.org/10.1016/j.jsat.2015.09.006

Quinn, A. E., Hodgkin, D., Perloff, J. N., Stewart, M. T., Brolin, M., Lane, N., & Horgan, C. M. (2017a). Design and impact of bundled payment for detox and follow-up care. *Journal of Substance Abuse Treatment, 82,* 113–121. https://doi.org/10.1016/j.jsat.2017.09.012

Quinn, A. E., Reif, S., Merrick, E. L., Horgan, C. M., Garnick, D. W., & Stewart, M. T. (2017b). How do private health plans manage specialty behavioral health treatment entry and continuing care? *Psychiatric Services, 68*(9), 931–937. https://doi.org/10.1176/appi.ps.201600081

Reif, S., Horgan, C. M., Hodgkin, D., Matteucci, A.-M., Creedon, T. B., & Stewart, M. T. (2016). Access to addiction pharmacotherapy in private health plans. *Journal of Substance Abuse Treatment, 66*, 23–29. https://doi.org/10.1016/j.jsat.2016.03.001

Rice, A. N., & Harris, S. C. (2021). Issues of cultural competence in mental health care. *Journal of the American Pharmacies Association, Science and Practice Commentary, 61*(1), E65–E68. https://doi.org/10.1016/j.japh.2020.10.015

Robinson, J. C. (2001). Theory and practice in the design of physician payment incentives. *The Milbank Quarterly, 79*(2), 149–177. https://doi.org/10.1111/1468-0009.00202

Roby, D. H., & Jones, E. E. (2016). Limits on same-day billing in Medicaid hinders integration of behavioral health into the medical home model. *Psychological Services, 13*(1), 110–119. https://doi.org/10.1037/ser0000044

Roman, P. M., Abraham, A. J., & Knudsen, H. K. (2011). Using medication-assisted treatment for substance use disorders: Evidence of barriers and facilitators of implementation. *Addictive Behaviors, 36*(6), 584–589. https://doi.org/10.1016/j.addbeh.2011.01.032

Saunders, H., & Rudowitz, R. (2022). *Demographics and health insurance coverage of nonelderly adults with mental illness and substance use disorders in 2020.* [Issue brief]. KFF. https://www.kff.org/mental-health/issue-brief/demographics-and-health-insurance-coverage-of-nonelderly-adults-with-mental-illness-and-substance-use-disorders-in-2020/

Shen, Y.-C. (2003). The effect of financial pressure on the quality of care in hospitals. *Journal of Health Economics, 22*(2), 243–269. https://doi.org/10.1016/S0167-6296(02)00124-8

Sinaiko, A. D., Bambury, E., & Chien, A. T. (2021). *Consumer choice in U.S. health care: Using Insights from the past to inform the way forward.* [Fund Report]. The Commonwealth Fund. https://doi.org/10.26099/7xbc-sb06

Steenhuis, S., Struijs, J., Koolman, X., Ket, J., & Van Der Hijden, E. (2020). Unraveling the complexity in the design and implementation of bundled payments: A scoping review of key elements from a payer's perspective. *The Milbank Quarterly, 98*(1), 197–222. https://doi.org/10.1111/1468-0009.12438

Stein, B. D., Pacula, R. L., Gordon, A. J., Burns, R. M., Leslie, D. L., Sorbero, M. J., Bauhoff, S., Mandell, T. W., & Dick, A. W. (2015). Where is buprenorphine dispensed to treat opioid use disorders? The role of private offices, opioid treatment programs, and substance abuse treatment facilities in urban and rural counties. *Milbank Quarterly, 93*(3), 561–583. https://doi.org/10.1111/1468-0009.12137

Stewart, R. E., Lareef, I., Hadley, T. R., & Mandell, D. S. (2017). Can we pay for performance in behavioral health care? *Psychiatric Services, 68*(2), 109–111. https://doi.org/10.1176/appi.ps.201600475

Stewart, M. T., Reif, S., Dana, B., Nguyen, A., Torres, M., Davis, M. T., Ritter, G., Hodgkin, D., & Horgan, C. M. (2018). Incentives in a public addiction treatment system: Effects on waiting time and selection. *Journal of Substance Abuse Treatment, 95*, 1–8. https://doi.org/10.1016/j.jsat.2018.09.002

Stuart, E. A., Barry, C. L., Donohue, J. M., Greenfield, S. F., Duckworth, K., Song, Z., Kouri, E. M., Ebnesajjad, C., Mechanic, R., Chernew, M. E., & Huskamp, H. A. (2017a). Effects of accountable care and payment reform on substance use disorder treatment: Evidence from the initial three years of the alternative quality contract. *Addiction (Abingdon, England), 112*(1), 124–133. https://doi.org/10.1111/add.13555

Stuart, E. A., McGinty, E. E., Kalb, L., Huskamp, H. A., Busch, S. H., Gibson, T. B., Goldman, H., & Barry, C. L. (2017b). Increased service use among children with autism spectrum disorder associated with mental health parity law. *Health Affairs, 36*(2), 337–345. https://doi.org/10.1377/hlthaff.2016.0824

Substance Abuse and Mental Health Services Administration. (2018). *Medicaid coverage of medication-assisted treatment for alcohol and opioid use disorders and of medication for the reversal of opioid overdose*. [Report; HHS Publication No. SMA-18-5093]. https://store.samhsa.gov/sites/default/files/d7/priv/medicaidfinancingmatreport_0.pdf

Substance Abuse and Mental Health Services Administration. (2022). *Key substance use and mental health indicators in the United States: Results from the 2021 National Survey on Drug Use and Health*. [Report; HHS Publication No. PEP22-07-01-005, NSDUH Series H-5]. SAMHSA, Center for Behavioral Health Statistics and Quality. https://www.samhsa.gov/data/sites/default/files/reports/rpt39443/2021NSDUHFFRRev010323.pdf

Substance use disorder prevention that promotes opioid recovery and treatment for Patients and Communities Act or the SUPPORT for Patients and Communities Act, Pub. L. No. 115–271. (2018). https://www.govinfo.gov/content/pkg/PLAW-115publ271/pdf/PLAW-115publ271.pdf

Thomeer, M. B., Moody, M. D., & Yahirun, J. (2023). Racial and ethnic disparities in mental health and mental health care during the COVID-19 pandemic. *Journal of Racial Ethnic Disparities, 10*(2), 961–976. https://doi.org/10.1007/s40615-022-01284-9

Thornicroft, G., Sunkel, C., Alikhon Aliev, A., Baker, S., Brohan, E., el Chammay, R., Davies, K., Demissie, M., Duncan, J., Fekadu, W., Gronholm, P. C., Guerrero, Z., Gurung, D., Habtamu, K., Hanlon, C., Heim, E., Henderson, C., Hijazi, Z., Hoffman, C., et al. (2022). The Lancet Commission on ending stigma and discrimination in mental health. *The Lancet, 400*(10361), 1438–1480. https://doi.org/10.1016/S0140-6736(22)01470-2

Tracking Accountability in Government Grants System (TAGGS). (2023). *Block grants for community mental health services*. [Web page]. U.S. Department of Health & Human Services. https://taggs.hhs.gov/Detail/CFDADetail?arg_CFDA_NUM=93958

United States Census Bureau. (2022). *Current population survey, 2021 and 2022 annual social and economic supplements (CPS ASEC)*. United States Census Bureau. https://www.census.gov/content/dam/Census/library/visualizations/2022/demo/p60-278/figure1.pdf

Wakeman, S. E., & Rich, J. D. (2018). Barriers to medications for addiction treatment: How stigma kills. *Substance Use & Misuse, 53*(2), 330–333. https://doi.org/10.1080/10826084.2017.1363238

Walker, E. R., Cummings, J. R., Hockenberry, J. M., & Druss, B. G. (2015). Insurance status, use of mental health services, and unmet need for mental health care in the United States. *Psychiatric Services, 66*(6), 578–584. https://doi.org/10.1176/appi.ps.201400248

Weber, E., & Steinberg, D. G. (2021). *Medicare coverage of substance use disorder: A landscape review of benefit coverage, service gaps and a path to reform*. [Report]. Legal Action Center. https://www.lac.org/resource/medicare-coverage-of-substance-use-disorder-care-a-landscape-review-of-benefit-coverage-service-gaps-and-a-path-to-reform

White, A. (2020). Gender differences in the epidemiology of alcohol use and related harms in the United States. *Alcohol Research: Current Reviews, 40*(2), 01. https://doi.org/10.35946/arcr.v40.2.01

Williams, E. C., Gupta, S., Rubinsky, A. D., Glass, J. E., Jones-Webb, R., Bensley, K. M., & Harris, A. H. S. (2017). Variation in receipt of pharmacotherapy for alcohol use disorders across racial/ethnic groups: A national study in the U.S. Veterans Health Administration. *Drug and Alcohol Dependence, 178*, 527–533. https://doi.org/10.1016/j.drugalcdep.2017.06.011

Xu, W. Y., Song, C., Li, Y., & Retchin, S. M. (2019). Cost-sharing disparities for out-of-network care for adults with behavioral health conditions. *JAMA Network Open, 2*(11), e1914554. https://doi.org/10.1001/jamanetworkopen.2019.14554

Zhu, J. M., Renfro, S., Watson, K., Deshmukh, A., & McConnell, K. J. (2023). Medicaid reimbursement for psychiatric services: Comparisons across states and with Medicare. *Health Affairs (Project Hope), 42*(4), 556–565. https://doi.org/10.1377/hlthaff.2022.00805

Zuckerman, S., Skopec, L., & Epstein, M. (2017). *Medicaid physician fees after the ACA primary care fee bump* (pp. 1–13). Urban Institute.

Chapter 11
Implementation Science to Promote Equity in Women's Behavioral Health

Enya Vroom and Amanda Sharp

Introduction

The scientific process is intentionally methodical and orderly, especially in fields where scientific discovery means the difference between life and death or well-being and suffering. However, the time lag between translating research findings to everyday practice remains problematic (Morris et al., 2011). The process of successfully implementing new strategies may be overlooked, even though the application of innovation is what creates meaningful and effective solutions to real-world problems. Implementation science has emerged in response to this research-to-practice gap, formalizing the application of innovation as an equal part of the scientific process, particularly in biomedical and behavioral sciences. While implementation science research and practice may be commonplace in many areas of health, such as medicine and nursing, implementation science has the potential to play a unique role in women's behavioral health.

We begin by exploring the inequities women have faced in scientific research and the emergence of a focus on women's issues in behavioral health over time. Next, we explore the history and development of implementation science. Finally, we will identify areas in extant literature that effectively utilize implementation science in women-focused interventions globally and identify where these approaches are specifically lacking for women's behavioral health issues. This chapter intends to

E. Vroom (✉)
Department of Medicine, University of Texas Health Science Center at San Antonio, San Antonio, TX, USA
e-mail: vroom@uthscsa.edu

A. Sharp
Department of Psychiatry, Harvard Medical School, Boston, MA, USA
e-mail: asharp@challiance.org

© The Author(s), under exclusive license to Springer Nature Switzerland AG 2024
A. Hanson, B. L. Levin (eds.), *Women's Behavioral Health*,
https://doi.org/10.1007/978-3-031-58293-6_11

provide a broad lens of both implementation science and women's behavioral health, focusing on how women's behavioral health issues may be more equitably addressed.

A Historical Lens on Evidence-Based Women's Behavioral Health Services

Historically, women's needs have been disproportionately affected by societal disparities, a result likely tied to their unequal representation in and engagement with the scientific community. Barely three decades ago, the National Institutes of Health (NIH, n.d.) established a policy advising the inclusion of women in clinical studies. However, it was not until 1993 that women as required participants in NIH research became law (NIH Revitalization Act, Pub. L. No. 103-43, 1993). However, the continued underrepresentation of women in behavioral health services research, delivery, and policy leads to fewer policies, programs, and research with a gender-specific focus (Gupta, 2020).

Societal biases and stereotypes continue to affect timely and appropriate access to and utilization of treatment (Becker & Lynn, 2020; GBD 2016 and HALE Collaborators, 2017; Terlizzi & Zablotsky, 2020). Women are affected disproportionately by the prevalence, incidence, and presentation of behavioral health disorders. For instance, women are twice as likely as men to have major depression or anxiety disorders (Kessler et al., 2005; Substance Abuse and Mental Health Services Administration (SAMHSA), 2018) and up to three times as likely to have post-traumatic stress disorder (PTSD) (Olff, 2017). Certain types of depression are unique only to women, such as premenstrual dysphoric disorder, perinatal depression, and perimenopausal depression (Kessler, 2006; Zhou et al., 2019). Additionally, the rate of women reporting substance use disorders (SUDs) has increased (Back et al., 2011). Women experience a more rapid progression in illicit drug use and have higher rates of drug-related overdose deaths when compared to men (Marsh et al., 2018). Women's behavioral health issues also result in heavier social consequences, medical vulnerabilities, and risks during pregnancy (Erol & Karpyak, 2015; Weiss-Laxer et al., 2021). Despite earlier policy-based mitigation efforts, the persistence of these disparities in current times signals that more specific attention should be given to sex- and gender-related research, training, and practice.

Rise of Evidence-Based Behavioral Health Practices

Due to the significant prevalence of behavioral health problems and the need for highly effective services in the U. S., the push for developing and implementing evidence-based practices (EBPs) has risen exponentially in the last 30 years (Southam-Gerow et al., 2012). Evidence-based practices can be described as activities, protocols, and/or frameworks that have demonstrated effectiveness empirically through research (American Psychological Association, 2006; Sackett et al., 1996). They have evolved to prioritize client and provider values (Spring et al., 2012), for example, prioritizing individualized treatment planning for SUD services (Gruman et al., 2010). Although the number of EBPs increased during the 1990s, at the end of that decade, the US Surgeon General reported the majority of individuals with behavioral health disorders were not receiving evidence-based health services, despite the establishment of EBPs in the scientific community (Office of the Surgeon General, 1999). This research-to-practice gap has resulted in federal and state initiatives and legislation mandating the utilization of empirical evidence in all clinical practices to enhance the effectiveness of services. Although significant strides have occurred in behavioral health services (Hyde & Enomoto, 2015), there remains a gap within research and service provision directed toward women's behavioral health (Ponce et al., 2014; Tuchman, 2010).

As previously mentioned, the NIH in 1993 was mandated to include women and minority groups in all NIH-funded clinical research. The goal of this policy was to determine if the variables in a clinical study affected women or members of minority groups differently than other trial participants (i.e., males and/or White individuals), and researchers were required to provide a rationale for the exclusion of women or members of minority groups (NIH Revitalization Act, Pub. L. No. 103-43, 1993). In 2010, the Patient Protection and Affordable Care Act (PPACA, 2010) and the Health Care and Education Reconciliation Act of 2010 (HCER, 2010) (which comprise the Affordable Care Act [ACA]) continued this shift toward a prioritization of EBPs in behavioral health treatment. The ACA not only expanded the scope of mental health and substance use parity, but it also incorporated EBPs into allowable reimbursements, with the intention of restructuring service systems to prioritize quality and effectiveness. As the importance of and access to equitable behavioral health care have increased, so has the demand for effective services.

Although there has been a steady increase in the availability and use of EBPs, issues related to the effective translation of programs into real-world settings persist (Massey & Vroom, 2020). Past research has estimated that a significant amount of research dollars aimed at clinical innovation have failed to make a public health impact (Bauer & Kirchner, 2020). Further, a large percentage of EBPs never make it into routine practice, as there are numerous challenges in navigating the adoption, implementation, and sustainability of EBPs within behavioral health services delivery. In response to these barriers, evidence-based behavioral health services expanded to prioritize the importance of the implementation process, and the field of implementation science emerged.

The Emergence of Implementation Science in Behavioral Health

In response to the emphasis on local, state, and federal guidelines requiring the use of EBPs, the field of behavioral health uses implementation science as a vehicle to enhance the successful adoption and utilization of evidence-based services. However, innovation development in other fields, such as biomedical sciences, agriculture, and industry, has shown that evidence of efficacy does not ensure uptake. The lack of adaptation of scientifically established "best practices" is grounded in the research fallacy that what works in a lab will work outside of the lab (Bauer & Kirchner, 2020). It has only been in the last several decades the field of implementation science has linked societal and contextual factors with the application of knowledge and technology (Rogers, 2010). Implementation science promotes the tailoring of research findings to improve their application in real-world settings, emphasizing patient-centered outcomes and quality of life.

There are now dozens of theories, models, and frameworks that attempt to support implementation research and practice within different behavioral health service settings (Nilsen, 2015; Damschroder et al., 2009). The implementation science field continues to establish not only specific components of implementation success (e.g., organizational readiness) but also relevant strategies, techniques for evaluation, and critical determinants of outcomes (e.g., fidelity) (Birken et al., 2017; Nilsen, 2015). In addition to frameworks and conceptual models, new research designs have been proposed for implementation research, including user-centered designs (Lyon & Koerner, 2016) and hybrid trials (Landes et al., 2019). These approaches not only highlight effectiveness but also incorporate implementation science research to best understand how, why, and in what settings EBPs are effective (Barwick et al., 2020; Vroom & Massey, 2022).

However, the sheer number of methods and approaches available may impede the selection of an implementation strategy for an EBP. This challenge may be heightened by the interdisciplinary conceptualization of frameworks and strategies across health disciplines, limited collaboration, and nominal guidance selecting methods that guarantee stakeholder's needs are addressed (Lyon & Koerner, 2016). This lack of transparency and cohesion among the research community has led to a "knowledge to practice gap" (Barwick et al., 2020; Vroom & Massey, 2022; Westerlund et al., 2019).

Increasing Health Equity Through Implementation Science

Attention should be paid to effective interventions as well as those interventions that reduce inequities. Healthy People 2030 supports the implementation of effective, scalable, and sustainable EBPs. In addition, state governments are urged to consider Healthy People 2030's recommendations as an important part of government budget priorities to reduce population health burden and reduce inequities in diagnosis, treatment, and access and utilization of services delivery (U.S. Department of Health and Human Services, 2021). However, the continued underrepresentation of vulnerable populations in clinical research, which is responsible for shaping and developing EBPs, has been attributed to contextual economic, social, historical, and/or political factors which may influence or perpetuate inequalities (Baumann & Cabassa, 2020).

Clinical research requires both internal and external validity to ensure the study results are trustworthy and meaningful. While internal validity relates to how well a study is conducted (i.e., its structure), external validity relates to how applicable the findings are to the real world. The emphasis on internal validity potentially affects universal interventions being universally applicable. Since external validity requires research findings from one study generalizes to or across groups of people, settings, treatments, and time periods, generalizability to vulnerable populations may be difficult to establish. However, the generalizability of research may not lend itself to specific populations.

Vulnerable populations often have a variety of health conditions exacerbated by unnecessarily inadequate health care. Further, they are at higher risk for inequities in health-care access and outcomes associated with race, ethnicity, gender, disability, environment, socioeconomic status (SES), geography, access, sociocultural factors, and individuals who lack adequate access to care (e.g., uninsured, underinsured, or those without a regular source of care). Implementation science can inform the development of critical partnerships with key stakeholders in high-income and low-income communities and countries to develop implementation strategies aimed at addressing health equity (Baumann & Cabassa, 2020).

Equity requires that we move beyond "business as usual" and adapt methods, interventions, and implementation strategies to best address patient needs. However, this has caused tension in the research community. Researchers are divided between adapting interventions to meet the needs of a specific setting or population sufficiently and equitably (e.g., gender or race/ethnicity) and leaving the intervention as originally designed. It is argued that an adapted EBP may compromise its essential or "core components," resulting in reduced effectiveness (Carvalho et al., 2013; Chambers & Norton, 2016). Although fidelity is considered the "gold standard" for successful implementation, it may not account for how an EBP fits within a specific context (Vroom & Massey, 2022). An adapted EBP may create a new standard of fidelity for a particular intervention for a specific population. However, continuous adaptations may eventually contradict the intended standardization and accountability efforts of original EBPs. This may result in extremely narrow interventions for increasingly segmented populations, which, in turn, risk failing to meet evidence-based gold standards.

Implementation science has the potential to expedite advancements in improving health equity by seeking to understand the process by which science is successfully brought to practice. Brownson et al. (2021) offer several recommendations to address the research-to-practice challenge. These include incorporating the social determinants of health (SDOH) and equity into health outcomes, systems, sectors, and policy. One such example is the Health Equity Implementation Framework (HEIF), which highlights SDOH factors related to adopting an EBP and increasing equity in health care (Woodward et al., 2019).

The foundation of HEIF is based on domains from the Integrated Promoting Action on Research in Implementation in Health Services (i-PARIHS), including innovation, recipients (i.e., patient and provider), context, and facilitation/process. However, the HEIF incorporated three additional health equity domains to the i-PARIHS: culturally relevant factors (i.e., demographics, medical mistrust, or bias), clinical encounter (i.e., patient-provider interaction), and societal context (i.e., sociopolitical forces, physical structures, and economies). These domains were informed by research that showed strong and explicit relationships with disparities in health care. This framework contrasts with the status quo of casually adding a disparity component to pre-existing frameworks (Brownson et al., 2021) as it accounts for factors at multiple levels in health-care disparities (Woodward et al., 2019). Implementation science frameworks that casually add a disparity component tend to do so in a vague manner, resulting in strategies that are too ambiguous to be meaningful (Woodward et al., 2021).

Although these inclusive strategies and conceptual frameworks are predominantly geared toward general health-care interventions, these strategies can combat inequities explicitly found in women's behavioral health. For example, research has shown a relationship between gender disparities in psychiatric disorders and social inequalities globally (Yu, 2018). Implementation frameworks which aid systems, organizations, and providers in identifying and providing strategies that address SDOH have the potential to improve access and outcomes within women's behavioral health care.

The Role of Implementation Science in Women's Behavioral Health

While the scientific community has been normed primarily by White male contributions, a shift in attention to promoting women in science and their needs in health care has been initiated. This concept has developed alongside the standardization and normalization of implementation science in behavioral health. In attempts to make more equitable contributions to EBPs and their adoption, implementation science asserts a consideration for environmental and societal contexts and diversity. Specifically, the utilization of implementation science in women's behavioral health provides a more equitable opportunity to explore and address the population's unique needs rather than assuming homogeneous approaches would be effective.

Despite the theoretical appropriateness of implementation science as a mechanism for women's behavioral health, few existing studies demonstrate the utilization of implementation frameworks and strategies for gender-specific applications in the U. S. Globally, implementation science has been used predominantly in the development and utilization of solutions for conventional somatic health issues, such as cancer, maternal health, HIV, and diabetes.

For example, a study in Australia used an implementation science approach for developing and implementing a dietitian-led model of care for gestational diabetes using the i-PARIHS framework to develop, implement, and evaluate the model of care (Meloncelli et al., 2020). Another study focused on the prevention of mother-to-child HIV transmission in Mozambique used the Reach, Effectiveness, Adoption, Implementation, and Maintenance (RE-AIM) framework, the Organizational Readiness for Implementing Change (ORIC) tool, and the Consolidated Framework for Implementation Research (CFIR) to guide the evaluation of the intervention, to examine readiness for the adoption of the intervention, and to determine the elements of success (Sherr et al., 2019). The implementation science frameworks in these global examples allowed the researchers to ensure the accurate adoption of person-centered and culturally competent interventions within the context of their specific settings. These studies exemplify the usefulness of implementation science for gender-specific health interventions, setting precedence for which gender-specific behavioral health interventions may build upon in the future.

Despite the lag, implementation science and practice are becoming more integrated into behavioral health research and intervention designs both in the U. S. and globally. As a result, the field of implementation science has developed several mechanisms to assist with the translation of research into real-world practice.

Mechanisms for Translating Research to Practice

Frequently referred to as the "funnel of attrition," there are multiple phases and activities necessary to obtain positive outcomes in real-world settings informed by research that potentially dwindles over time due to barriers (Albers et al., 2020; Colditz & Emmons, 2018). In the last 15 years, the field of implementation science has prioritized understanding the theoretical foundation of how and why the implementation of EBPs may succeed or fail (Nilsen, 2015). The need for better understanding has led the field to develop theoretical bases and explore barriers to and facilitators of implementation. As previously mentioned, there are multiple implementation models, frameworks, and strategies that can be used to plan how an EBP will be adopted, implemented, and/or sustained, to identify determinants that influence implementation, and to evaluate whether implementation was successful (Kirchner et al., 2018; Nilsen, 2015). These tools assist with consolidating findings from implementation science research and aid in working toward definitions, operationalizing implementation science concepts, and developing theory (Damschroder, 2020).

Frameworks now exist that assist with multiple different aspects of implementation, including planning, strategies, and evaluation. One of the most frequently used and cited frameworks is the Consolidated Framework for Implementation Research (CFIR) (Damschroder et al., 2009). The CFIR is a determinant framework that assists with identifying barriers and facilitators and how they may affect implementation outcomes. The CFIR provides an overview of common constructs present in implementation science theory and frameworks and outlines a list of domains that are believed to affect implementation. It is comprised of five domains (i.e., intervention characteristics, outer setting, inner setting, characteristics of individuals involved, and the process of implementation). Each CFIR domain includes multiple constructs (e.g., adaptability, external policies and incentives, implementation climate, self-efficacy, and planning).

Frequently, the CFIR is used in conjunction with the Expert Recommendations for Implementing Change (ERIC) (Powell et al., 2015). The ERIC is a compilation of implementation strategies and definitions gathered from implementation science experts. Many studies use the CFIR to identify implementation determinants (i.e., facilitators or barriers) and then match determinants to different implementation science strategies informed by ERIC. However, more research is needed to adequately prioritize and tailor implementation strategies for specific EBPs, such as intervention mapping (Waltz et al., 2019). There is also a need to incorporate the stakeholder voice in implementation science work.

AcademyHealth's 2021 and 2022 conferences on the Science of Dissemination and Implementation in Health highlighted the importance of stakeholder involvement, reconfiguring power imbalances (i.e., between researchers and community) and focusing on real-world practice. Many researchers and practitioners are familiar with the CFIR, which has been widely cited since its publication in 2009. Despite this, the developers of the CFIR have come to understand the need to capture the nuances of the implementers and intervention recipients to fully inform the implementation process (Damschroder et al., 2021).

The updated CFIR, released in October 2022, includes an Outcomes Addendum, more construct description, an emphasis on operationalizing adapted constructs, measuring constructs both qualitatively and quantitatively, and introduces new constructs related to equity in implementation (Damschroder et al., 2022a). The Outcomes Addendum presents explicit conceptual distinctions between CFIR outcome types. The updated CFIR also introduces new constructs to examine determinants related to equity more successfully and encourages users to utilize equity and social justice theories and collaborate with equity experts (Damschroder et al., 2022a). This will provide clarity for researchers who are considering what outcomes are the most applicable to evaluate and assist in centering outcomes to different individual priorities/interests (e.g., patient, clinician, system). The goal is to "help researchers and organizations orient to values of humanism and equity" (Damschroder et al., 2022b, p. 7).

The welcomed additions and modifications of the CFIR mark an important transition for the field, especially with its strong focus on inequity. We need to critique frameworks and tools to modify and improve them for use so they may be utilized in the most effective ways. This is particularly important for women's behavioral health as the field moves toward implementation frameworks and strategies that are sensitive not only to the unique needs of women but also to the organizations and providers that facilitate women's services provision. These implementation tools can provide needed guidance in certain aspects of service provision. For example, the Implementation Climate Scale (ICS) can be used to assess the implementation climate of an organization. Examining implementation climate can provide insight into how employees perceive the adoption, implementation, and use of an EBP and if the organizational change is expected, rewarded, and prioritized by the organization (Ehrhart et al., 2014). Utilizing comprehensive measures to assess organizational and implementation climates can assist in identifying barriers and facilitators to EBP use that may, directly and indirectly, affect client outcomes.

The field has also come to recognize that implementation is a dynamic process, often being conducted in stages or phases. Implementation process models describe/guide the process of translating research into practice and include different factors that may affect success at different stages or phases of implementation (Nilsen, 2015). The Exploration, Adoption/Preparation, Implementation, and Sustainment (EPIS) framework, a very well-known implementation process model, highlights factors that are particularly important during different stages of implementation in both outer (i.e., service system) and inner (i.e., organization) contexts (Aarons et al., 2011). For example, client advocacy led by organizations at the sociopolitical level (i.e., outer context) may be particularly important for women receiving gender-specific care (inner context, e.g., trauma-informed care), as these organizations can influence policy related to the adoption of specific EBPs.

To successfully utilize evidence-based services and approaches, all components of implementation science (methods, concepts, tools, and measurement) must be considered. For example, measuring implementation outcomes is essential. If implementation outcomes are not measured, it makes it difficult to determine if strong or poor clinical outcomes are related to the intervention or to its implementation (Albers et al., 2020). Hence, researchers may not be capturing the whole picture regarding fidelity or success of implementation.

Utilizing implementation science frameworks allows for research to be replicable and assists with guiding data collection, analysis, and interpretation. These frameworks aid in the establishment of external validity and the ability of implementation research to be generalized across different contexts (Kirk et al., 2016). Utilizing implementation frameworks and tools may shorten the gap between research and practice by enabling knowledge translation, as these frameworks and tools can assist in the development, maintenance, and evaluation of implementation initiatives (Tabak et al., 2018).

The following case studies show how implementation science was integrated at the conceptualization phase and beyond to comprehensively explore the contextual factors that influence the adoption, adaptation, implementation, and sustainability of programs, protocols, and strategies.

Novel Implementation Research Designs

Meffert et al. (2016) utilized a type 1 implementation-effectiveness hybrid research design to determine the effectiveness of interpersonal psychotherapy (IPT) in the treatment of emotional distress among HIV+ female survivors of gender-based violence (GBV) in Kenya. A type 1 hybrid study design seeks to determine the effectiveness of an intervention with broad eligibility, approximate real-world use, and a better understanding of the implementation context. This design contrasts with the traditional model of research, where the main aim is to establish interval validity (i.e., efficacy). Using data from their needs assessment, Meffert et al. (2016) adapted the IPT intervention to better fit the context and target population, focusing on clinician training and the IPT manual. The type 1 study design allowed for adaptations to be made on-site during training and piloting IPT cases to enhance fit while simultaneously preserving fidelity to the IPT protocol.

The type 1 study design allowed for the scale-up and delivery of the adapted IPT with the simultaneous collection of individual clinical outcomes. Not only does this specific design emphasize evaluating effectiveness while allowing for client-level randomization, but it also emphasizes collecting data related to implementation factors (e.g., staff involvement). The design can be critical for the successful scale-up of mental health services within low- and middle-income countries, where female survivors of GBV are at high risk of developing mental disorders (e.g., PTSD) but rarely access the services they need.

Implementing and Sustaining Recovery for Survivors Healing from Abuse

To improve women's outcomes related to sexual violence sequela (e.g., drug use, mental illness, sex work) and reduce recidivism in the criminal justice system is a complex undertaking. Zielinski et al. (2021) implemented an exposure-based group therapy program, known as the Survivors Healing from Abuse: Recovery through Exposure (SHARE) program, with incarcerated women who have been victims of sexual violence. This innovative program began through a partnership between a clinical psychology program, a women's prison in Kentucky (US), and a domestic violence shelter. A retrospective process evaluation using the EPIS and ERIC frameworks was conducted to evaluate the program to examine potential barriers and facilitators to implementing and sustaining SHARE.

The EPIS framework (Aarons et al., 2011) guided the researchers in the development of the qualitative interview guide, which elicited implementation information, including organizational, implementer, and intervention characteristics. To analyze the qualitative interviews, EPIS phases were assigned to segments of data. In addition, the ERIC was used to identify and code implementation strategies within the interviews. Utilizing different implementation frameworks, such as EPIS and ERIC, allowed for a closer examination of characteristics and strategies that may be unique to violence programs implemented for women. Key findings highlighted crucial factors of successful implementation: mutually beneficial partnerships, collaborators sharing similar values, program champions, and training for implementers. From an implementation practice standpoint, the nontraditional, integrated use of partnerships seemed to be a key element to the successful implementation and sustainability of a behavioral health intervention focused on treating female victims of sexual violence.

Development and Pilot Test of an Adaptable Protocol to Address Postpartum Depression

Although PPD affects approximately 25% of women in lower-income and minority populations, less than half of pediatricians serving these populations screen or refer for PPD in the first 6 months postpartum. To address this inequity in service, Goff et al. (2020) developed and piloted a PPD screening protocol in safety-net pediatric care practices in Massachusetts (US). The CFIR was used to guide the conceptual and analytic framework for the two-phase pilot study. Phase 1 saw the development of a focus group interview guide as well as the codebook development and data analysis. Data from Phase 1 focus groups informed not only the development of the PPD screening and referral protocol but also provided strategies tailored to implement the protocol across the safety-net practices.

Goff et al. (2020) also formed an advisory board with members from a community health setting, a behavioral health system, and a perinatal depression coalition to assist in developing the protocol. The advisory board's workgroup discussions were guided by the CFIR and aided the advisory board in identifying potential barriers to implementation and developing implementation strategies (e.g., creating a PPD toolkit that includes resources and reminders for providers). Results provided insight into barriers and facilitators that may be experienced when implementing evidence-based PPD screening, such as difficulties coordinating care when the mother is not the patient or privacy regulations.

The development of this PPD screening protocol was conducted in a flexible setting, with the goal of the screening tool to be adaptable in different settings to best suit the needs of the provider and client. The study aimed to develop implementation strategies that were informed by key stakeholders (i.e., providers). The goal was not to test the effectiveness of said strategies but instead to use a layered approach to inform the implementation of future testing.

As demonstrated by these case studies, implementation science frameworks and study designs can provide structure to identify factors that may influence implementation. Stakeholders should consider that different barriers and facilitators may present based on the implementation outcome being targeted. In other words, implementation science frameworks and study designs may need to be tailored to fit the organization, clients, and intended outcomes.

Need for Improvement: Women's Substance Use and Implementation Science

Substance use is one area of behavioral health for women that would benefit from a stronger foothold in implementation science. Research has shown that substance use is, in fact, "gendered," with men being twice as likely as women to have a substance use disorder (Marsh et al., 2018). However, women increase their rate of substance use at a more rapid pace when compared to men once use has been initiated (Meyer et al., 2019), and they are at a greater risk for nonmedical prescription opioid use than men (Back et al., 2011; Marsh et al., 2018). In addition, illicit drug use contributes to both men's and women's involvement in the criminal legal system (Bennett et al., 2008); however, women in drug courts identify opioids as their preferred drug of choice more often than men (Shannon et al., 2020).

Despite women's gender-specific risks and needs, access to gender-specific substance use treatment services is limited. In the USA, approximately 32% of all substance use treatment facilities offer gender-tailored treatment for women, and only 13% provide treatment services for pregnant and postpartum women (Evans et al., 2013; SAMHSA, 2011). Approximately 4–5% of pregnant women ages 15–44 report illicit drug use while pregnant; however, they are less likely to receive drug treatment than nonpregnant women (Mozurkewich & Rayburn, 2014; Stone, 2015).

A specific area of women's substance use treatment that would benefit from the integration of implementation science is medication for opioid use disorder (MOUD). MOUD is a method of treatment shown to effectively improve recovery outcomes, such as improved treatment retention, reduced relapse, and reduced overdose (Fullerton et al., 2014; Hser et al., 2014; Pierce et al., 2016; Sullivan et al., 2019). MOUD treatment for pregnant women is more complicated than treating nonpregnant women or men to prevent the child from being born with neonatal abstinence syndrome. The medication must be carefully chosen with a close assessment of the mother and child during induction, stabilization, and after delivery (Jones et al., 2008). While clinically relevant solutions exist, the implementation of best practices remains limited.

Challenges in accessing treatment arise due to fewer MOUD prescribers willing to accept pregnant patients (Patrick et al., 2019), the stigma associated with mothers with opioid use disorder, and the mother's fear of child welfare involvement should she admit to having a drug use problem during pregnancy (Kremer & Arora, 2015). Solutions for these barriers involve tailoring existing MOUD programs to accommodate pregnant women and applying person-centered care to establish trust between the mother and provider, solutions that would benefit from an implementation science approach (Preis et al., 2020; Sutter et al., 2017).

Substance use interventions are one area where women's needs would be better served by carefully considering the implementation process. However, there remains a dearth of strategies and implementation research in other women's behavioral health areas, such as gender-specific crisis intervention and mental health treatment for depression and trauma. More thorough integration of implementation science in women's behavioral health would create a firmer foundation for equitable and equal representation of women's issues in the behavioral health field (for more about substance use, see Chap. 5 in this volume).

Implications for Women's Behavioral Health

Implementation science has been shown to be effective, particularly in adopting and using evidence-based practices to improve women's health across the lifespan. However, with any initiative to reduce health inequities, there are issues of fidelity, appropriateness, and buy-in from stakeholders who receive or provide services that affect behavioral health research, practice, and policy.

Implementation science can be used as a tool to accelerate the successful adoption of EBPs into routine care (Hamilton et al., 2017). However, implementation science research is often something that is done to key stakeholders (i.e., end-users and consumers) rather than in collaboration with them. Stakeholder perspectives on EBP implementation, including barriers and facilitators, are often disregarded because research suggests that quantitative methods and models may be superior (Last et al., 2021; Vroom et al., 2021). The lack of incorporation of the stakeholder's voice may result in frameworks and strategies that are highly effective in controlled settings but less effective in practice because the approaches do not consider real-world application.

The field of implementation science has created a bridge from research to practice, but the complexities of these strategies may convolute the innate translation of EBPs. The field of implementation science has realized that scientific theory, coupled with stakeholder perspectives, can illuminate why or why not certain implementation strategies are successful. Lived experience, working in tandem with scientific theory, can aid the development and organization of implementation science concepts that are sensitive to the unique demands of organizations serving women's behavioral health needs (Last et al., 2021; Vroom et al., 2021). Future researchers would benefit from embedding implementation science into the development stages of behavioral health innovation and interventions for women.

Women's needs are different from men's needs. Therefore, we must consider the role that gender-specific physiological, hormonal, and societal and culturally normed expectations play in determining best practices for service delivery. In more recent history, women have advocated for equal treatment among men, but the next step is to achieve equitable treatment that considers and tailors to the unique needs of women. Implementation science de-emphasizes the determination of the effectiveness of services to a more comprehensive consideration of not only "what works" but also how it works for whom (Barwick et al., 2020; Lyon & Koerner, 2016; Vroom & Massey, 2022). This shift toward leveraging the appropriate fit for interventions promotes the implementation of targeted treatments that are gender-specific.

Given the evolution and existing research on implementation science and EBP in behavioral health, there is precedent for the strategic and systematic integration of implementation science for women's behavioral health. As shown in the ACA, the WHO Sustainable Development Goals, and Healthy People 2030, national and global policy presents an opportunity for codifying the prioritization, adoption, and thoughtful implementation of EBPs for women. Future policy would benefit from the standardization of measurements, mandated implementation science-related requirements, and evaluation of the implementation processes. Continuing to develop policy and funding strategies that place value on implementation science would promote a more thoroughly equitable systems approach to behavioral health-care delivery for women.

In summary, implementation science provides tools for practitioners and researchers to navigate how to best integrate EBPs into real-world health-care settings. The inclusion of implementation science in women's behavioral health professional education, both pre-service and in-service, will ensure that future researchers and practitioners clearly understand how to identify research to practice gaps, design appropriate interventions, and meaningfully evaluate the outcomes of programs/interventions.

References

Aarons, G. A., Hurlburt, M., & McCue Horwitz, S. (2011). Advancing a conceptual model of evidence-based practice implementation in public service sectors. *Administration and Policy in Mental Health and Mental Health Services Research, 38*(1), 4–23. https://doi.org/10.1007/s10488-010-0327-7

Albers, B., Shlonsky, A., & Mildon, R. (2020). En route to implementation science 3.0. In B. Albers, A. Shlonsky, & R. Mildon (Eds.), *Implementation science 3.0* (pp. 1–38). Springer. https://doi.org/10.1007/978-3-030-03874-8

American Psychological Association, & APA Presidential Task Force on Evidence-Based Practice. (2006). Evidence-based practice in psychology. *American Psychologist, 61*(4), 271–285. https://www.apa.org/pubs/journals/features/evidence-based-statement.pdf

Back, S. E., Payne, R. L., Wahlquist, A. H., Carter, R. E., Stroud, Z., Haynes, L., Hillhouse, M., Brady, K. T., & Ling, W. (2011). Comparative profiles of men and women with opioid dependence: Results from a national multisite effectiveness trial. *The American Journal of Drug and Alcohol Abuse, 37*(5), 313–323. https://doi.org/10.3109/00952990.2011.596982

Barwick, M., Dubrowski, R., & Damschroder, L. (2020). Factors associated with effective implementation: Research and practical implications. In B. Albers, A. Shlonsky, & R. Mildon (Eds.), *Implementation science 3.0* (pp. 81–100). Springer Nature. https://doi.org/10.1007/978-3-030-03874-8

Bauer, M. S., & Kirchner, J. (2020). Implementation science: What is it and why should I care? *Psychiatry Research, 283*, 112376. https://doi.org/10.1016/j.psychres.2019.04.025

Baumann, A. A., & Cabassa, L. J. (2020). Reframing implementation science to address inequities in healthcare delivery. *BMC Health Services Research, 20*(190). https://doi.org/10.1186/s12913-020-4975-3

Becker, M. A., & Lynn, V. A. (2020). Women's behavioral health needs. In B. L. Levin & A. Hanson (Eds.), *Foundations of behavioral health* (pp. 183–204). Springer. https://doi.org/10.1007/978-3-030-18435-3_9

Bennett, T., Holloway, K., & Farrington, D. (2008). The statistical association between drug misuse and crime: A meta-analysis. *Aggression and Violent Behavior, 13*(2), 107–118. https://doi.org/10.1016/j.avb.2008.02.001

Birken, S. A., Powell, B. J., Shea, C. M., Haines, E. R., Kirk, M. A., Leeman, J., Rohweder, C., Damschroder, L., & Presseau, J. (2017). Criteria for selecting implementation science theories and frameworks: Results from an international survey. *Implementation Science, 12*(124). https://doi.org/10.1186/s13012-017-0656-y

Brownson, R. C., Kumanyika, S. K., Kreuter, M. W., & Haire-Joshu, D. (2021). Implementation science should give higher priority to health equity. *Implementation Science, 16*(28). https://doi.org/10.1186/s13012-021-01097-0

Carvalho, M. L., Honeycutt, S., Escoffery, C., Glanz, K., Sabbs, D., & Kegler, M. C. (2013). Balancing fidelity and adaptation: Implementing evidence-based chronic disease prevention. *Journal of Public Health Management and Practice, 19*(4), 348–356. https://doi.org/10.1097/PHH.0b013e31826d80eb

Chambers, D. A., & Norton, W. E. (2016). The Adaptome: Advancing the science of intervention adaptation. *American Journal of Preventive Medicine, 51*(4 Suppl 2), S124–S131. https://doi.org/10.1016/j.amepre.2016.05.011

Colditz, G. A., & Emmons, K. M. (2018). The promise and challenges of dissemination and implementation research. In R. C. Brownson, G. A. Colditz, & E. K. Proctor (Eds.), *Dissemination and implementation research in health: Translating science to practice* (2nd ed., pp. 1–18). Oxford University Press. https://doi.org/10.1093/acprof:oso/9780199751877.001.0001

Damschroder, L. J. (2020). Clarity out of chaos: Use of theory in implementation research. *Psychiatry Research, 283*, 112461. https://doi.org/10.1016/j.psychres.2019.06.036

Damschroder, L. J., Aron, D. C., Keith, R. E., Kirsh, S. R., Alexander, J. A., & Lowery, J. C. (2009). Fostering implementation of health services research findings into practice: A consolidated framework for advancing implementation science. *Implementation Science, 4*(50). https://doi.org/10.1186/1748-5908-4-50

Damschroder, L. J., Reardon C. M., Opra Widerquist, M. A., & Lowery, J. C. (2021, December 14–16). *Introduction and application of the consolidated framework for implementation research (CFIR): Version 2.0 (CFIR V2)* [Conference session]. 14th Annual Conference on the Science of Dissemination and Implementation in Health, Virtual Conference.

Damschroder, L. J., Reardon, C. M., Opra Widerquist, M. A., & Lowery, J. (2022a). The updated Consolidated Framework for Implementation Research based on user feedback. *Implementation Science, 17*(1), 75. https://doi.org/10.1186/s13012-022-01245-0

Damschroder, L. J., Reardon, C. M., Opra Widerquist, M. A., & Lowery, J. (2022b). Conceptualizing outcomes for use with the Consolidated Framework for Implementation Research (CFIR): The CFIR Outcomes Addendum. *Implementation Science, 17*(7). https://doi.org/10.1186/s13012-021-01181-5

Ehrhart, M. G., Aarons, G. A., & Farahnak, L. A. (2014). Assessing organizational context for EBP implementation: The development and validity testing of the Implementation Climate Scale (ICS). *Implementation Science, 9*(157). https://doi.org/10.1186/s13012-014-0157-1

Erol, A., & Karpyak, V. M. (2015). Sex and gender-related differences in alcohol use and its consequences: Contemporary knowledge and future research considerations. *Drug and Alcohol Dependence, 156*, 1–13. https://doi.org/10.1016/j.drugalcdep.2015.08.023

Evans, E., Li, L., Pierce, J., & Hser, Y.-I. (2013). Explaining long-term outcomes among drug dependent mothers treated in women-only versus mixed-gender programs. *Journal of Substance Abuse Treatment, 45*(3), 293–301. https://doi.org/10.1016/j.jsat.2013.04.003

Fullerton, C. A., Kim, M., Thomas, C. P., Lyman, D. R., Montejano, L. B., Dougherty, R. H., Daniels, A. S., Ghose, S. S., & Delphin-Rittmon, M. E. (2014). Medication-assisted treatment with methadone: Assessing the evidence. *Psychiatric Services, 65*(2), 146–157. https://doi.org/10.1176/appi.ps.201300235

GBD 2016 and HALE Collaborators. (2017). Global, regional, and national disability-adjusted life-years (DALYs) for 333 diseases and injuries and healthy life expectancy (HALE) for 195 countries and territories, 1990–2016: A systematic analysis for the Global Burden of Disease Study 2016. *The Lancet, 390*(10100), 1260–1344. https://doi.org/10.1016/S0140-6736(17)32130-X

Goff, S. L., Moran, M. J., Szegda, K., Fioroni, T., DeBanate, M. A., & Byatt, N. (2020). Development and pilot testing of an adaptable protocol to address postpartum depression in pediatric practices serving lower-income and racial/ethnic minority families: Contextual considerations. *Implementation Science Communications, 1*(66). https://doi.org/10.1186/s43058-020-00049-x

Gruman, J., Rovner, M. H., French, M. E., Jeffress, D., Sofaer, S., Shaller, D., & Prager, D. J. (2010). From patient education to patient engagement: Implications for the field of patient education. *Patient Education and Counseling, 78*(3), 350–356. https://doi.org/10.1016/j.pec.2010.02.002

Gupta, N. (2020). *Women in science and technology: Confronting inequalities*. Sage Publications.

Hamilton, A. B., Farmer, M. M., Moin, T., Finley, E. P., Lang, A. J., Oishi, S. M., Huynh, A. K., Zuchowski, J., Haskell, S. G., & Bean-Mayberry, B. (2017). Enhancing mental and physical health of women through engagement and retention (EMPOWER): A protocol for a program of research. *Implementation Science, 12*(127). https://doi.org/10.1186/s13012-017-0658-9

Health Care and Education Reconciliation Act, Pub. L. No. 111–152, U.S.C. 42 § 1305. (2010). https://www.congress.gov/111/plaws/publ152/PLAW-111publ152.pdf

Hser, Y.-I., Saxon, A. J., Huang, D., Hasson, A., Thomas, C., Hillhouse, M., Jacobs, P., Teruya, C., McLaughlin, P., Wiest, K., Cohen, A., & Ling, W. (2014). Treatment retention among patients randomized to buprenorphine/naloxone compared to methadone in a multi-site trial. *Addiction, 109*(1), 79–87. https://doi.org/10.1111/add.12333

Hyde, P. S., & Enomoto, K. (2015). What is behavioral health worth? *Public Health Reports, 130*(1), 6–9. https://doi.org/10.1177/003335491513000103

Jones, H. E., Martin, P. R., Heil, S. H., Kaltenbach, K., Selby, P., Coyle, M. G., Stine, S. M., O'Grady, K. E., Arria, A. M., & Fischer, G. (2008). Treatment of opioid-dependent pregnant women: Clinical and research issues. *Journal of Substance Abuse Treatment, 35*(3), 245–259. https://doi.org/10.1016/j.jsat.2007.10.007

Kessler, R. C. (2006). The epidemiology of depression among women. In C. L. M. Keyes & S. H. Goodman (Eds.), *Women and depression: A handbook for the social, behavioral, and biomedical sciences* (pp. 22–37). Cambridge University Press. https://doi.org/10.1017/CBO9780511841262.004

Kessler, R. C., Chiu, W. T., Demler, O., Merikangas, K. R., & Walters, E. E. (2005). Prevalence, severity, and comorbidity of 12-month DSM-IV disorders in the National Comorbidity Survey Replication. *Archives of General Psychiatry, 62*(6), 617–627. https://doi.org/10.1001/archpsyc.62.6.617

Kirchner, J. E., Waltz, T. J., Powell, B. J., Smith, J. L., & Proctor, E. K. (2018). Implementation strategies. In R. C. Brownson, G. A. Colditz, & E. K. Proctor (Eds.), *Dissemination and implementation research in health: Translating science to practice* (2nd ed., pp. 245–266). Oxford University Press. https://doi.org/10.1093/acprof:oso/9780199751877.001.0001

Kirk, M. A., Kelley, C., Yankey, N., Birken, S. A., Abadie, B., & Damschroder, L. (2016). A systematic review of the use of the consolidated framework for implementation research. *Implementation Science, 11*(72). https://doi.org/10.1186/s13012-016-0437-z

Kremer, M. E., & Arora, K. S. (2015). Clinical, ethical, and legal considerations in pregnant women with opioid abuse. *Obstetrics and Gynecology, 126*(3), 474–478. https://doi.org/10.1097/AOG.0000000000000991

Landes, S. J., McBain, S. A., & Curran, G. M. (2019). An introduction to effectiveness-implementation hybrid designs. *Psychiatry Research, 280*, 112630. https://doi.org/10.1016/j.psychres.2019.112513

Last, B. S., Schriger, S. H., Timon, C. E., Frank, H. E., Buttenheim, A. M., Rudd, B. N., Fernandez-Marcote, S., Comeau, C., Shoyinka, S., & Beidas, R. S. (2021). Using behavioral insights to design implementation strategies in public mental health settings: A qualitative study of clinical decision-making. *Implementation Science Communications, 2*(6). https://doi.org/10.1186/s43058-020-00105-6

Lyon, A. R., & Koerner, K. (2016). User-centered design for psychosocial intervention development and implementation. *Clinical Psychology: Science and Practice, 23*(2), 180–200. https://doi.org/10.1111/cpsp.12154

Marsh, J. C., Park, K., Lin, Y. A., & Bersamira, C. (2018). Gender differences in trends for heroin use and nonmedical prescription opioid use, 2007–2014. *Journal of Substance Abuse Treatment, 87*, 79–85. https://doi.org/10.1016/j.jsat.2018.01.001

Massey, O. T., & Vroom, E. B. (2020). The role of implementation science in behavioral health. In B. L. Levin & A. Hanson (Eds.), *Foundations of behavioral health* (pp. 101–118). Springer. https://doi.org/10.1007/978-3-030-18435-3

Meffert, S. M., Neylan, T. C., Chambers, D. A., & Verdeli, H. (2016). Novel implementation research designs for scaling up global mental health care: Overcoming translational challenges to address the world's leading cause of disability. *International Journal of Mental Health Systems, 10*(19). https://doi.org/10.1186/s13033-016-0049-7

Meloncelli, N., Barnett, A., & de Jersey, S. (2020). An implementation science approach for developing and implementing a dietitian-led model of care for gestational diabetes: A pre-post study. *BMC Pregnancy and Childbirth, 20*(1). https://doi.org/10.1186/s12884-020-03352-6

Meyer, J. P., Isaacs, K., El-Shahway, O., Burlew, A. K., & Wechsberg, W. (2019). Research on women with substance use disorders: Reviewing progress and developing a research and implementation roadmap. *Drug and Alcohol Dependence, 197*, 158–163. https://doi.org/10.1016/j.drugalcdep.2019.01.017

Morris, Z. S., Wooding, S., & Grant, J. (2011). The answer is 17 years, what is the question: Understanding time lags in translational research. *Journal of the Royal Society of Medicine, 104*(12), 510–520. https://doi.org/10.1258/jrsm.2011.110180

Mozurkewich, E. L., & Rayburn, W. F. (2014). Buprenorphine and methadone for opioid addiction during pregnancy. *Obstetrics and Gynecology Clinics, 41*(2), 241–253. https://doi.org/10.1016/j.ogc.2014.02.005

National Institutes of Health. (n.d.). *History of women's participation in clinical research.* https://orwh.od.nih.gov/toolkit/recruitment/history

National Institutes of Health Revitalization Act [Women and Minorities as Subjects in Clinical Research], Pub. L. No. 103-43. (1993). https://www.govinfo.gov/content/pkg/STATUTE-107/pdf/STATUTE-107-Pg122.pdf

Nilsen, P. (2015). Making sense of implementation theories, models and frameworks. *Implementation Science, 10*, 53. https://doi.org/10.1186/s13012-015-0242-0

Office of the Surgeon General. (1999). *Mental health: A report of the Surgeon General.* U.S. Department of Health and Human Services. https://www.loc.gov/item/2002495357/

Olff, M. (2017). Sex and gender differences in post-traumatic stress disorder: An update. *European Journal of Psychotraumatology, 8*(sup4), 1351204. https://doi.org/10.1080/20008198.2017.1351204

Patient Protection and Affordable Care Act, Pub. L. No. 111–148, U.S.C. 42 §18001. (2010). https://www.congress.gov/111/plaws/publ148/PLAW-111publ148.pdf

Patrick, S. W., Buntin, M. B., Martin, P. R., Scott, T. A., Dupont, W., Richards, M., & Cooper, W. O. (2019). Barriers to accessing treatment for pregnant women with opioid use disorder in Appalachian states. *Substance Abuse, 40*(3), 356–362. https://doi.org/10.1080/08897077.2018.1488336

Pierce, M., Bird, S. M., Hickman, M., Marsden, J., Dunn, G., Jones, A., & Millar, T. (2016). Impact of treatment for opioid dependence on fatal drug-related poisoning: A national cohort study in England. *Addiction, 111*(2), 298–308. https://doi.org/10.1111/add.13193

Ponce, A. N., Lawless, M. S., & Rowe, M. (2014). Homelessness, behavioral health disorders and intimate partner violence: Barriers to services for women. *Community Mental Health Journal, 50*(7), 831–840. https://doi.org/10.1007/s10597-014-9712-0

Powell, B. J., Waltz, T. J., Chinman, M. J., Damschroder, L. J., Smith, J. L., Matthieu, M. M., Proctor, E. K., & Kirchner, J. E. (2015). A refined compilation of implementation strategies: Results from the Expert Recommendations for Implementing Change (ERIC) project. *Implementation Science, 10*(21). https://doi.org/10.1186/s13012-015-0209-1

Preis, H., Garry, D. J., Herrera, K., Garretto, D. J., & Lobel, M. (2020). Improving assessment, treatment, and understanding of pregnant women with opioid use disorder: The importance of life context. *Women's Reproductive Health, 7*(3), 153–163. https://doi.org/10.1080/2329369 1.2020.1780395

Rogers, E. M. (2010). *Diffusion of innovations*. Simon and Schuster.

Sackett, D. L., Rosenberg, W. M., Gray, J. A., Haynes, R. B., & Richardson, W. S. (1996). Evidence based medicine: What it is and what it isn't. *BMJ, 312*(7023), 71–72. https://doi.org/10.1136/bmj.312.7023.71

Shannon, L., Jones, A., Newell, J., & Nichols, E. (2020). Examining predisposing factors and program performance indicators associated with program completion: A comparison of opioid and non-opioid preferring participants in drug court. *International Journal of Offender Therapy and Comparative Criminology, 64*(12), 1236–1257. https://doi.org/10.1177/0306624X19866130

Sherr, K., Ásbjörnsdóttir, K., Crocker, J., Coutinho, J., de Fatima Cuembelo, M., Tavede, E., Manaca, N., Ronen, K., Murgorgo, F., Barnabas, R., John-Stewart, G., Holte, S., Weiner, B. J., Pfeiffer, J., & Gimbel, S. (2019). Scaling-up the systems analysis and improvement approach for prevention of mother-to-child HIV transmission in Mozambique (SAIA-SCALE): A stepped-wedge cluster randomized trial. *Implementation Science, 14*, 41. https://doi.org/10.1186/s13012-019-0889-z

Southam-Gerow, M. A., Rodriguez, A., Chorpita, B. F., & Daleiden, E. L. (2012). Dissemination and implementation of evidence based treatment for youth: Challenges and recommendations. *Professional Psychology: Research and Practice, 43*(5), 527–534. https://doi.org/10.1037/a0029101

Spring, B., Neville, K., & Russell, S. W. (2012). Evidence-based practice. In V. S. Ramachandran (Ed.), *Encyclopedia of human behavior* (2nd ed., pp. 86–93). Academic Press. https://doi.org/10.1016/B978-0-12-375000-6.00155-5

Stone, R. (2015). Pregnant women and substance use: Fear, stigma, and barriers to care. *Health and Justice, 3*, 2. https://doi.org/10.1186/s40352-015-0015-5

Substance Abuse and Mental Health Services Administration. (2011). *National Survey of Substance Abuse Treatment Services (N-SSATS): 2010. Data on substance abuse treatment facilities* (DASIS Series S-59, HHS Publication No [SMA] 11–4665). Center for Behavioral Health Statistics and Quality. https://wwwdasis.samhsa.gov/dasis2/nssats/2010_nssats_rpt.pdf

Substance Abuse and Mental Health Services Administration. (2018). *Key substance use and mental health indicators in the United States: Results from the 2017 National Survey on Drug Use and Health (NSDUH Series H-53, HHS Publication No. PEP18-5068)*. Center for Behavioral Health Statistics and Quality. https://www.samhsa.gov/data/sites/default/files/cbhsq-reports/NSDUHFFR2017/NSDUHFFR2017.pdf

Sullivan, M. A., Bisaga, A., Pavlicova, M., Carpenter, K. M., Choi, C. J., Mishlen, K., Levin, F. R., Mariani, J. J., & Nunes, E. V. (2019). A randomized trial comparing extended-release injectable suspension and oral Naltrexone, both combined with behavioral therapy, for the treatment of opioid use disorder. *American Journal of Psychiatry, 176*(2), 129–137. https://doi.org/10.1176/appi.ajp.2018.17070732

Sutter, M. B., Gopman, S., & Leeman, L. (2017). Patient-centered care to address barriers for pregnant women with opioid dependence. *Obstetrics and Gynecology Clinics, 44*(1), 95–107. https://doi.org/10.1016/j.ogc.2016.11.004

Tabak, R. G., Chambers, D. A., Hook, M., & Brownson, R. C. (2018). The conceptual basis for dissemination and implementation research: Lessons from existing models and frameworks. In R. C. Brownson, G. A. Colditz, & E. K. Proctor (Eds.), *Dissemination and implementation research in health: Translating science to practice* (2nd ed., pp. 1–18). Oxford University Press. https://doi.org/10.1093/acprof:oso/9780199751877.001.0001

Terlizzi, E. P., & Zablotsky, B. (2020). *Mental health treatment among adults: United States, 2019* (NCHS Data Brief no. 380). National Center for Health Statistics. https://www.cdc.gov/nchs/data/databriefs/db380-H.pdf

Tuchman, E. (2010). Women and addiction: The importance of gender issues in substance abuse research. *Journal of Addictive Diseases, 29*(2), 127–138. https://doi.org/10.1080/10550881003684582

U. S. Department of Health and Human Services. (2021). *Secretary's Advisory Committee on National Health Promotion and Disease Prevention Objectives for 2030 report #2: Recommendations for developing objectives, setting priorities, identifying data needs, and involving stakeholders for Healthy People 2030.* Office of Disease Prevention and Health Promotion, U.S. Department of Health and Human Services. https://www.healthypeople.gov/sites/default/files/Advisory_Committee_Objectives_for_HP2030_Report.pdf

Vroom, E. B., & Massey, O. T. (2022). Moving from implementation science to implementation practice: The need to solve practical problems to improve behavioral health services. *Journal of Behavioral Health Services and Research, 49*(1), 106–116. https://doi.org/10.1007/s11414-021-09765-1

Vroom, E. B., Massey, O. T., Martinez Tyson, D., Levin, B. L., & Green, A. L. (2021). Conceptualizing implementation practice capacity in community-based organizations delivering evidence-based behavioral health services. *Global Implementation Research and Applications, 1*(4), 246–257. https://doi.org/10.1007/s43477-021-00024-1

Waltz, T. J., Powell, B. J., Fernandez, M. E., Abadie, B., & Damschroder, L. J. (2019). Choosing implementation strategies to address contextual barriers: Diversity in recommendations and future directions. *Implementation Science, 14*(42). https://doi.org/10.1186/s13012-019-0892-4

Weiss-Laxer, N. S., Johnson, S. B., & Riley, A. W. (2021). Variation of behavioral health care by behavioral health symptom profile among a diverse group of pregnant and parenting mothers. *Journal of Behavioral Health Services and Research, 48*(1), 36–49. https://doi.org/10.1007/s11414-020-09701-9

Westerlund, A., Nilsen, P., & Sundberg, L. (2019). Implementation of implementation science knowledge: The research practice gap paradox. *Worldviews on Evidence-based Nursing, 16*(5), 332–334. https://doi.org/10.1111/wvn.12403

Woodward, E. N., Matthieu, M. M., Uchendu, U. S., Rogal, S., & Kirchner, J. E. (2019). The health equity implementation framework: Proposal and preliminary study of hepatitis C virus treatment. *Implementation Science, 14*, 26. https://doi.org/10.1186/s13012-019-0861-y

Woodward, E. N., Singh, R. S., Ndebele-Ngwenya, P., Castillo, A. M., Dickson, K. S., & Kirchner, J. E. (2021). A more practical guide to incorporating healthy equity domains in implementation determinant frameworks. *Implementation Science, 2*, 61. https://doi.org/10.1186/s43058-021-00146-5

Yu, S. (2018). Uncovering the hidden impacts of inequality on mental health: A global study. *Translational Psychiatry, 8*, 98. https://doi.org/10.1038/s41398-018-0148-0

Zhou, J., Ko, J. Y., Haight, S. C., & Tong, V. T. (2019). Treatment of substance use disorders among women of reproductive age by depression and anxiety disorder status, 2008–2014. *Journal of Women's Health, 28*(8), 1068–1076. https://doi.org/10.1089/jwh.2018.7597

Zielinski, M. J., Allison, M. K., Roberts, L. T., Karlsson, M. E., Bridges, A. J., & Kirchner, J. E. (2021). Implementing and sustaining SHARE: An exposure-based psychotherapy group for incarcerated women survivors of sexual violence. *American Journal of Community Psychology, 67*(1–2), 76–88. https://doi.org/10.1002/ajcp.12461

Chapter 12
The Role of Pharmacists in the Intersection of Women's Health and Mental Health

Carol A. Ott and Carolanne C. Wartman

Introduction

Pharmacists have often been defined as "the most accessible health-care professional" due to their direct service presence in the community. People are most familiar with pharmacists in these dispensing roles (e.g., within drug stores or local grocery stores). However, the role of the pharmacist has grown exponentially over the years. Pharmacists are now integral components of the interdisciplinary team in hospital or clinic settings, in addition to interacting with patients directly. In these settings, pharmacists assist patients and the health-care team by providing comprehensive medication management; assisting with transitions of care by completing medication reconciliations, ensuring appropriate medication coverage, and facilitating patient assistance programs; and providing person-centered care to ensure all aspects of the patient's life are factored into their care. Social determinants of health (SDOH) are now taught in most pharmacy curricula, and guidance has been published by multiple organizations, such as the Pharmacy Quality Alliance (2022, January), to aid pharmacists in implementing these principles into practice. With these principles, pharmacists have many opportunities to assist mental health in the context of women's health.

This chapter will focus on three primary areas: comprehensive medication and collaborative drug therapy management, opioid use disorder (OUD) and medications for OUD (MOUD) in pregnancy, and mental health medications with recommendations and caveats for use. The authors also provide a women's health checklist from a pharmacist's perspective and end with implications for women's behavioral

C. A. Ott (✉)
College of Pharmacy, Purdue University, West Lafayette, IN, USA
e-mail: caott@iupui.edu

C. C. Wartman
College of Pharmacy, University of Arizona, Tucson, USA
e-mail: carolanne.wartman@gmail.com

© The Author(s), under exclusive license to Springer Nature Switzerland AG 2024
A. Hanson, B. L. Levin (eds.), *Women's Behavioral Health*,
https://doi.org/10.1007/978-3-031-58293-6_12

health. In keeping with pharmacy practice for this chapter, the term "mental" will be used as the umbrella term for mental illnesses and substance use disorders in lieu of the term "behavioral." "Behavioral" is considered to be stigmatizing, inferring that there is a behavioral control that the person has over his/her disorder.

Comprehensive Medication and Collaborative Drug Therapy Management

In community pharmacy settings, pharmacists provide comprehensive medication management (CMM) and drug therapy reviews that have been shown to improve adherence to medication and enhanced quality of life (Jokanovic et al., 2017). In community pharmacies, CMM roles allow pharmacists to provide education to patients and recommendations to health-care providers to decrease drug interactions and side effects. Drug regimens can be streamlined to incorporate the patient lifestyle and needs while improving therapeutic relationships.

Clinical pharmacists who have completed 1–2 years of postgraduate residency training are able to implement collaborative drug therapy management (CDTM) agreements with health-care providers in outpatient clinic settings. Pharmacists may elect to become board-certified in pharmacy practice areas to signify areas of proficiency. In mental health practice, psychiatric clinical pharmacists have developed CDTMs for a range of services, including metabolic monitoring for antipsychotic medications, monitoring and dose adjustment for clozapine, mood disorder medication management, and treatment of medical illnesses for mental health patients (Silvia et al., 2020; Tewksbury et al., 2018).

AbuNaba'a and Basheti (2020) evaluated the impact of a pharmacist intervention for medication management for women diagnosed with anxiety and depression. The pharmacist intervention was a medication management review service with patient education and psychiatrist recommendations related to possible treatment-related problems. Study participants randomized to the intervention were compared with participants who did not receive the intervention. There was significant improvement in medication adherence in the intervention group compared to the control group (88.9% and 51.4%, respectively), along with a decline in the number of treatment-related problems. Anxiety and depression rating scores also significantly improved with the pharmacist intervention (AbuNaba'a & Basheti, 2020).

Pharmacists and Practice Settings (Community and Clinical Pharmacy)

Pharmacists provide services across numerous practice settings, ranging from community health centers, health centers for residents of public housing, pharmacies and drug stores, hospitals, federal government, and physician offices. These practice sites expand across rural and urban areas, as well as at local, state, regional, national, and international levels, such as Doctors Without Borders/Médecins Sans Frontières. Each setting has its unique challenges and opportunities.

Federally Qualified Health Centers (FQHCs)

FQHCs are federally funded outpatient, community-based clinics that provide primary care services to underserved communities or areas (such as people experiencing housing difficulties or persons living in rural areas) specific to the U. S. The clinics are in turn provided with specific funding and reimbursements through the Health Resources and Services Administration (HRSA, 2022b, June). The HRSA funds approximately 1400 health centers across the nation and served more than 30 million people in 2021 (HRSA, 2022a, August).

Not only have pharmacists been integrated into FQHCs, but they also continue to expand further within these clinics by promoting quality care for the population. The Uniform Data System found that the total staffing full-time equivalent (FTE) for pharmacy personnel (i.e., pharmacists, pharmacy technicians) grew from 21.8% to 25.2% from 2016 to 2020 (Rodis et al., 2022). Pharmacists provide comprehensive services for chronic disease state management, such as patients with diabetes, hypertension, pain management, preventative care, and mental health conditions. Although pharmacists can see patients independently under a collaborative agreement, they are unable to bill for services since they are not recognized as providers under Medicare. Despite this, pharmacists have been shown to provide positive process and clinical outcomes for FQHCs through quicker time to appointment visits, reduction in depressive symptoms among patients, and improving safety and monitoring of psychotropic medications (Rodis et al., 2022).

Community Mental Health Centers (CMHCs)

The original goal of CMHCs was to develop an alternative to institutionalization by creating locations within the community to provide mental health services (American Psychological Association, 2022). Pharmacists may be integrated into CMHCs in a variety of ways. The CMHC itself could have a pharmacy located within the clinic or it may partner with community pharmacies to provide a pharmacy location within the clinic. Certain companies, like Genoa Healthcare, specialize in this approach. Pharmacies under Genoa Healthcare's umbrella can provide the patient with refill reminders, medication delivery, and specialized packaging. Although the pharmacy is located within a clinic specializing in mental health care, its pharmacists can also fill prescriptions for other disease states outside of psychiatry.

Within the clinic itself, a pharmacist may be a part of the treatment team providing clinical services such as patient education and medication reviews. A retrospective study was conducted assessing medication adherence and Medicaid claims between pharmacies within CMHCs and traditional community pharmacies. The study found that patients who utilized CMHC pharmacies had higher medication adherence, decreased emergency department use, and decreased rates of hospitalization. In turn, this improved patient care while also decreasing health care use and costs (Wright et al., 2016).

Medical Home Model

The medical home model, or patient-centered medical home (PCMH), incorporates a team of health-care providers, such as nurses, physicians, pharmacists, and social workers, to provide primary care services. In the U. S., the Agency for Healthcare Research and Quality (2022, August) defines the five functions and attributes of the PCMH as accessible services, comprehensive care, coordinated care, patient-centered, and quality and safety. Through these principles, the hope is that the PCMH will lead to lower costs and deliver a high quality of care by improving patient experiences and health outcomes. In Europe, the PCMH is seen as a potential model for improving primary care, particularly for chronically ill patients (Faber et al., 2013) as well as patients with multi-morbidity (Kuipers et al., 2019).

Pharmacists can be incorporated into the medical home team physically or virtually, through telehealth services. Some pharmacists use an embedded approach where they may see patients independently or as a shared visit with the team within the clinic. A different off-site approach incorporates community pharmacists into the PCMH team to provide coordinated services outside of the clinic (Schnur et al., 2014). Having these different options available increases the accessibility to care for the population.

Rural Health

There are many definitions for the term "rural." According to the U.S. Census Bureau (n.d.), rural regions are all areas and populations not included within an urban area or cluster (<2500 people). Based on various government agencies to date, about 15–19% of the total U.S. population is categorized as rural (Rural Health Information Hub, 2022, January 27). The Substance Abuse and Mental Health Services Administration's (SAMHSA) *National Survey on Drug Use and Health* found approximately 20% of nonmetropolitan adults reported they had a mental illness, which is similar to what is reported in non-rural areas (SAMHSA, 2022, January 11). However, rural areas experience disproportionate challenges with accessibility, affordability, and provider availability. These populations also experience inequities due to the SDOH, such as fewer resources, higher rates of poverty, and barriers to housing, transportation, and food access, compared to the nation as a whole. The U. S. Census Bureau estimated the 2021 nonmetro poverty rate to be 14% compared to 11.1% for metro areas (Creamer et al., 2022, September 13), which is down slightly from the start of the COVID-19 pandemic (Economic Research Service, 2022, March 7). Pharmacists can serve as available resources to assist with access and availability of care through in-person and telehealth visits.

With the limited accessibility in the rural setting, it may be advantageous to incorporate mental health care through primary care clinics. One study, assessing the integration of a psychiatric pharmacist into a rural internal medicine clinic, found that many of the patients seen by the pharmacist were women (Doughty et al., 2023). Additionally, despite only being in clinic 2 days a week, integration of a psychiatric pharmacist added an overall benefit to the clinic patients (increase in guideline-driven treatments, improved depression screening scores, and decrease in health-care utilization) and to the clinic (increase in provider time to see other patients, estimated reimbursement rate of $29,600 for the health system, and positive perceptions of pharmacist integration by the clinic staff) over a 3-year time frame. These are examples of the positive outcomes a pharmacist can offer to the rural health-care team (for more on rural health, see Chap. 7 in this volume).

Global Health

Global health aims to achieve equity, improve health, unite disciplines, and build partnerships across the world (Rutgers Global Health Institute, 2022, June 23). Historically, the pharmacist's role was covered by other health-care professionals in countries with lower income; however, there has been an increase in pharmacists practicing in the global health environment (Allayla et al., 2018; Center for Global Health, 2022). Pharmacists are now assisting with disaster preparedness and post-disaster relief; delivering immunization and treatment for acute and chronic diseases; collaborating with other countries and disciplines on research; and providing preventative measures (Steeb & Ramaswamy, 2019). Although the role of pharmacists in mental health care is increasing globally, the need for pharmacist involvement is still needed. A Jordanian study assessing control of psychiatric symptoms and referral to a pharmacist in rural areas of Jerash found suboptimal control of psychiatric symptoms in addition to minimal use of pharmacy services (Qunaibi et al., 2021). Many current global and local practices can easily be replicated worldwide.

Mental health transcends borders and faces a number of challenges including stigma, accessibility concerns, human rights violations, and general disparities between countries and regions. Globally, one in four people will experience a mental health condition throughout their lifetime, with depression described as a leading cause of disability worldwide. This prevalence has likely increased following the aftermath of the COVID-19 pandemic. The World Health Organization (WHO) recognizes these challenges and has created multiple initiatives. To date, the WHO has incorporated mental health into the United Nations Sustainable Development Goals to decrease suicide rates (United Nations, 2022a). An additional initiative included the publication of the *World Mental Health Report*, to highlight where change is needed and actionable steps to achieve them (WHO, 2022a, June 16). Finally, the WHO created a global initiative for universal mental health coverage with a goal to provide access for 100 million more people by 2023 (WHO, 2019b) (for more on global health, see Chap. 1 in this volume).

Motivational Interviewing/Shared Decision-Making

Health care has moved from a generalized medical approach to a person-centered model, which focuses on creating an individualized and collaborative approach to treatment. Two techniques for achieving this approach are motivational interviewing and shared decision-making. Motivational interviewing is a counseling technique that guides a patient toward a behavior change, such as smoking cessation, medication adherence, or general lifestyle changes. This focuses on the individual patient's goals and willingness to change. Shared decision-making allows the provider and the patient to come to a reasonable treatment plan as a team. The provider will use patient-specific factors to display assorted options, educating the patient on the positives and negatives of each choice and acknowledging the patient's concerns. Thus, it empowers the patient to make an informed decision, build rapport, and create a healthy therapeutic relationship.

These approaches are commonly used by pharmacists when completing individual visits in the office or at community pharmacies. Aljumah and Hassali (2015) found that patients undergoing pharmacist intervention with shared decision-making had significantly favorable outcomes on their depression treatment compared to the group that did not receive shared decision-making. Participants in the study received either pharmacist intervention using a shared decision-making approach to patient counseling that engaged the patients in appraising their knowledge and attitudes about antidepressant medications or standard medication information. Increased adherence to antidepressant medication, belief about the effectiveness of medication, and treatment satisfaction over time were found in the intervention group versus the standard patient counseling group (Aljumah & Hassali, 2015). This approach is now taught to all pharmacy students, and utilizing these skills is an expectation of the profession.

Opioid Use Disorder (OUD) and Medications for Opioid Use Disorder (MOUD) in Pregnancy

Treatment Guidelines and Access to MOUD

The WHO antenatal care recommendations suggest that health-care providers should screen for past and present substance use at the first antenatal visit and at each visit thereafter (WHO, 2016). Counseling and brief interventions should be provided to all pregnant women about the effects of substance use on the fetus, as well as medical and medication options for treatment during pregnancy. In 2020, the American Society of Addiction Medicine (ASAM) published a focused update on the treatment of opioid use disorders (OUD) revising recommendations for when to offer medications (ASAM, 2020). Previously, clinical practice dictated that medications be offered to patients based upon their engagement in other forms of treatment, including psychotherapy and support groups. The ASAM-focused update recommended that medications were a first-line treatment regardless of other forms of treatment for all people with OUD, specifically for pregnant women based on the risks for negative pregnancy outcomes associated with opioid use. The American College of Obstetricians and Gynecologists (ACOG) recommends that screening for opioid use disorder should be undertaken for all pregnant women in partnership with the woman in a comprehensive, inclusive manner (ACOG, 2017). Taken together, these evidence-based guidelines advocate for early screening and treatment of OUD in pregnant women with early use of medications and routine antenatal appointments.

Racial and ethnic disparities, as well as stigma, exist in access to MOUD for pregnant women. Stigma experienced by pregnant women with OUD from health-care providers can relate to negative perceptions of women as "bad parents," not listening to them, judgmental language, and a lack of interest in the evidence base for medical treatment (Crawford et al., 2022). Pregnant women who use substances often avoid antenatal care because of fear of health-care provider judgment and blame of the mother for any potential negative pregnancy outcomes (Schiff et al., 2022). Since Black and Latina women may seek prenatal care later in pregnancy, they may be diagnosed an average of 37 days later in pregnancy compared with White women, leading to a more problematic pregnancy and poorer outcomes for the infant (Gao et al., 2022). A policy of screening all pregnant women for substance use disorders and training health-care professionals about the impact of stigma on pregnancy outcomes is necessary to improve pregnancy outcomes in a diverse population of women.

Pharmacists are in an opportune position among health-care professionals to engage with pregnant women with OUD due to their community accessibility. Assessment for OUD, patient education about the effects of OUD on pregnancy outcomes, safe breastfeeding, linkage to health-care services, medication management, and harm reduction interventions are roles that the pharmacist can fill to address the public health needs of this population (Muzzy Williamson et al., 2022).

Unfortunately, while increased education is being provided in schools and colleges of pharmacy in the U. S., pharmacist stigma continues to be a barrier to access to medication and inclusive patient interactions. Pharmacists may distance themselves personally from people who may be perceived as misusing opioids, which may then be reflected in pharmacist-patient interactions in the pharmacy setting. In a study by Nichols et al. (2022), pharmacists endorsed providing less medication education for MOUD in the community pharmacy setting and negatively perceiving the effectiveness of buprenorphine and methadone for OUD treatment, considering this to be "substituting one addiction for another" (Nichols et al., 2022).

Treatment Options in the Prenatal/Antenatal Care Setting

MOUD is the first-line recommended treatment for OUD in pregnancy. This modality is preferred over opioid detoxification due to the risks for setback to opioid use during pregnancy and potential for withdrawal symptoms that can negatively affect the fetus. Buprenorphine, methadone, and naltrexone are the medications most used to treat OUD (ACOG, 2017; ASAM, 2020). Screening tools, such as the 5Ps (parents, peers, partner, during pregnancy, past), National Institute on Drug Abuse (NIDA) Quick Screen, and CRAFFT tools, can be used to assess antenatal substance use and need for referral for treatment (ACOG, 2017). The 5Ps tool is specifically used to identify substance use in the prenatal period and is the most commonly recommended tool in the outpatient clinic setting. The NIDA Quick Screen tool is validated for use in all populations. The CRAFFT rating scale includes questions about the use of substances related to riding in a *Car*, using substances to *Relax*, using substances *Alone*, *Forgetting* activities while using substances, having *Family* or friends say that the person should reduce substance use, and getting in *Trouble* when using substances; this tool is validated for adolescents and young adults (ACOG, 2017).

Methadone and buprenorphine are opioid agonist medications that decrease cravings for opioids and reduce the risk of withdrawal symptoms. Methadone is available for OUD treatment in the U. S. only in federally certified opioid treatment programs (OTP) that require daily in-person dosing. Providers should assess the availability of transportation for pregnant women as well as the travel distance to the OTP to ensure compliance with treatment. There are eligibility requirements for OTP services; however, many of these requirements are waived for pregnant women to increase immediate access to care (Rodriguez & Klie, 2019).

Buprenorphine is available with or without naloxone in the sublingual tablet. Naloxone is present to decrease the risk of misuse of buprenorphine; this has allowed physicians, physician assistants, and nurse practitioners to prescribe buprenorphine in a primary care or obstetric health-care practice, eliminating the need for travel to an OTP. Previously, prescribers were required to participate in training established through the Drug Addiction Treatment Act of 2000 (Pub. L. No. 106-310) in order to prescribe buprenorphine in the outpatient setting. However, this requirement has been eliminated as of January 2023, further increasing access to this medication. Both methadone and buprenorphine are considered effective medications and safe for use in pregnancy when compared to opioid misuse. ACOG (2017) endorses the use of these medications for treatment and supplies guidance for obstetricians and gynecologists for prescribing and monitoring. Increased doses of buprenorphine and methadone may be needed relative to increased body volume in later stages of pregnancy.

Naltrexone is used in the general population for the treatment of OUD. It is an opioid antagonist that blocks the opioid receptor to decrease the effects of opioids. Naltrexone is not currently recommended in treatment guidelines for pregnant women due to limited knowledge of birth defects and safety concerns (Ecker et al., 2019). If a woman becomes pregnant when receiving naltrexone, informed consent should be obtained. The consent process should ensure the patient receives education about the unknowns of treatment and potential pregnancy outcomes. However, two recent studies of pregnant women and mother/infant dyads suggest naltrexone may be safe for use in pregnancy (Towers et al., 2020; Wachman et al., 2019). There are concerns for the use of naltrexone for pain management in labor and delivery because naltrexone blocks the opioid receptors and decreases effectiveness of pain management as well as an increased risk for setback to opioid use due to rapid maternal clearance of naltrexone. Both issues require further research.

Naloxone is a medication used to rapidly reverse opioid overdose in medical settings and in the community. Since naloxone may precipitate withdrawal in the mother and cause fetal distress, the smallest dose of naloxone necessary to reverse an overdose should be used while calling for emergency services. It is recommended that take-home doses of naloxone be provided to pregnant women and their families regardless of their desire to engage in MOUD. Appropriate education should be given about how to administer the intranasal dose and when to call an ambulance (Blandthorn et al., 2018).

Labor and Delivery: MOUD and Pain Management

Pregnant women with OUD are often concerned about pain management during labor and delivery, and a plan should be developed with their involvement to ensure appropriate pain relief (SAMHSA, 2018). If women are taking buprenorphine or methadone as MOUD, their current dose should be maintained during labor and delivery, and additional pain management modalities should be provided. Medications, which may precipitate withdrawal (e.g., butorphanol, nalbuphine), are contraindicated for use. Epidural or spinal analgesia, nonsteroidal anti-inflammatory drugs, and opioids such as morphine are appropriate with careful monitoring for respiratory depression or sedation (Ecker et al., 2019; Roper & Cox, 2017). Higher doses of opioids may be needed for pain relief in labor and delivery, as well as Cesarean section.

Continuation of Care: Postpartum Use of MOUD

In the time immediately after birth, the mother should be monitored for sedation, as well for any needed dose adjustments for MOUD. MOUD should be continued postpartum in the same dose ranges used preconception and in the antenatal period. Attention should be given to transitions of care to ensure there are no missed doses of MOUD. Breastfeeding should be encouraged for mother/infant bonding and as appropriate nutrition for the infant. Methadone and buprenorphine are secreted in breast milk in small amounts that are not considered to be adverse for the infant (Roper & Cox, 2017). Screening for co-occurring mental health disorders should be undertaken as a part of maternal discharge planning (SAMHSA, 2018). Ensuring a mother/infant bond and a safe, stable home environment are paramount; rates of setback for opioid use disorder increase in the postpartum period.

Mental Health Medications and Women's Health

Medications play an integral role in the treatment of mental health disorders, but they are not devoid of risks. There are various times throughout a woman's lifecycle where the risks of treatment need to be weighed against the benefit, such as during childbearing age, pregnancy, and postpartum and in older age. Each medication has its own specific concerns and monitoring recommendations. This section will review common psychotropic medications and their risks to women.

Mood Stabilizers

Antiseizure mood stabilizers: teratogenicity, polycystic ovarian syndrome, vitamin D deficiency, and drug interactions This section focuses on antiseizure medications (ASMs), formerly called antiepileptics. Of note, there is a current systemic change in nomenclature from antiepileptics to ASMs, so both terms may be used throughout (French & Perucca, 2020). ASM mood stabilizers consist of valproate, carbamazepine, oxcarbazepine, lamotrigine, and topiramate. These medications may be used in a variety of disease states, including bipolar disorder, epilepsy, and migraine prophylaxis, all of which commonly occur in women. Teratogenicity, polycystic ovarian syndrome (PCOS), vitamin D deficiency, and drug interactions are issues associated with the use of these agents as it relates to women.

Teratogenicity is defined as the ability of a substance to cause developmental malformations or some other harm to a fetus when exposed in utero (Merriam-Webster, 2022). These abnormalities can include structural or functional congenital malformations (such as cleft plate/palate, heart defects, and neural tube defects) or neurodevelopmental disorders (such as attention deficit/hyperactivity disorder, autism spectrum disorder, intellectual disabilities, and tic disorder) (Morris-Rosendahl & Crocq, 2020). Valproate and topiramate are both teratogenic when taken by pregnant women. Specifically, topiramate should be avoided in the first trimester due to a two- to five-fold increased risk of developing a cleft plate/palate, while valproate should be avoided in all trimesters since it can cause a much wider range of malformation and disorders (Hernandez-Diaz et al., 2018; Mulryan et al., 2018).

Since there are known significant risks to offspring, pregnancy registries have been created to monitor and evaluate the risk. The North American Antiepileptic Drug Pregnancy Registry (n.d.) was established to monitor pregnant women in the U. S. and Canada who are, and are not, on ASMs. As of May 2022, the registry reported the risk of malformation in the first trimester as 9.2% in 336 women on valproate alone, with the next highest being 5.1% in 509 women on topiramate alone. Unfortunately, this does not show the true population risk since this registry is specific to use in epilepsy and the requirement of women to self-enroll into the program.

Two other resources are the National Institute for Health and Care Excellence (NICE) in the United Kingdom and the American Epilepsy Society (2021), who have put forth guidance on valproate use and risk during pregnancy. The NICE Guidance has been incorporated into national practice by the UK National Health Service (Medicines and Healthcare Products Regulatory Agency, 2021, February 11). The risks and benefits of treatment with these agents needs to be heavily weighed in people of childbearing age since many individuals do not discover they are pregnant until well into the first trimester. There also needs to be comprehensive education and emphasis on this risk when prescribing these agents, considering other social determinants of health principles such as health care and education access and quality and social support, specific to the patient (World Health Organization, 2022b). In addition to the teratogenic effects, valproate has been linked to causing PCOS. On its own, PCOS variably affects about 4–20% of reproductive age women globally (Deswal et al., 2020). In addition to the physical disturbances that can accompany PCOS (missed or irregular periods, unwanted hair growth, acne), if untreated, PCOS could lead to cardiovascular events, diabetes, and endometrial cancer. With the number one cause of death in women being heart disease, it is imperative to prevent this from developing. Although data was previously conflicting on whether valproate was the link to PCOS symptoms or if it was the disease state itself, two 2006 studies conducted by the same research team attempted to answer this question. These studies found more women on valproate experienced PCOS symptoms compared to the non-valproate group (10.5% vs 1.4%) (Joffe et al., 2006). The team also found discontinuing valproate therapy resulted in a resolution of symptoms for most women, while continuing therapy led to persistent symptoms (Joffe et al., 2006). If discontinuing valproate therapy is not in the best interest of the patient, PCOS treatment may be needed to prevent further complications.

In addition, carbamazepine and oxcarbazepine carry a risk of vitamin D deficiency. Normal vitamin D levels are imperative in women to prevent osteoporosis and muscle weakness, to support levels in the fetus during pregnancy, and to prevent symptoms of depression (Khadilkar, 2013). The development of osteoporosis can lead to falls which may be potentially fatal, especially in the elderly. A recent meta-analysis found that individuals taking carbamazepine had an average lower vitamin D level across all studies compared to those not on carbamazepine (LoPinto-Khoury et al., 2021). It was found that age, sex, and duration of therapy did not have a significant impact on the finding.

Current data is more prominent for carbamazepine, but since oxcarbazepine is structurally similar, it is thought to produce a deficiency similar to that of carbamazepine. Of note, valproate is also associated with vitamin D deficiency, but the deficiency is found more commonly in the pediatric population. The pharmacist could assist by recommending or ordering a vitamin D level on all women, especially those receiving either of these medications. If supplementation is needed, the pharmacist can recommend the appropriate dosage and assist with any cost considerations or concerns since there are differing dosage formulations depending on the vitamin D level. By obtaining baseline values, the pharmacist may be able to prevent further life-altering complications.

Lastly, drug interactions are common and can change the metabolism and concentrations of medications in the body. Pharmacists are trained in analyzing drug therapy regimens and ensuring there are no concerning interactions. A common interaction that may have detrimental effects is with lamotrigine and estrogen. Normally there is concern for certain medications, like antibiotics, which may decrease the effectiveness of oral contraceptives; however, the concern here is the opposite. It has been found that estrogens substantially reduce the concentrations of lamotrigine in the body by about 50–60% (Reimers, 2017). The reduction of lamotrigine may lead to destabilization in mood or loss of seizure control depending on the indication. Since many providers may not be aware of this interaction, adding a pharmacist to the team could be advantageous to mitigate these types of interactions.

Lithium Lithium receives its own category because, although it is a mood stabilizer, it is not categorized as an ASM. Similar to valproate, lithium has considerations that affect pregnant women. However, unlike valproate, it is less detrimental to a child. First, lithium requires blood level monitoring to ensure effectiveness and prevent toxicity. These levels may fluctuate during pregnancy given the changes occurring to the body. Lithium levels need to be monitored more frequently as the woman progresses through different stages of the pregnancy (Wesseloo et al., 2017). Additionally, lithium carries a risk of cardiac malformation, called Ebstein's anomaly, when exposure occurs in the first trimester (remembering that women may be unaware of their pregnancy until well into the first trimester). Unlike some of the malformations that may occur with valproate use, Ebstein's anomaly is considered to be mild, and many children may not need to undergo surgery (American Heart Association, 2021, May 11). However, if surgery is needed, it is considered to be a simple surgery and many children will recover and live a healthy life. Although both surgical or nonsurgical considerations are benign and may just require additional monitoring, the treatment team, including the pharmacist, need to consider the potential direct and indirect costs to the patient. It is imperative to ensure adequate transportation, a support system, and the means to continue treatment during this time.

Lithium is also associated with hypothyroidism or an underactive thyroid gland. Common symptoms of hypothyroidism may include constipation, fatigue, hair loss, and/or weight gain (American Thyroid Association, 2015, August). It is also considered to be more common in women. Lithium has been known to cause thyroid dysfunction at variable degrees with prevalence estimates ranging from 14% to 35% (Lieber et al., 2020). Patients diagnosed with lithium-induced hypothyroidism may need to receive synthetic thyroid supplementation or discontinuation of lithium treatment. Similar to all of the previously discussed implications, the woman's voice needs to be heard, and a shared decision approach between the treatment team and the patient is essential to determine the best course for each woman individually.

Antipsychotics

Hyperprolactinemia, menstrual cycles, and osteoporosis   Although antipsychotics can be used in a variety of disease states, they are considered the treatment of choice in schizophrenia. Side effects associated with antipsychotics include weight gain, elevated blood glucose, sexual dysfunction, and involuntary movements. In general, women have been found to experience side effects more frequently than men, especially weight gain, sexual dysfunction, and cardiovascular disease (Barker & Vigod, 2020). Studies have shown that women with schizophrenia experience symptoms of sexual dysfunction more frequently than healthy controls (Dumontaud et al., 2020). Unfortunately, this is compounded by the side effects of antipsychotics themselves, with some medications worse than others.

The primary mechanism of antipsychotic-induced sexual dysfunction in women is thought to be due to the increase of prolactin, a hormone released in our bodies which is mostly known for breast milk development (Barker & Vigod, 2020). Elevated prolactin levels are beneficial for breastfeeding mothers, but in all other circumstances, hyperprolactinemia can disrupt menstrual cycles, cause acne, increase hair growth on the face, and lead to osteoporosis by decreasing bone mineral density. Multiple studies have found that sexual health is not a topic that is commonly discussed during mental health visits (Barker & Vigod, 2020). Pharmacists can help bridge this gap by communicating with clients about sexual dysfunction, checking prolactin levels, and mitigating side effects by adjusting the dose, discontinuing treatment, or adding supportive medications.

Safety in pregnancy Antipsychotics are not necessarily overtly teratogenic but may cause complications. Women with schizophrenia have been found to experience more unintended pregnancies and rapid repeat pregnancies than women without schizophrenia, which is why it is imperative for providers and patients to understand the risks of antipsychotic use in pregnancy (Gupta et al., 2019; Miller, 1997). For all antipsychotic in utero exposure, there is an increased risk of involuntary movements and withdrawal symptoms in the newborn, especially if exposure occurred in the third trimester. Withdrawal symptoms may include agitation, tremor, somnolence, or changes in muscle tone; these symptoms are normally benign and can be easily managed in the hospital. Congenital malformations have also been described but found to occur less commonly. Antipsychotic exposure is associated with a higher risk of adverse birth outcomes including decreased birth weight, heart defects, major malformations, and preterm delivery (Coughlin et al., 2015). However, it is not recommended for women with schizophrenia to discontinue their treatment when they become pregnant. Abrupt discontinuation of treatment can lead to a higher risk of symptomatic relapses during pregnancy (Tosato et al., 2017).

Atypical (second-generation) antipsychotics are used more frequently than typical (first-generation) antipsychotics due to less movement side effects. The main concern with the atypical agents is the risk of metabolic syndrome, a group of conditions that increase the risk of cardiovascular disease (e.g., diabetes, hypertension, and weight gain). There is also an elevated risk of gestational diabetes and neonatal complications for women and their infants. A Finnish population-based cohort study of over one million pregnant women found a significantly increased risk for gestational diabetes among women exposed to second-generation antipsychotics compared to the unexposed control group related to impaired glucose metabolism (Ellfolk et al., 2020). The study also found increased risks of cesarean section, infants born large for their gestational age, and preterm births. Pregnant women should be advised to enroll in their local pregnancy registry if available, such as the National Pregnancy Registry for Atypical Antipsychotics in the U. S. (MGH Center for Women's Mental Health, 2018b).

Antidepressants

Treatment of premenstrual dysphoric disorder (PMDD) PMDD is thought to be considered a more severe form of premenstrual syndrome (PMS). Per the *Diagnostic and Statistical Manual of Mental Disorders, Fifth Edition (DSM-5)*, there must be a total of five symptoms (e. g., marked irritability, marked depression mood, sleep disturbances, concentration difficulties, fatigue) that occur in the week before the onset of menses and improve a few days after the onset of menses (American Psychiatric Association, 2013). PMDD is often associated with a combination of physical and emotional symptoms (Johns Hopkins Medicine, 2019, November 19). Unfortunately, menstruation is highly stigmatized. A 2017 poll of

1500 women across the U. S. found more than half (58%) of women felt embarrassed while having their period and 42% endured period shaming in their life (Thinx Inc. & PERIOD, 2019). This stigmatization can lead to less women seeking treatment for their symptoms.

The American Family Physician guidelines for treatment of PMDD start with non-pharmacologic options through lifestyle changes (Bhatia & Bhatia, 2002). Although the ideal situation is to eliminate PMDD symptoms by promoting regular exercise, changing to a healthy, balanced diet, and sleeping 7–8 hours every night, this is not always practical or possible for all women; pharmacists may need to consider outside influences from the SDOH (Healthy People 2030, n.d.). Outside of lifestyle changes, antidepressants are the treatment of choice for PMDD, specifically agents that increase levels of serotonin, a chemical messenger found in our body. These antidepressants provide rapid relief, unlike the medications used in major depressive disorder, so they can be dosed 2 weeks prior to menses or when symptoms begin (Steiner et al., 2006). This may be advantageous for women who are apprehensive to taking medications or who wish to minimize the side effects to medications.

Safety in pregnancy US-based studies show that approximately 6% of pregnant women are prescribed antidepressants (Ailes et al., 2016; Andrade et al., 2008). The most used agents are selective serotonin reuptake inhibitors (SSRIs) due to their relatively benign safety profile; thus, they are also the most well studied. The risk of birth defects with SSRIs are thought to be similar to nonexposed women (Reefhuis et al., 2015). However, one SSRI in particular, paroxetine, has been linked to septal and atrial heart defects during first trimester exposure.

Birth defects and malformations are normally linked to exposure during the first trimester, when organ formation is occurring. Poor neonatal adaptation syndrome (PNAS) occurs in about 30% of newborns exposed to serotonergic antidepressants, primarily during the third trimester (Grigoriadis et al., 2013). It is thought to be due to either antidepressant withdrawal or toxicity of serotonin (Hendson et al., 2021). Symptoms of PNAS include sleep disturbances, feeding difficulties, respiratory distress, and irritability, which are considered self-limiting and usually resolve with supportive care.

Similar to use of antipsychotics in pregnancy, women should be advised to enroll in a local pregnancy registry, like the National Pregnancy Registry for Antidepressants in the U.S., to assist in further monitoring and safety of antidepressant use in pregnancy (MGH Center for Women's Mental Health, 2018a). Although there are risks with antidepressant use in pregnancy, it is difficult to establish causality between antidepressant use itself versus worsening of the untreated disease state.

Postpartum depression Postpartum depression (PPD) is generally thought of as the presence of depressive symptoms following childbirth. With the release of the *DSM-5*, the name was changed to peripartum depression to emphasize the fact that the onset may occur during pregnancy (APA, 2013). Hence, peripartum and postpartum depression may be used interchangeably in this chapter. Postpartum depression is extremely common; globally, the prevalence of PPD was found to be approximately 17% (Wang et al., 2021) and the prevalence of PPD in the U. S. was 13.2% (Bauman et al., 2020). Like PMDD, it is important to decrease the stigma surrounding peripartum depression because, if left untreated, it can lead to adverse consequences for the mother, infant, and family. Studies have shown women often do not receive treatment, even when a depressive episode occurs (Flynn et al., 2006; Yonkers et al., 2009).

The first-line treatment for peripartum depression is psychotherapy and/or pharmacotherapy, depending on the severity of disease and the woman's preference. Aside from the medication safety considerations during pregnancy, an additional consideration for peripartum depression is medication safety during lactation. The relative infant dose (RID) is the estimated drug exposure to the baby via breast milk. In general, a RID of <10% is considered acceptable and clinically insignificant, while anything >10% should be used with caution or avoided (Hotham & Hotham, 2015). To some degree, all antidepressants pass through breast milk, which is why psychotherapy is usually considered as the first option (Sriraman et al., 2015). There are many antidepressant options, and each antidepressant passes through breast milk at different rates. The pharmacist can help determine the RID for each medication and can provide recommendations on overall safety of the agent chosen.

Brexanolone (Zulresso®) was approved in 2019 specifically for the treatment of postpartum depression, but it comes with multiple restrictions for use in the U. S. (Morrison et al., 2019). Unlike other antidepressant options, Brexanolone is a 60-hour infusion given following childbirth, which poses significant risks to the patient (excessive sedation, loss of consciousness, and loss of oxygen). The US Food and Drug Administration (2022, June 16) allows administration of the drug only through a Risk Evaluation and Mitigation Strategy (REMS) program. REMS requires a health-care provider in a certified health-care facility to administer the drug. Lastly, there is a significant cost (approximately $34,000 US) associated with the inpatient hospitalization, fees, and the medication itself (Morrison et al., 2019).

Women's Health Checklist: A Role for Pharmacists

Pregnancy Planning/Contraception Counseling

Women with mental health conditions often do not receive adequate reproductive services (Barker & Vigod, 2020). An unwanted pregnancy prevalence of 24.3–47.5% has been described in women with schizophrenia in Colombia (Posada Correa et al., 2020). Despite this increased risk and the various medications that affect fetal development, pregnancy planning and sexual health discussions are not standard of care in psychiatric practice. It is advantageous for behavioral health providers to collaborate with pharmacists and other disciplines to help bridge this gap and coordinate the delivery of care.

Pharmacists can assist with this need by meeting with patients to discuss pregnancy planning and educate on contraceptive options. Pharmacists in the community are equipped to provide counseling on these topics as well as those in the clinic setting. One UK study found a significant increase in contraception education when physicians and pharmacists collaborated to provide such information to women of childbearing age taking valproate following clinical guidelines (Mace & Taylor, 2011).

Vaccinations

Primary series and booster vaccine recommendations are important to address for women and girls across their lifespans. ACOG (2022) recommends the minimum vaccinations for women of childbearing age to be human papillomavirus (HPV); tetanus toxoid, diphtheria toxoid, acellular pertussis (Tdap); and influenza. The US Centers for Disease Control and Prevention (CDC) recommends the measles-mumps-rubella (MMR) vaccine should be given to women of child-bearing age and pregnancy should be avoided for at least 1 month after vaccination (CDC, 2020, December 31). The HPV vaccination has been shown to be effective in reducing the risk of invasive cervical cancer by approximately 90% in girls and women aged 10–30 years (Lei et al., 2020). Neonatal tetanus is primarily caused by a lack of hygiene during delivery and has an 80–100% mortality rate (Kanu et al., 2022). Rubella infection early in pregnancy can lead to congenital rubella syndrome, miscarriage, and stillbirth. Because the rubella vaccine is live and attenuated, there is a risk of passing the virus to the fetus from the vaccine (CDC, 2020, December 31).

Since 2020, US pharmacists may immunize in the community pharmacy setting in all 50 states, as well as Washington, DC, Puerto Rico, and the US territories. Since immunization practices are not regulated by federal law, statutes governing the breadth of the pharmacist scope of practice vary by state and territory and can include restrictions on types of vaccines and age ranges for immunization in community settings. Pharmacists must also be certified in immunization administration to provide this service. The National Alliance of State Pharmacy Associations (NASPA) is an authoritative resource to verify state requirements (NASPA, 2022).

Laboratory Monitoring

Specific laboratory monitoring is required and encouraged depending on the psychotropic agents, described in this chapter. In general, it is recommended to obtain baseline laboratory values when starting psychotropic medications to assess organ function. After completion of baseline values, additional values can be repeated annually or more frequently if clinically necessary. Common levels obtained include vitamin D levels, pregnancy tests, electrocardiogram (ECG), and thyroid function tests.

Implications for Women's Behavioral Health

Forty years after the adoption of a global document empowering women to have the right to health care, women's right and access to care remain problematic. In 1979, the United Nations General Assembly adopted the Convention on the Elimination of All Forms of Discrimination against Women (UN General Assembly, 1979, December 18). The Committee on the Elimination of Discrimination against Women (CEDAW) is empowered to monitor state bodies who have ratified the treaty and their implementation of the articles (UN, 2022b, October 31). Article 12 of the Convention states that discrimination against women in health care should be eliminated by ensuring equal access to health care and reproductive health care. Women suffer from mental health issues at a higher rate than men, often related to traumatic experiences, domestic and sexual violence, and gender discrimination (Lan et al., 2022). Increased rates of poverty derive from the fact that women are often at the mercy of men who control the household finances. Women can feel cultural shame and stigma related to mental health symptoms and experience misinterpretation and somatization of their symptoms (Lan et al., 2022).

Women comprise approximately 70% of the global health workforce but are not often in leadership positions and face sexual harassment that increases stress and mental health issues (World Health Organization, 2019a). According to the American Association of Colleges of Pharmacy, in 2019, 61.8% of pharmacists were women, compared with 52.7% in 2014; of the 2100 cases of pharmacist discrimination reported in 2019, 74.7% were made by female pharmacists who experienced gender discrimination (Arya et al., 2020, January 10).

The prioritization of women's health has been championed across the globe. Empowering women with increased access to high-quality health care improves not only their mental health but also the health of her family, community, and country (Partners in Health, 2022). Although no specific objective for mental health for women exists in Healthy People 2030, the broad goal of promoting health and well-being for women is evidenced through objectives for reproductive health and substance use that then impact mental health (U.S. Department of Health and Human Services, 2020). The UN Sustainable Development Goal (SDG) 5 specifically focuses on women: "Achieve gender equality and empower all women and girls." However, currently, only 57% of women in their reproductive years are able to make their own decisions about reproductive health (United Nations, 2022a, b).

The role of the pharmacist in the intersection between women's health and mental health continues to expand. CMM and CDTM protocols allow the pharmacist to go beyond medication review and dispensing into collaborative practices that advance mental health outcomes for women. The next challenge for pharmacists is to incorporate the social determinants of health, Healthy People 2030 goals, and SDGs to assess a woman's access more broadly to both primary and mental health care and provide appropriate interventions.

References

AbuNaba'a, Y., & Basheti, I. A. (2020). Assessing the impact of medication management review service for females diagnosed with depression and anxiety: A randomized control trial. *Journal of Evaluation in Clinical Practice, 26*(5), 1478–1489. https://doi.org/10.1111/jep.13314

Agency for Healthcare Research and Quality. (2022, August). *Defining the PCMH* [Web page]. AHRQ. https://www.ahrq.gov/ncepcr/research/care-coordination/pcmh/define.html

Ailes, E. C., Simeone, R. M., Dawson, A. L., Petersen, E. E., & Gilboa, S. M. (2016). Using insurance claims data to identify and estimate critical periods in pregnancy: An application to antidepressants. *Birth Defects Research. Part A: Clinical and Molecular Teratology, 106*(11), 927–934. https://doi.org/10.1002/bdra.23573

Aljumah, K., & Hassali, M. A. (2015). Impact of pharmacist intervention on adherence and measurable patient outcomes among depressed patients: A randomised controlled study. *BMC Psychiatry, 15*, 219. https://doi.org/10.1186/s12888-015-0605-8

Allayla, T., Nouri, A., & Hassali, M. (2018). Pharmacist role in global health: A review of literature. *Malaysian Journal of Pharmaceutical Sciences, 16*(1), 45–54. https://doi.org/10.21315/mjps2018.16.1.4

American College of Obstetricians and Gynecologists. (2017). Committee Opinion No. 711: Opioid use and opioid use disorder in pregnancy. *Obstetrics and Gynecology, 130*(2), e81–e94. https://doi.org/10.1097/aog.0000000000002235

American College of Obstetricians and Gynecologists. (2022). *Increasing adult immunization rates through obstetrician-gynecologist partnerships* [Report]. https://www.acog.org/-/media/project/acog/acogorg/files/pdfs/reports/integrating-immunizations-final-report.pdf?la=en&hash=584914CCF90A5265467753DC5817BA35

American Epilepsy Society. (2021, June 8). *Position statement on the use of valproate by women of childbearing potential* [Webpage]. AES. https://www.aesnet.org/about/about-aes/position-statements/position-statement-on-the-use-of-valproate-by-women-of-childbearing-potential

American Heart Association. (2021, May 11). *Ebstein's anomaly* [Web page]. AHA. https://www.heart.org/en/health-topics/congenital-heart-defects/about-congenital-heart-defects/ebsteins-anomaly

American Psychiatric Association. (2013). *Diagnostic and statistical manual of mental disorders (DSM-5)*. APA.

American Psychological Association. (2022). *Community mental health center (CMHC)* [Web page]. APA. https://dictionary.apa.org/community-mental-health-center

American Society of Addiction Medicine. (2020). The ASAM national practice guideline for the treatment of opioid use disorder: 2020 focused update. *Journal of Addiction Medicine, 14*(2S Suppl 1), 1–91. https://doi.org/10.1097/adm.0000000000000633

American Thyroid Association. (2015). Hypothyroidism. *Clinical Thyroidology for the Public, 8*(8), 3–4. https://www.thyroid.org/wp-content/uploads/publications/ctfp/volume8/issue8/ct_public_v88_3_4.pdf

Andrade, S. E., Raebel, M. A., Brown, J., Lane, K., Livingston, J., Boudreau, D., Rolnick, S. J., Roblin, D., Smith, D. H., Willy, M. E., Staffa, J. A., & Platt, R. (2008). Use of antidepressant medications during pregnancy: A multisite study. *American Journal of Obstetrics and Gynecology, 198*(2), 194.e191–194.e195. https://doi.org/10.1016/j.ajog.2007.07.036

Arya, V., Bakken, B. K., Doucette, W. R., Gaither, C. A., Kreling, D. H., Mott, D. A., Schommer, J. C., & Witry, M. J. (2020, January 10). *Final report of the National Pharmacist Workforce Study 2019* [Report]. Pharmacy Workforce Center, Inc. https://www.aacp.org/sites/default/files/2020-03/2019_NPWS_Final_Report.pdf

Barker, L. C., & Vigod, S. N. (2020). Sexual health of women with schizophrenia: A review. *Frontiers in Neuroendocrinology, 57*, 100840. https://doi.org/10.1016/j.yfrne.2020.100840

Bauman, B. L., Ko, J. Y., Cox, S., D'Angelo Mph, D. V., Warner, L., Folger, S., Tevendale, H. D., Coy, K. C., Harrison, L., & Barfield, W. D. (2020). Vital Signs: Postpartum depressive symptoms and provider discussions about perinatal depression – United States, 2018. *MMWR: Morbidity and Mortality Weekly Report, 69*(19), 575–581. https://doi.org/10.15585/mmwr.mm6919a2

Bhatia, S. C., & Bhatia, S. K. (2002). Diagnosis and treatment of premenstrual dysphoric disorder. *American Family Physician, 66*(7), 1239–1248.

Blandthorn, J., Bowman, E., Leung, L., Bonomo, Y., & Dietze, P. (2018). Managing opioid overdose in pregnancy with take-home naloxone. *Australian and New Zealand Journal of Obstetrics and Gynaecology, 58*(4), 460–462. https://doi.org/10.1111/ajo.12761

Center for Global Health. (2022). *Expanding the role of pharmacists in global health* [Web page]. Massachusetts General Hospital. https://globalhealth.massgeneral.org/expanding-the-role-of-pharmacists-in-global-health/

Centers for Disease Control and Prevention. (2020, December 31). *Pregnancy and rubella* [Web page]. CDC. https://www.cdc.gov/rubella/pregnancy.html#:~:text=Vaccine%20Recommendations&text=Because%20MMR%20vaccine%20is%20an,weeks%20after%20receiving%20MMR%20Vaccine

Coughlin, C. G., Blackwell, K. A., Bartley, C., Hay, M., Yonkers, K. A., & Bloch, M. H. (2015). Obstetric and neonatal outcomes after antipsychotic medication exposure in pregnancy. *Obstetrics and Gynecology, 125*(5), 1224–1235. https://doi.org/10.1097/aog.0000000000000759

Crawford, A. D., McGlothen-Bell, K., Recto, P., McGrath, J. M., Scott, L., Brownell, E. A., & Cleveland, L. M. (2022). Stigmatization of pregnant individuals with opioid use disorder. *Women's Health Report, 3*(1), 172–179. https://doi.org/10.1089/whr.2021.0112

Creamer, J., Shrider, E. A., Burns, K., & Chen, F. (2022, September 13). *Poverty in the United States: 2021* [Report Number P60-277; Table C-1. People in Poverty by Selected Characteristics: 2020 Estimates Using 2010 Census-Based Population Controls and 2020 Census-Based Population Controls]. U.S. Census Bureau. https://www.census.gov/library/publications/2022/demo/p60-277.html

Deswal, R., Narwal, V., Dang, A., & Pundir, C. S. (2020). The prevalence of polycystic ovary syndrome: A brief systematic review. *Journal of Human Reproductive Sciences, 13*(4), 261–271. https://doi.org/10.4103/jhrs.JHRS_95_18

Doughty, B., Fink, A., Sellaouti, B., Stasko, J., Surdi, H., & Prabhu, S. (2023). Assessment of an integrated psychiatric pharmacy practice within a rural internal medicine clinic. *Journal of the American Pharmacists Association, 63*, 655–660. https://doi.org/10.1016/j.japh.2022.09.014

Drug Addiction Treatment Act (DATA), Pub. L. No. 106-310, 114 U.S.C. § 3501. (2000). https://www.congress.gov/106/plaws/publ310/PLAW-106publ310.pdf

Dumontaud, M., Korchia, T., Khouani, J., Lancon, C., Auquier, P., Boyer, L., & Fond, G. (2020). Sexual dysfunctions in schizophrenia: Beyond antipsychotics: A systematic review. *Progress in Neuro-Psychopharmacology and Biological Psychiatry, 98*, 109804. https://doi.org/10.1016/j.pnpbp.2019.109804

Ecker, J., Abuhamad, A., Hill, W., Bailit, J., Bateman, B. T., Berghella, V., Blake-Lamb, T., Guille, C., Landau, R., Minkoff, H., Prabhu, M., Rosenthal, E., Terplan, M., Wright, T. E., & Yonkers,

K. A. (2019). Substance use disorders in pregnancy: Clinical, ethical, and research imperatives of the opioid epidemic: A report of a joint workshop of the Society for Maternal-Fetal Medicine, American College of Obstetricians and Gynecologists, and American Society of Addiction Medicine. *American Journal of Obstetrics and Gynecology, 221*(1), B5–B28. https://doi.org/10.1016/j.ajog.2019.03.022

Economic Research Service. (2022, March 7). *Rural poverty & well-being* [Web page]. U.S. Department of Agriculture. https://www.ers.usda.gov/topics/rural-economy-population/rural-poverty-well-being/

Ellfolk, M., Leinonen, M. K., Gissler, M., Lahesmaa-Korpinen, A. M., Saastamoinen, L., Nurminen, M. L., & Malm, H. (2020). Second-generation antipsychotics and pregnancy complications. *European Journal of Clinical Pharmacology, 76*(1), 107–115. https://doi.org/10.1007/s00228-019-02769-z

Faber, M., Voerman, G., Erler, A., Eriksson, T., Baker, R., De Lepeleire, J., Grol, R., & Burgers, J. (2013). Survey of 5 European countries suggests that more elements of patient-centered medical homes could improve primary care. *Health Affairs, 32*(4), 797–806. https://doi.org/10.1377/hlthaff.2012.0184

Flynn, H. A., O'Mahen, H. A., Massey, L., & Marcus, S. (2006). The impact of a brief obstetrics clinic-based intervention on treatment use for perinatal depression. *Journal of Women's Health, 15*(10), 1195–1204. https://doi.org/10.1089/jwh.2006.15.1195

French, J. A., & Perucca, E. (2020). Time to start calling things by their own names? The case for antiseizure medicines. *Epilepsy Currents, 20*(2), 69–72. https://doi.org/10.1177/1535759720905516

Gao, Y. A., Drake, C., Krans, E. E., Chen, Q., & Jarlenski, M. P. (2022). Explaining racial-ethnic disparities in the receipt of medication for opioid use disorder during pregnancy. *Journal of Addiction Medicine, 16*, e356. https://doi.org/10.1097/adm.0000000000000979

Grigoriadis, S., VonderPorten, E. H., Mamisashvili, L., Eady, A., Tomlinson, G., Dennis, C. L., Koren, G., Steiner, M., Mousmanis, P., Cheung, A., & Ross, L. E. (2013). The effect of prenatal antidepressant exposure on neonatal adaptation: A systematic review and meta-analysis. *Journal of Clinical Psychiatry, 74*(4), e309–e320. https://doi.org/10.4088/JCP.12r07967

Gupta, R., Brown, H. K., Barker, L. C., Dennis, C. L., & Vigod, S. N. (2019). Rapid repeat pregnancy in women with schizophrenia. *Schizophrenia Research, 212*, 86–91. https://doi.org/10.1016/j.schres.2019.08.007

Health Resources & Services Administration. (2022a, August). *Health Center Program: Impact and growth* [Web page]. HRSA. https://bphc.hrsa.gov/about-health-centers/health-center-program-impact-growth

Health Resources & Services Administration. (2022b, June). *Health Center Program award recipients* [Web page]. HRSA. https://www.hrsa.gov/opa/eligibility-and-registration/health-centers/fqhc

Healthy People 2030. (n.d.). *Social determinants of health* [Web page]. Office of Disease Prevention and Health Promotion, Office of the Assistant Secretary for Health, Office of the Secretary, U.S. Department of Health and Human Services. https://health.gov/healthypeople/objectives-and-data/social-determinants-health

Hendson, L., Shah, V., & Trkulja, S. (2021). Selective serotonin reuptake inhibitors or serotonin-norepinephrine reuptake inhibitors in pregnancy: Infant and childhood outcomes. *Paediatrics & Child Health, 26*(5), 321–322. https://doi.org/10.1093/pch/pxab021

Hernandez-Diaz, S., Huybrechts, K. F., Desai, R. J., Cohen, J. M., Mogun, H., Pennell, P. B., Bateman, B. T., & Patorno, E. (2018). Topiramate use early in pregnancy and the risk of oral clefts: A pregnancy cohort study. *Neurology, 90*(4), e342–e351. https://doi.org/10.1212/wnl.0000000000004857

Hotham, N., & Hotham, E. (2015). Drugs in breastfeeding. *Australian Prescriber: An Independent Review, 38*(5), 156–159. https://doi.org/10.18773/austprescr.2015.056

Joffe, H., Cohen, L. S., Suppes, T., McLaughlin, W. L., Lavori, P., Adams, J. M., Hwang, C. H., Hall, J. E., & Sachs, G. S. (2006). Valproate is associated with new-onset oligomenorrhea with hyperandrogenism in women with bipolar disorder. *Biological Psychiatry, 59*(11), 1078–1086. https://doi.org/10.1016/j.biopsych.2005.10.017

Johns Hopkins Medicine. (2019, November 19). *Premenstrual dysphoric disorder (PMDD)* [Web page]. https://www.hopkinsmedicine.org/health/conditions-and-diseases/premenstrual-dysphoric-disorder-pmdd

Jokanovic, N., Tan, E. C., Sudhakaran, S., Kirkpatrick, C. M., Dooley, M. J., Ryan-Atwood, T. E., & Bell, J. S. (2017). Pharmacist-led medication review in community settings: An overview of systematic reviews. *Research in Social & Administrative Pharmacy, 13*(4), 661–685. https://doi.org/10.1016/j.sapharm.2016.08.005

Kanu, F. A., Yusuf, N., Kassogue, M., Ahmed, B., & Tohme, R. A. (2022). Progress toward achieving and sustaining maternal and neonatal tetanus elimination – Worldwide, 2000-2020. *MMWR: Morbidity and Mortality Weekly Report, 71*(11), 406–411. https://doi.org/10.15585/mmwr.mm7111a2

Khadilkar, S. S. (2013). The emerging role of vitamin D3 in women's health. *Journal of Obstetrics and Gynaecology of India, 63*(3), 147–150. https://doi.org/10.1007/s13224-013-0420-4

Kuipers, S. J., Cramm, J. M., & Nieboer, A. P. (2019). The importance of patient-centered care and co-creation of care for satisfaction with care and physical and social well-being of patients with multi-morbidity in the primary care setting. *BMC Health Services Research, 19*(1), 13. https://doi.org/10.1186/s12913-018-3818-y

Lan, L., Borba, C. P. C., Crist, K. D., Patel, J. G., & Jain, S. (2022, January 31). Perspectives on global women's mental health. *Psychiatric Times* [HTML]. https://www.psychiatrictimes.com/view/perspectives-on-global-womens-mental-health

Lei, J., Ploner, A., Elfström, K. M., Wang, J., Roth, A., Fang, F., Sundström, K., Dillner, J., & Sparén, P. (2020). HPV vaccination and the risk of invasive cervical cancer. *New England Journal of Medicine, 383*(14), 1340–1348. https://doi.org/10.1056/NEJMoa1917338

Lieber, I., Ott, M., Öhlund, L., Lundqvist, R., Eliasson, M., Sandlund, M., & Werneke, U. (2020). Lithium-associated hypothyroidism and potential for reversibility after lithium discontinuation: Findings from the LiSIE retrospective cohort study. *Journal of Psychopharmacology, 34*(3), 293–303. https://doi.org/10.1177/0269881119882858

LoPinto-Khoury, C., Brennan, L., & Mintzer, S. (2021). Impact of carbamazepine on vitamin D levels: A meta-analysis. *Epilepsy Research, 178,* 106829. https://doi.org/10.1016/j.eplepsyres.2021.106829

Mace, S., & Taylor, D. (2011). Improving adherence to NICE guidance for bipolar illness: Valproate use in women of childbearing potential. *The Psychiatrist, 35*(2), 63–67. https://doi.org/10.1192/pb.bp.110.030106

Medicines and Healthcare Products Regulatory Agency. (2021, February 11). *Guidance: Valproate use by women and girls* [Web page]. GOV.UK. https://www.gov.uk/guidance/valproate-use-by-women-and-girls

Merriam-Webster. (2022). *Teratogenic* [Web page; Dictionary]. Author. https://www.merriam-webster.com/dictionary/teratogenic

MGH Center for Women's Mental Health. (2018a). *National Pregnancy Registry for antidepressants* [Web page]. Massachusetts General Hospital & Harvard Medical Center. https://womensmentalhealth.org/research/pregnancyregistry/antidepressants/

MGH Center for Women's Mental Health. (2018b). *National Pregnancy Registry for atypical antipsychotics* [Web page]. Massachusetts General Hospital & Harvard Medical Center. https://womensmentalhealth.org/research/pregnancyregistry/atypicalantipsychotic/

Miller, L. J. (1997). Sexuality, reproduction, and family planning in women with schizophrenia. *Schizophrenia Bulletin, 23*(4), 623–635. https://doi.org/10.1093/schbul/23.4.623

Morrison, K. E., Cole, A. B., Thompson, S. M., & Bale, T. L. (2019). Brexanolone for the treatment of patients with postpartum depression. *Drugs of Today, 55*(9), 537–544. https://doi.org/10.1358/dot.2019.55.9.3040864

Morris-Rosendahl, D. J., & Crocq, M. A. (2020). Neurodevelopmental disorders: The history and future of a diagnostic concept. *Dialogues in Clinical Neuroscience, 22*(1), 65–72. https://doi.org/10.31887/DCNS.2020.22.1/macrocq

Mulryan, D., McIntyre, A., McDonald, C., Feeney, S., & Hallahan, B. (2018). Awareness and documentation of the teratogenic effects of valproate among women of child-bearing potential. *BJPsych Bulletin, 42*(6), 233–237. https://doi.org/10.1192/bjb.2018.48

Muzzy Williamson, J. D., DiPietro Mager, N., Bright, D., & Cole, J. W. (2022). Opioid use disorder: Calling pharmacists to action for better preconception and pregnancy care. *Research in Social & Administrative Pharmacy, 18*(7), 3199–3203. https://doi.org/10.1016/j.sapharm.2021.08.004

National Alliance of State Pharmacy Associations. (2022, August 12). *Pharmacist immunization authority* [Web page]. NASPA. https://naspa.us/resource/pharmacist-authority-to-immunize/

Nichols, M. A., Kepley, K. L., Rosko, K. S., Hudmon, K. S., Curran, G. M., Ott, C. A., Snyder, M. E., & Miller, M. L. (2022). Community pharmacist-provided opioid intervention frequencies and barriers. *Journal of the American Pharmacists Association, 63*, 336. https://doi.org/10.1016/j.japh.2022.10.004

North American Antiepileptic Drug Pregnancy Registry. (n.d.). *History* [Web page]. The Massachusetts General Hospital; Harvard Medical School. https://www.aedpregnancyregistry.org/history/

Partners in Health. (2022). *Gender equity* [Web page]. PIH. https://www.pih.org/programs/gender-equity

Pharmacy Quality Alliance. (2022, January). *PQA social determinants of health (SDOH) resource guide* [Report]. PQA. https://issuu.com/pqaalliance/docs/pqa_sdoh_resource_guide

Posada Correa, A. M., Andrade Carrillo, R. A., Suarez Vega, D. C., Gómez Cano, S., Agudelo Arango, L. G., Tabares Builes, L. F., Agudelo García, Á. M., Uribe Villa, E., Aguirre-Acevedo, D. C., & López-Jaramillo, C. (2020). Sexual and reproductive health in patients with schizophrenia and bipolar disorder. *Revista Colombiana de Psiquiatría, 49*(1), 15–22. https://doi.org/10.1016/j.rcp.2018.04.007

Qunaibi, E. A., Afeef, M. M., Othman, B., Al-Zoubani, A. Z., & Basheti, I. A. (2021). Perspectives of psychiatric patients in rural areas of Jordan: Barriers to compliance and pharmacist role. *International Journal of Clinical Practice, 75*(10), e14575. https://doi.org/10.1111/ijcp.14575

Reefhuis, J., Devine, O., Friedman, J. M., Louik, C., & Honein, M. A. (2015). Specific SSRIs and birth defects: Bayesian analysis to interpret new data in the context of previous reports. *BMJ: British Medical Journal, 351*, h3190. https://doi.org/10.1136/bmj.h3190

Reimers, A. (2017). Hormone replacement therapy with estrogens may reduce lamotrigine serum concentrations: A matched case-control study. *Epilepsia, 58*(1), e6–e9. https://doi.org/10.1111/epi.13597

Rodis, J. L., Irwin, A. N., Valentino, A. S., & Erdmann, A. M. (2022). Pharmacist care in federally qualified health centers: A narrative review. *JACCP: Journal of the American College of Clinical Pharmacy, 15*, 1297–1306. https://doi.org/10.1002/jac5.1696

Rodriguez, C. E., & Klie, K. A. (2019). Pharmacological treatment of opioid use disorder in pregnancy. *Seminars in Perinatology, 43*(3), 141–148. https://doi.org/10.1053/j.semperi.2019.01.003

Roper, V., & Cox, K. J. (2017). Opioid use disorder in pregnancy. *Journal of Midwifery & Women's Health, 62*(3), 329–340. https://doi.org/10.1111/jmwh.12619

Rural Health Information Hub. (2022, January 27). *What is rural? Overview* [Web page]. RHIH. https://www.ruralhealthinfo.org/topics/what-is-rural

Rutgers Global Health Institute. (2022, June 23). *What is global health?* [Web page]. Rutgers University. https://globalhealth.rutgers.edu/what-we-do/what-is-global-health/

Schiff, D. M., Stoltman, J. J. K., Nielsen, T. C., Myers, S., Nolan, M., Terplan, M., Patrick, S. W., Wilens, T. E., & Kelly, J. (2022). Assessing stigma towards substance use in pregnancy: A randomized study testing the impact of stigmatizing language and type of opioid use on attitudes toward mothers with opioid use disorder. *Journal of Addiction Medicine, 16*(1), 77–83. https://doi.org/10.1097/adm.0000000000000832

Schnur, E. S., Adams, A. J., Klepser, D. G., Doucette, W. R., & Scott, D. M. (2014). PCMHs, ACOs, and medication management: Lessons learned from early research partnerships. *Journal of Managed Care Pharmacy, 20*(2), 201–205. https://doi.org/10.18553/jmcp.2014.20.2.201

Silvia, R. J., Lee, K. C., Bostwick, J. R., Cobb, C. D., Goldstone, L. W., Moore, T. D., Payne, G. H., & Ho, J. L. (2020). Assessment of the current practice of psychiatric pharmacists in the United States. *Mental Health Clinician, 10*(6), 346–353. https://doi.org/10.9740/mhc.2020.11.346

Sriraman, N. K., Melvin, K., & Meltzer-Brody, S. (2015). ABM Clinical Protocol #18: Use of antidepressants in breastfeeding mothers. *Breastfeeding Medicine, 10*(6), 290–299. https://doi.org/10.1089/bfm.2015.29002

Steeb, D. R., & Ramaswamy, R. (2019). Recognizing and engaging pharmacists in global public health in limited resource settings. *Journal of Global Health, 9*(1), 010318. https://doi.org/10.7189/jogh.09.010318

Steiner, M., Pearlstein, T., Cohen, L. S., Endicott, J., Kornstein, S. G., Roberts, C., Roberts, D. L., & Yonkers, K. (2006). Expert guidelines for the treatment of severe PMS, PMDD, and comorbidities: The role of SSRIs. *Journal of Women's Health, 15*(1), 57–69. https://doi.org/10.1089/jwh.2006.15.57

Substance Abuse and Mental Health Services Administration. (2018). *Clinical guidance for treating pregnant and parenting women with opioid use disorder and their infants* [Report; HHS Publication No. (SMA) 18-5054]. SAMHSA. https://store.samhsa.gov/sites/default/files/d7/priv/sma18-5054.pdf

Substance Abuse and Mental Health Services Administration. (2022, January 11). *Results from the 2020 National Survey on Drug Use and Health: Detailed tables* [Web site; Data Tables]. SAMHSA. https://www.samhsa.gov/data/report/2020-nsduh-detailed-tables

Tewksbury, A., Bozymski, K. M., Ruekert, L., Lum, C., Cunningham, E., & Covington, F. (2018). Development of collaborative drug therapy management and clinical pharmacy services in an outpatient psychiatric clinic. *Journal of Pharmacy Practice, 31*(3), 272–278. https://doi.org/10.1177/0897190017710521

Thinx Inc., & PERIOD. (2019). *State of the period: The widespread impact of period poverty on US students* [White paper]. The Policy Project. https://thepolicyproject.org/wp-content/uploads/2019/10/State-of-the-Period-white-paper_Thinx_PERIOD.pdf

Tosato, S., Albert, U., Tomassi, S., Iasevoli, F., Carmassi, C., Ferrari, S., Nanni, M. G., Nivoli, A., Volpe, U., Atti, A. R., & Fiorillo, A. (2017). A systematized review of atypical antipsychotics in pregnant women: Balancing between risks of untreated illness and risks of drug-related adverse effects. *Journal of Clinical Psychiatry, 78*(5), e477–e489. https://doi.org/10.4088/JCP.15r10483

Towers, C. V., Katz, E., Weitz, B., & Visconti, K. (2020). Use of naltrexone in treating opioid use disorder in pregnancy. *American Journal of Obstetrics and Gynecology, 222*(1), 83.e81–83.e88. https://doi.org/10.1016/j.ajog.2019.07.037

U.S. Census Bureau. (n.d.). *How does the U.S. Census Bureau define "rural?"* [Web page]. Author. https://mtgis-portal.geo.census.gov/arcgis/apps/MapSeries/index.html?appid=49cd4bc9c8eb444ab51218c1d5001ef6

U.S. Department of Health and Human Services. (2020). *Women – Healthy People 2030* [Web page]. US DHHS. https://health.gov/healthypeople/objectives-and-data/browse-objectives/women

U.S. Food and Drug Administration. (2022, June 16). *Approved Risk Evaluation and Mitigation Strategies (REMS): Zulresso* [Web page]. FDA. https://www.accessdata.fda.gov/scripts/cder/rems/index.cfm?event=IndvRemsDetails.page&REMS=387#tabs-2

United Nations. (2022a). *The sustainable development goals report 2022* [Web page]. UN. https://unstats.un.org/sdgs/report/2022/

United Nations. (2022b, October 31). *Committee on the elimination of discrimination against women* [Web page]. OHCHR. https://www.ohchr.org/en/treaty-bodies/cedaw

United Nations General Assembly. (1979, December 18). *Convention on the elimination of all forms of discrimination against women New York, 18 December 1979* [Web page]. United Nations. https://www.ohchr.org/en/instruments-mechanisms/instruments/convention-elimination-all-forms-discrimination-against-women

Wachman, E. M., Saia, K., Miller, M., Valle, E., Shrestha, H., Carter, G., Werler, M., & Jones, H. (2019). Naltrexone treatment for pregnant women with opioid use disorder compared with matched buprenorphine control subjects. *Clinical Therapeutics, 41*(9), 1681–1689. https://doi.org/10.1016/j.clinthera.2019.07.003

Wang, Z., Liu, J., Shuai, H., Cai, Z., Fu, X., Liu, Y., Xiao, X., Zhang, W., Krabbendam, E., Liu, S., Liu, Z., Li, Z., & Yang, B. X. (2021). Mapping global prevalence of depression among postpartum women. *Translational Psychiatry, 11*(1), 543. https://doi.org/10.1038/s41398-021-01663-6

Wesseloo, R., Wierdsma, A. I., van Kamp, I. L., Munk-Olsen, T., Hoogendijk, W. J. G., Kushner, S. A., & Bergink, V. (2017). Lithium dosing strategies during pregnancy and the postpartum period. *British Journal of Psychiatry, 211*(1), 31–36. https://doi.org/10.1192/bjp.bp.116.192799

World Health Organization. (2016). *WHO recommendations on antenatal care for a positive pregnancy experience* [Book]. Author. https://apps.who.int/iris/rest/bitstreams/1064182/retrieve

World Health Organization. (2019a). *Delivered by women, led by men: A gender and equity analysis of the global health and social workforce* (Author, Ed.) [Book; Human Resources for Health Observer Series No. 24]. WHO. https://apps.who.int/iris/bitstream/handle/10665/311322/9789241515467-eng.pdf?ua=1

World Health Organization. (2019b). *The WHO special initiative for mental health (2019–2023): Universal health coverage for mental health* [Report; WHO/MSD/19.1]. Author. https://apps.who.int/iris/handle/10665/310981

World Health Organization. (2022a, June 16). *World mental health report: Transforming mental health for all* [Report]. Author. https://apps.who.int/iris/rest/bitstreams/1433523/retrieve

World Health Organization. (2022b). *Social determinants of health* [Web page]. WHO. https://www.who.int/health-topics/social-determinants-of-health#tab=tab_1

Wright, W. A., Gorman, J. M., Odorzynski, M., Peterson, M. J., & Clayton, C. (2016). Integrated pharmacies at community mental health centers: Medication adherence and outcomes. *Journal of Managed Care & Specialty Pharmacy, 22*(11), 1330–1336. https://doi.org/10.18553/jmcp.2016.16004

Yonkers, K. A., Smith, M. V., Lin, H., Howell, H. B., Shao, L., & Rosenheck, R. A. (2009). Depression screening of perinatal women: An evaluation of the healthy start depression initiative. *Psychiatric Services, 60*(3), 322–328. https://doi.org/10.1176/appi.ps.60.3.322

Chapter 13
Behavioral Health Data: Addressing Women's Needs

Ardis Hanson, Bruce Lubotsky Levin, and Kimberly Menendez

Introduction

Just as women are underrepresented in research studies, women are underrepresented in the collection of data to answer research, practice, and policy questions. Gender data gaps have been identified in behavioral health (alcohol use, drug use, and mental disorders) and other elements of the social determinants or sociostructural components of both behavioral health and health. These gaps contribute to the global burden of disease and affect an individual's functional and societal outcomes.

The 2030 Sustainable Development Goals address the potential for collecting accurate data, and using comparative indicators to addressing global was adopted by all United Nations Member States in 2015. However, with such a wide global initiative, three questions emerge. First, how do we document and categorize the knowledge base of prevention and intervention efforts within and across countries, continents, and worldwide to improve women's behavioral health? Second, how do we identify and select criteria for prevention priorities, within and across nations?

A. Hanson (✉)
USF Health Libraries and the College of Public Health, University of South Florida, Tampa, FL, USA
e-mail: hanson@usf.edu

B. L. Levin
College of Behavioral and Community Sciences, College of Public Health, University of South Florida, Tampa, FL, USA
e-mail: levin@usf.edu

K. Menendez
College of Behavioral and Community Sciences, University of South Florida, Tampa, FL, USA
e-mail: kmenendez@usf.edu

Finally, having documented, categorized, identified, and prioritized behavioral health initiatives, how can we best ensure agreement on global priorities?

To place these questions in context, it is critical to understand the organization, financing, and delivery of behavioral health services and systems, as well as the implications for access, cost, outcomes, and quality. However, the complexity and amount of data generated within behavioral health services research, although significant, are not comparable to current data generated and used within somatic health.

The purpose of this chapter is twofold. It addresses what data are routinely (or not) collected globally and in the United States on women's behavioral health and the effects this absence of data has on the development and delivery of effective provision of services for women. To do so, we describe the effects of gender gap data in the provision, planning, and evaluation and assessment of these services.

Challenges for Global and U. S. Behavioral Health Systems

During the past 30 years, major global and national reports have repeatedly prioritized women's behavioral health services as an essential element of health. In 2001, the World Health Organization (WHO) published its *World Health Report (WHR): Mental Health: New Understanding, New Hope*. This report provided the first comprehensive description of how small percentages of the health risks associated with death, disability, and disease were associated with a significant amount of morbidity and mortality. In 2001, the top 10 global health risks accounted for more than one-third of all deaths (WHO, 2001). Today, the health risks have changed, but they still account for the majority of deaths. The WHO also noted that these risk factors could be reversed relatively quickly and, by addressing these risk factors, could also reduce societal inequities.

The *WHR* referenced findings from the U. S. Office of the Surgeon General's *Mental Health* report (1999). The *Report* concluded that mental illnesses are influenced by a combination of biological (sex), psychological, and social (gender, cultural) factors. The WHO also strongly reiterated the influence of gender (i.e., gender itself is affected by biopsychosocial factors). Most importantly, it described two pillars of a community care paradigm. The first pillar is based on the respect of the human rights of individuals with behavioral disorders; the second pillar emphasizes the use of current interventions and techniques.

To successfully create and sustain a community care paradigm (i.e., the public sector), the World Health Assembly supported an intersectoral approach, partnering with nongovernmental organizations, local government, and private sector organizations to develop a working scientific framework. This framework would be comprised of a shared language, standard taxonomies, methods, and assessments to address the underlying determinants and risks to health from both communicable (CD) and noncommunicable diseases (NCDs). The 2001 report concluded with three recommendations for national governments: (1) formulating risk prevention policies; (2) prioritizing prevention and early intervention; and (3) implementing cost-effective and affordable interventions.

Twenty years later, the 2022 *World Mental Health Report: Transforming Mental Health for All* (*WMHR*) continues to emphasize an intersectoral approach and the two pillars of care (WHO, 2022). The *WMHR* calls for reforming mental health systems to promote equity and reduce disparities in the provision of, access to, and utilization of behavioral health services. The 2022 report also emphasizes the extent of inequities and disparities in the receipt of health and behavioral care by women, gender-based, and other socially marginalized groups.

The Grand Challenges in Global Mental Health Initiative was part of a U. S. National Institute of Mental Health's (NIMH) effort to address the global effects of mental, neurological, and substance use (MNS) disorders (Collins et al., 2011). In addition, the Initiative addressed cross-national influences on mental health using a "global" definition which included both environmental concerns (climate change) and macroeconomic policies. The six overarching Grand Challenges goals (see Table 13.1) complement elements within the framework of the social determinants of health within the global Sustainable Development Goals and support ongoing "health in all policies" and "whole-of-society" initiatives across the world (Castillo-Carandang et al., 2020; World Health Organization & Ministry of Social Affairs and Health, 2014). All six Grand Challenges elements are dependent upon accurate data collection, analysis, and dissemination.

Considering the effects of NCDs, potential infectious disease outbreaks, and pandemics on women, international agreements are essential to ensure national efforts support improvements for behavioral health across all sectors, populations, and settings. In short, it requires a continued commitment to global behavioral health. Whether countries develop these agreements as global action plans, frameworks, goals, or regulations, intersectoral engagement is key. However, nations will need to show how they will measure the goals, what data are available, and how the action plans may need to be implemented in phases. All countries, regardless of economic status, can show their progress in reaching these goals. These types of initiatives require nations to address the implications data may have on resource allocation and quality of life, across local and regional levels, and perhaps national levels.

Table 13.1 Grand challenges in global mental health initiative goals (NIMH, n.d.)	
	1. Identify root causes, risk, and protective factors
	2. Advance prevention and implementation of early interventions
	3. Improve treatments and expand access to care
	4. Raise awareness of the global burden
	5. Build human resource capacity
	6. Transform health system and policy responses

From a data perspective, elements, such as global health regulations, health metrics, disease surveillance systems, data architectures, standards, and information systems, need to be monitored. This should happen, at a minimum, by country and local levels. For example, four types of tools that could be used to assess and determine response to national or global behavioral health issues, especially for women, include disease surveillance, laboratory assessment, and service, and facility or system capacity reviews.

Behavioral Health Services Research Data

Although countries are encouraged to develop national health information systems, nevertheless, how data is defined and collected differs across each agency, organization, and delivery system. These differences affect data collection, database design, formatting structure, and reporting requirements, which may or may not be categorized by population demographics (e.g., age, ethnicity, and gender). Further, each reporting stream from these agencies, organizations, or delivery systems may not be relevant to each of the data users and collectors across the variety of health and mental health-care settings.

As behavioral health services research continues to evolve across countries, the amount and type of data, including private and public sector research, have grown exponentially. Data are gathered using different formats, forms, levels, and types and are then translated into information. Agencies and governments collect sociodemographic or disease surveillance data to help them decide how to best address behavioral health from a population-level perspective. Researchers use data to describe, evaluate, and/or substantiate interventions and practice. Policymakers use data to support their decisions on which policies or programs to implement. Epidemiologists and community planners use spatial data to address neighborhood-based health inequities from a social determinants of health (SDOH) perspective or to analyze the best site to place a new treatment center.

Although behavioral health data comes in many formats, data are often classed as primary, secondary, or tertiary data. Primary data are original unprocessed data. The data may be quantitative (e.g., numeric, spatial) or qualitative (e.g., textual or interview data). The data may differ in the composition of the population, the structure of the data, the granularity of the data collected, the intended use of the data, the magnitude and scope of the data collected, and the methodological rigor by which it is collected.

Primary data is specific since it was collected to answer a specific question(s). An example of primary data is "big data," which are unstructured data in large data sets that require computational analysis to reveal statistical correlations, as well as other patterns, relationships, and trends. An example of big data is the data collected for the Global Burden of Disease (GBD) study. Considered to be the most comprehensive global observational epidemiological study to date, the GBD data started as a methodological question on how to best quantify the health consequences of the years of life lived with disabilities (Murray & Lopez, 1994).

The analyses of primary data result in secondary (processed) data which are interpretative syntheses from the analysis of raw data. Secondary data analyses from the GBD have been published in multiple formats for almost 30 years (GBD 2019 Diseases and Injuries Collaborators, 2020; GBD 2019 Risk Factors Collaborators, 2020; Murray & Lopez, 1996) or aggregated in platforms, such as the GBD Cause and Risk Summaries website (The Lancet, 2022). The 2019 GBD analysis, for example, created secondary data in the form of 450 cause and risk summaries of global trends in disease, injury, impairments, and health risks.

Tertiary data, the synthesis of data and secondary reports, often are repurposed for a specific use within behavioral health services research, such as reference works providing background information or topical compilations. An example would be The Lancet (2022) GBD summaries site or infographics provided by the Institute for Health Metrics and Evaluation GBD site (Institute for Health Metrics and Evaluation, 2022). These sources may be good for a quick distillation but often do not provide full citations to the actual published works. These examples illustrate the importance of how data are used.

Data standards are constantly evolving due to the increased accountability for behavioral health services and the inclusion of women-focused outcomes. Hence, what is measured, what is counted, what is assessed, and what are the outcomes continue to change to ensure equity, quality, and effectiveness of services. As data are created, extracted, or repurposed, there are significant challenges in defining and structuring specific types of data. These include the following types of data: definitional; system (administrative); clinical (patient); and public access-funded research.

Definitional Data

Definition and contextualization of terms is the first step in behavioral health data collection. Developed by the WHO, the international standards for defining behavioral health disorders are the *International Classification of Diseases and Related Health Problems (ICD-11)* and the *International Classification of Functioning, Disability and Health (ICF)* to determine burden of disease (WHO, 2017, 2018). The *ICD* and the *ICF* are complementary standards, as the *ICD* is used for the diagnosis and etiology of disorders and to report baseline statistics, diseases, and health conditions. The *ICF* is used to classify the functional components of health conditions vis-à-vis diagnoses. The *ICF* is especially useful from social and behavioral determinants of health or sociostructural perspectives. It provides a crosswalk between the clinical components of mental disorders and the contexts of disability that affect individuals' level of functioning across interpersonal, family, social, educational, occupational, and/or environmental domains.

New approaches in the diagnosis and classification of behavioral health disorders within the *ICD* and the *ICF* to address psychological factors and sex differences should lead to more accurate diagnoses and effective treatment of women across their lifespan (Dalgleish et al., 2020; Keeley et al., 2016; Levin et al., 2014; Reed et al., 2019; Ruisoto et al., 2022; Yücel et al., 2019). For example, correlating the presentation of stigma to specific areas of the ICF provided insights into the treatment and rehabilitation of women living with HIV in Zambia. As part of a larger longitudinal study (Stevens et al., 2019), women with HIV were interviewed about their daily activities, social activities, and the future. Using three ICF domains (environmental factors, participation restrictions, and personal factors), researchers were able to better understand how stigma affected the ability of women to become more functional across these domains (Stevens et al., 2021).

The *Diagnostic and Statistical Manual* (*DSM*), published in the United States since 1952, is the primary diagnostic tool for behavioral health disorders across the lifespan (American Psychiatric Association, 2022). Now in its 5th edition, the *DSM-5-TR* addresses behavioral health disorders in North America only. Although there is some relationship between the *DSM* and the *ICF* (the *DSM* utilizes the *ICD* codes from the *ICD-10-CM*), there is little if any use of the *ICF* in tandem with the *DSM* to determine domains or levels of functioning. Unlike the ICD/ICF, the *DSM-5-TR* makes correlating diagnosis and burden of disease very difficult.

Behavioral Health System Data (Administrative)

Behavioral health system (BHS) data, often considered administrative data, spans private and public providers across all phases of care (e.g., diagnosis and treatment), financing, legislation, and regulation. BHS data involves all levels of organizational and individual providers, from systems to licensed health-care professionals and peer support workers. It captures acute (crisis) or long-term (maintenance) care delivered in any setting, from institutional to noninstitutional, including academic health centers, clinics, community mental health centers, alcohol and drug use facilities, hospitals, jails and prisons, peer-run centers, private facilities, private providers' offices, religious organizations (pastoral care), or state or local government facilities. However, two major caveats to administrative data. First, there are different reporting rules regarding which provider or facility receives or supplies what data. Second, the granularity (details) of that data differs by provider of the data. Not all individual or organizational providers are required to collect or report their administrative data to local, state, regional, or national entities.

The most common behavioral health measures capture a patient's service (treatment) history, their level of disability, and assessment of their quality of care. It tracks their behavioral health treatment from diagnosis to the most current episode of care. Level of disability addresses the severity of their disorder and compares their everyday level of functioning before and after onset of disease (pre- and post-morbid). These data are then used to design their treatment protocol and connect them to any supportive services they may require. Finally, their diagnosis and treatment will be assessed against individual treatment and system performance indicators and measures. These measures are based on standards to ensure fidelity and quality of care.

One example is the study conducted in Portugal by Coelho et al. (2022) using Organization for Economic Co-operation and Development (OECD) measures and protocols (OECD Patient-reported Indicators Surveys and the OECD PaRIS (Patient-Reported Indicator Surveys) Mental Health Working Group 2021 protocol). Developed for international benchmarking, the OECD surveys and protocols allow data to be compared across other OECD member countries. The OECD recommends the use of the Patient-Reported Outcomes (PROMs) and the Patient-Reported Experiences (PREMs). These measures correlate with the national behavioral health reforms currently in process in Portugal across the micro (individual), meso (provider), and macro (system) levels. Women taking part in the study reported a lower overall satisfaction with the mental health services they received and lower well-being scores than men participating in the study. Although there is still a large gap in gender equality in Portugal, which affects sense of well-being, Portugal's score is improving steadily, which could result in an increase of overall well-being for women with mental illnesses. Coelho and colleagues suggest patient-reported metrics not only supply useful clinical information but also allow for cross-cultural comparisons of behavioral, health, and social outcomes.

Behavioral Health Clinical Data (Patient)

Behavioral health clinical data is derived from all types of data (e.g., best practices data, individual and aggregate patient data at the facility or system level, raw patient data, and surveillance data). Clinical data may be linked across a variety of health and behavioral health-care sectors and agencies. It is often reused for administrative and clinical data-based decision-making, evaluation (programmatic and outcomes), program planning, and research. It also is created and (re)used in a variety of settings, including clinical, governmental, research, and private sectors. Table 13.2 provides an example of the clinical data and where it may be used in community-based programs.

In 2006, the U. S. Institute of Medicine (IOM) recommended the electronic collection of patient data address the longitudinal collection of patient information and immediate 24/7 electronic access by all authorized parties. The use of this data would be to improve clinical decision-making, quality of care, and health care efficiency. Mental and substance use disorders were determined to be the leading cause of combined disability and death for American women, with unipolar major depression ranked second as the cause of DALYs (disability-adjusted life years), behind ischemic heart disease (IOM, 2006). The IOM's recommendation addressed issues surrounding behavioral health data due to federal and state constraints. Federal Health Insurance Portability and Accountability Act (HIPAA) laws governed patient privacy laws, and the transmission of individually identifiable protected health information could be disclosed for treatment purposes without patient consent (45

Table 13.2 Data and program types

Types of data	What, where, and how
Accreditation Administrative Admissions Caregiver/clinician reports Emergency/crisis Genomic profiles Medical records Medical/lab tests Patient assessment Patient history Patient-provided information Patient report cards Patient satisfaction surveys Programmatic outcomes Treatment	*Supported services*: Case management, hotline/crisis service, mobile care team, and supported employment/education/housing
	Evaluation: Consultation, client liaison, and referral to service/treatment
	Treatment: Emergency/crisis services, integrated care, rehabilitation (vocational, physical), and specialty care
	Research: Ambulatory care, case management, day program, hospital, peer-run programs

C.F.R. Parts 160 and 164). However, behavioral health treatment information was the exception to CFR 164. State laws also had exceptions to the use or transmission of behavioral health treatment information, regardless of inpatient or outpatient status or provider of care.

Today, electronic medical records (EMRs) or electronic health records (EHRs) are used by most practitioners. Simply a digital version of the paper charts, EMRs (or EHRs), have more than standard clinical data. Comprehensive lists of patient's medications and allergies, computerized orders for prescriptions, imaging results, laboratory tests, patient history and demographics, and physician clinical notes are central to a basic EHR system. In addition, an EMR also contains administrative and billing data (ICD or DPT codes), crosswalk tables for behavioral health diagnosis codes, data dictionaries of included variables, progress notes, and evidence-based tools, such as clinical texts and databases.

There are innovations in digital behavioral health technologies (DHTs) that not only address personalization of these tools but also workflow adoption and implementation concerns (Graham et al., 2020). Apps, social media, smartphones, and chatbots are increasingly used as adjuvant technologies, and clinical evidence-based uses of DHTs are used in health promotion and prevention as well as in disease management of long-term, chronic mental illnesses (Torous et al., 2021). Although these tools currently do not integrate easily into EHRs and are subject to privacy and confidentiality concerns, they may eventually become part of the evidence-base of care and play a role in how EHRs integrate with disease management and peer support tools.

Public Access-Funded Research

Both administrative data and patient data are used in "open access" (OA) databases that focus on women's health and behavioral health. These OA databases may be funded by federal or state agencies or private sector organizations. One example of a federal agency is the Centers for Disease Control and Prevention (CDC). The CDC supports a variety of public use data and statistics on mental health. The Behavioral Risk Factor Surveillance System, for example, collects data on adult health risk behaviors, health-care access, and preventive practices, while the Youth Risk Behavior Surveillance System focuses on students in grades 9 through 12. The Household Pulse Survey collects health insurance coverage, mental health, and problems accessing care post-COVID near real-time data collection. WISQARS™ is an interactive database for morbidity and mortality data. The School Health Policies and Programs Study (SHPPS) collects data at the classroom, school, and state levels including behavioral health and social service policies.

A grants-funded study, the Study of Women Across the Nation (SWAN, 2023), is a longitudinal study on mid-life experiences affecting health and quality of life women experience. Funded by NIH across six of its institutes and centers and the Department of Defense Congressionally Directed Medical Research Programs, SWAN has collected data since 1994 on the study participants: premenopausal women from five racial/ethnic groups, capturing diverse backgrounds and distinct cultures. In addition to core physical and laboratory measures and questionnaires, SWAN has added new measures of cardiovascular health, cognition, physical activity, sexual health, sleep, social functioning, and urogenital health, which have a role to play in women's behavioral health. In addition to its main database, SWAN also supplies data to the National Institute on Aging Biobank and the National Archive of Computerized Data on Aging.

From the private sector, there is the Kaiser Family Foundation Women's Health website (KFF, 2023b), which includes the State Profiles for Women's Health and the annual KFF Women's Health Surveys (WHS). The State Profiles provide national and state-specific data on health status, demographics, access and service utilization, insurance coverage (private and public), maternal and infant health, sexual health, and abortion policies. The WHS is a nationally representative survey of approximately 5000 self-identified women ages 18–64. In the 2022 WHS, 64% of young women (18–25), half of women (18–64), and a third of women (50–64) reported they needed mental health services. Although half of the women (18–64) were able to schedule an appointment, 40% failed to seek care, and 10% were unable to schedule appointments. The most common reasons for not accessing care were limited provider availability, provider's unwillingness to accept their insurance, and the cost of care. Longitudinal data, such as these, can be mined to show trends and to make recommendations to improve care.

Academic Behavioral Health Services Resource Data

Behavioral health data is complex; however, discovering and using behavioral health data is equally complex. A multitude of local, county, regional, state, national, and global health and behavioral health agencies gather and retain data on women with mental and substance use disorders. However, academia explores women's behavioral health, using a variety of print and online sources to provide to their findings. In addition to secondary and tertiary data, primary data is increasingly available as part of published research journal articles appended as supplemental material to the article within the journal. Academic behavioral health services resource data can also be found in academic institutional repositories.

Although the intent and use of data may change across private and public sectors, as well as across private and public spheres, data keeps evolving across media in format, structure, sources, and use. Data may now be found only in digital format, original source, repurposed adaptations, and mashups. It may also range from big data to real-time data. Public sector data and public domain data are essential sources for public sector behavioral health information. Public sector data are defined as "recorded information, such as facts, data, or opinions, created or received by a component of the federal government when conducting public business" (Stuessy, 2022, March 31, p. 2). Public sector data may either be protected data or exist in the public domain. Governmental and institutional policies of use and reuse, as well as constitutional, federal, or state law, vary widely. Changes to these laws and policies potentially affect content, use, and access to the data (Abresch et al., 2008). Public sector data are often proprietary, and portions of or all the data may be subject to release under specific government or agency conditions. However, elements of public sector data may also be released as part of the public domain. This allows for use and reuse of that data only.

As shown in Table 13.3, there are a variety of types of behavioral health data used in health-care systems that address both population and patient health within and across public and private sector systems. As shown in Fig. 13.1, the types of behavioral health data are interlinked across, within, and around sectors and uses of data.

Challenges in Reporting Behavioral Health Data

There are a variety of challenges in how policymakers understand and use measures to address complex issues in behavioral health. A simple response to a complex policy question may distort what is really happening or redirect focus to a tangential issue. Inappropriate reactions to standardized targets may be driven by fear of impossible targets based on distorted perceptions of measures. Measures focusing

Table 13.3 Uses of data across the hybrid public-private sectors in behavioral health systems (see Fig. 13.1)

Clinical care	*Private sector*
Comparative effectiveness research	Benefit management
Cost-effectiveness	Business development
Cost-efficacy	Cost-benefit analysis
Direct patient care	Drug development
Health behaviors	Health plans
Laboratory data	Marketing
Medication uses	Patient-generated health information
Patient safety	Patient safety
Risk assessment	Post-marketing surveillance
Patient-centered outcomes	Return on investment
Quality assurance	Risk assessment
Quality improvement	
Quality of Care	
Public sector	*Research*
Accountability	Clinical trials
Assessment/evaluation	Confidentiality
DALYS, YLD, and YLL	Data repositories
Epidemiology	Discovery
Human services	Health disparity
Immunization	Health equity
Morbidity/mortality	Patient safety
Patient-generated health information	Prediction
Population health	Recruitment
Public policy	Risk assessment
Regulation	Trial design
Safety/risk	
SDOH	
Surveillance	

more on outcomes rather than outputs are less vulnerable to distortion. Measures also may have diminished utility over time. Official policy benchmarks may have outlived their usefulness since what they were measuring may have changed over time.

Inconsistency in data collection measures affects data comparability and makes accuracy in data analysis and reporting more difficult. It also hinders the development of effective research, practice, and policies focused on improving the well-being of women with behavioral health disorders. For example, evolving indicators may outweigh the utility of consistency. Measures also may have limited relevance. While standard measurements may reflect the views of government officials, these measures may not be relevant to other stakeholders. Hence selecting the right structural, process, or outcome measure(s) is key in developing sustainable programs and systems to effectively address women's behavioral health needs.

Fig. 13.1 The interrelatedness of behavioral health data across research, policy, and practice

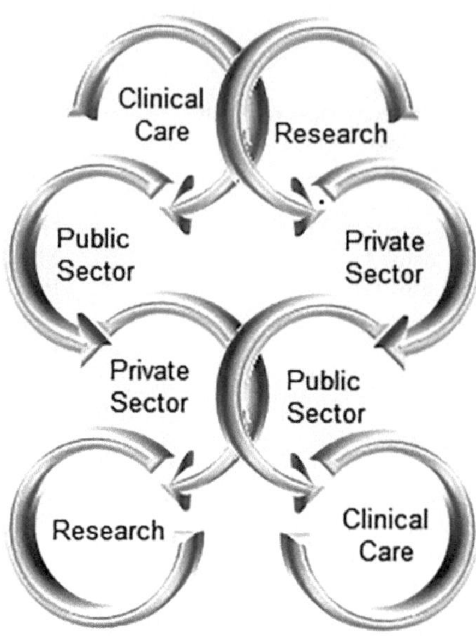

Understanding Measures and Standards in Data

Policymakers want established measures of quantities and qualities. They also need concepts and relationships that define these measures to better understand or predict outcomes. However, measurement is more than creating categories or assigning values. Measurement requires that values be assigned in a systematic and grounded way. Systematic measurement, therefore, requires standardization. There are three important aspects of standardization to consider in the collection of data: (1) characterization; (2) representation; and (3) procedures (Bradburn et al., 2016, September). *Characterization* begins with an ontology. An ontology describes the hierarchical relationship of a group of things, their relationships, and their attributes, usually in a well-bounded domain. *Representation* is a metrical system that represents a concept or a quantity. *Procedures* are the rules used to apply the specific metrical system to produce measurement results. These elements help to ensure that we know what we are measuring.

To create a measure, a concept must be chosen. That concept requires selection of a unit or units of observation or analysis. Once the unit has been selected, then a threshold level is selected for each unit. A threshold level also requires established parameters, so the threshold can be adjusted as necessary across units, time, and location. Finally, each unit is then compared to the resources being measured. If the threshold is higher than its comparison unit, the unit is in that concept.

Concepts are either absolute (e.g., single-value function) or relative (e.g., indicators or indices). Absolute (*aka* pinpoint) concepts are specific qualitative/quantitative features or functions of features, such as the gender and age of women receiving

Medicaid benefits. Relative (*aka* cluster) concepts are more ambiguous. Since relative features may be socially or relationally constructed, they are often loosely defined. However, a concept must have a metric, whether it is an explicit definition (e.g., formulas), an implicit definition (axiomatic or referential), or an operational definition (e.g., diagnostic). How that concept is metrically represented can be problematic.

Refinement of a measure may result in overly granular definitions, which could be either good or problematic. An overly granular definition is problematic when it loses associational components. These associational components may have equal value for that concept. Losing them can affect accuracy when measuring very specific factors, such as subcounty depression prevalence rates for women (Davidson et al., 2018). Finally, data collection procedures must be accurate and precise. Procedurally, accuracy means data reflects the true value of what factor needs measuring, while precision ensures there is a narrow range of estimation.

Why Standardize Data?

Estimating the true global burden of mental illness requires addressing how the concept is characterized, represented, and procedurally appropriate. There are measurement challenges for the GBD. One such example is the use of the *International Classification of Disease*, 10th edition (*ICD-10*), currently used by the GBD Group. The *ICD-10* establishes a common nosological language (WHO, 2018). However, the *ICD* does not address disease distribution or lifespan transitions, essential elements for the GBD's population-based perspective (Vigo et al., 2016). Additional elements, such as personal experiences, or recategorizations may be necessary to truly capture the burden of disease (Barra et al., 2020). Hence, representation may be problematic and affect data collection procedures.

Standardization is also critical if measures are for research (science), practice, or policy. Looking at standard measures also means one must accommodate for differences between women and men in the presentation of diseases, symptoms, triggers, and confounding factors. For example, although there is no single accepted disability measure, there are disability measures to evaluate health outcomes, evaluate employment outcomes, and evaluate adherence to disability legislation (National Research Council, 2011). These also affect our perspectives, in what we recognize and what we determine to be important enough to be counted. These differences in perspective affect how data is framed and treatment recommendations are prioritized. A major obstacle in data collection, for example, is the use of indicators over time. Indicators measuring effectiveness, structure, process, or other outcomes are often bounded by culture, society, or history. Indicators should be reevaluated as necessary to ensure they are capturing relevant data based on the current point in time and have value moving into the future. How data are measured and used varies across research, practice, and policy.

Measuring for research Since 2010, the Patient-Centered Outcomes Research Institute (PCORI), the Agency for Healthcare Research and Quality (AHRQ), and the U. S. Office of the Assistant Secretary for Planning and Evaluation (ASPE) have focused on improving the relevance and quality of the evidence generated by research initiatives funded through the Patient-Centered Outcomes Research Trust Fund (PCORTF) (NASEM, 2022b). Patient-Centered Outcomes Research (PCOR) ensures the research community is engaging effectively with all the stakeholder community(ies) most affected by federally funded research (i.e., patients, advocates, caregivers, community health/behavioral health providers, and health systems).

The intent of PCOR-based research is to increase patient decision-making capability, improve health equity, and lower health-care costs through comparative effectiveness research models (Sox et al., 2010). If researchers design studies for the people who will be receiving treatments with the people affected by the condition, the PCOR process ensures relevant stakeholders are included throughout the research process. Both parties are involved in making the study design, disseminating results, and recommending adoption and implementation of evidence-based results. However, standardized measures are essential, whether they are addressing nontraditional patient roles, reporting and handling missing outcome data, or establishing core outcome sets.

When patients, advocates, or caregivers take on the nontraditional role of patient research partner, they simultaneously could be advisor, research subject, or study personnel. A recent Delphi study produced three domains important for the conduct of patient-centered research (Gelinas et al., 2018). Domain 1 addresses patients in nontraditional study roles. The use of a formal taxonomy of research roles for patient research partners would ensure they receive the proper training for their roles. The taxonomy would also clarify permissions for patients with multiple simultaneous research roles, who switch between roles in the same study. Their duties as study personnel, for example, may conflict with the requirements of their role as research subject (e.g., blinding, randomization, and placebo). Domain 2 focuses on the oversight of emerging technologies focuses on data collection, participant privacy and confidentiality, use of social media for recruitment, and electronic consent. Domain 3 identifies and engages with patient research partners, using a variety of patient partners to ensure multiple perspectives on patient-preferred outcomes and patient concerns. This also include managing financial and nonfinancial conflicts of interest among patient partners, especially those with multiple research roles (Gelinas et al., 2018).

Measuring for practice A challenge for community-based "research to practice" partnerships is making the data available for community partners. Ideally, data should be in usable formats, identify both outcomes and processes, share common measures, crosswalk across data dictionaries, and standardize concepts and measures. However, the sheer complexity and size of behavioral health data, with the lack of crosswalks and little standardization of concepts, make it difficult to share data effectively across partners and providers.

Severity of disorder is a constant in any discussion on women's behavioral health. Not only can severity be based on presentation of disorder; it may also be based on basic levels of functioning (Sharp, 2022). However, severity is also a relative concept, grounded in the sociocultural norms within a particular society or cultural group (Barra et al., 2020). The literature clearly shows the intersectionality of trauma, violence, abuse, and the SDOH that affect women and girls disproportionately, placing them at greater risk for certain mental and substance use disorders. Women, who often are the primary caretakers of family members who suffer from behavioral health disorders, make most of the health decisions for family members. This may place an undue burden on them, increasing a women's risk of mental illnesses.

Mental illnesses also mimic intergenerational cycles. Maternal depression increases the risk of depression in children, who then become adults with depression, who increase their children's risk of depression. These cycles also perpetuate stigma, discrimination, social isolation, and poorer developmental and general health outcomes overall for women and their family members. However, there are few, if any, tools measuring all these elements (severity, functioning, SDOH, stigma, trauma, violence, and abuse) for use in diagnosis or treatment. Complex constructs for disorders with layers upon layers of intersectionality have no single measure.

Measures which can address disparities in diagnosis and intervention are critical but are difficult to standardize in practice. Diagnostic interviews or screening assessment tools have issues regarding validation, applicability to patient practice, and generalizability or transferability across populations. One example is the evaluation of the psychometric properties of self-reported measures of alcohol consumption. McKenna and colleagues (2018) used the transparent and validated COSMIN (COnsensus-based Standards for the selection of health Measurement INstruments) to assess reliability and validity of the measures. The team found problems with methodological quality and inconsistency in the assessment of psychometric properties. No study, for example, assessed all psychometric properties. A single measure, quantity-frequency, was determined to have the highest reliability and validity assessment for self-reported measures of alcohol consumption.

Measuring for policy Although standardized measures may not be perfect, perfect standardized measures may not be possible. Here is where researchers, policymakers, and statistical agencies need to work together to create standard measures using relevant and realistic indicators. Particularly for policy, explicit values may take precedence in a measure. However, there are challenges in setting explicit values because it is difficult to revise the measures once they are set. An explicit measure also may result in inequities among populations, giving one population an advantage over another. We see this in measures normed on men, such as cut points for alcohol abuse, which are less sensitive to screening for alcohol and drug use problems in women (Dhalla & Kopec, 2007; Grekin et al., 2010; Grella, 2008).

A common question is how indicators are accepted for use in policy. There are three main avenues for adoption: (1) public sector; (2) private sector; and (3) nonprofit organization. When a public sector agency has oversight for implementation of a new program or policy, that agency will take the initiative and create indicators for what it is required to measure, so the agency meets its legislative mandate. For example, U. S. federal statistical agencies follow *Principles and Practices for a Federal Statistical Agency* to ensure their indicators have "relevance to policy issues, credibility among data users, trust among data providers, independence from political and other undue external influence, and continual improvement and innovation" (National Academies of Sciences, Engineering, & Medicine, 2021, pp. 2–4). The operations of these agencies are overseen by the U. S. Office of Management and Budget and by additional legislation and guidance particular to that agency and its departments.

Private sector models and measures have been adopted differentially in the public and health system research sectors. Service quality measures, for example, are more than just quality of service; they also must address customer expectations, perceptions, and outcomes within and across the entire services delivery process (Black et al., 2001). Nonprofit organizations may also develop and adopt a new measure as a standard before an issue is widely accepted as something that needs to be measured. These issues, once identified and standardized, often are further developed into open resources. Two such examples are the "Medicaid Managed Care Market Tracker" and "Health Measures for the Developed World." The KFF, a U. S. nonprofit organization, created the Medicaid Managed Care Market Tracker (KFF, 2023a), which showcases data on women's health at the national- and state-specific level. One such indicator is for the average number of "poor mental health days" reported in the last 30 days for all women, stratified by race/ethnicity. The State of the USA's (2023) "Health Measures for the Developed World" is a collaboration with the U. S. National Academy of Sciences (a private nonprofit) to implement a Key National Indicator System (KNIS).

Temporal Caveats in Using Behavioral Health Data

A major consideration in the use of data is the release of that data. Time from creation to discovery (retrieval) may affect access to the data. Information derived from data can have entirely different meanings to its users based on the availability of the data. Many countries have "embargo" statutes which prohibit the disclosure of different categories of information for a restricted amount of time. Added issues regarding timing in the release of behavioral health data are the effects on governmental or agency decision-making, individual privacy or confidentiality, transparency, and archiving of the data. Therefore, both the timing of when information and what information is released matter in the dissemination and use of data.

A Cross-Cutting Measure for Behavioral Health Equity

A common discussion in public sector behavioral health is how equity is measured. Equity discussions affect decisions on what conditions will be funded for research, access to providers and health systems and other practice concerns, and prioritizing areas of population health through policymaking. Equity can be horizontal or vertical. Horizontal equity focuses on equal access or treatment based on equal need. Vertical equity focuses on ensuring that individuals with greater clinical needs (due to severity of disease) should have more intervention. Health state weight estimations, used in the WHO's Global Health Estimates, are useful to address vertical equity. The health state weight measure adjusts the time spent in a specific state of health vis-à-vis the level of health or impairment experienced by the person with the condition (WHO, 2020, December). An individual presenting with acute schizophrenia, the most impairing of health conditions, has a health state rate of 0.78. That individual has approximately one-fifth of the level of functioning and health status of a healthy person. Using a vertical equity perspective, severe mental illnesses should be a priority for research, practice, and policy due to the level of impairment experienced by the individual and the level of care needed (Barra et al., 2020; Sharp, 2022). The next step is to use this measure to address gender inequity when establishing women's behavioral health as a policy priority.

Gender Gaps in Behavioral Health Services Research Data

When behavioral health services research addresses the sociostructural and behavioral risk factors female patient populations experience, health systems are closer to improving individual and population health and outcomes, as well as supplying more cost-effective care and more effective service delivery. These outcomes are possible when examining population health analytic activities that incorporate both social and behavioral factors (Predmore et al., 2019). Evidence-based monitoring and assessment, health promotion, and inter- and multi-sectoral action are fast becoming essential components of behavioral health-care services research, practice, and policy, especially with responsive and accurate data collection and analysis.

O'Campo and Dunn (2012) suggest social epidemiology should focus on problem-identification (e.g., identifying social inequalities and their risk factors), problem-focused research (i.e., causes of these inequities), and solution-based research (i.e., the effectiveness of interventions to reduce them). However, as researchers begin to think and create new ways to measure and address gender gaps in behavioral health research, it is critical that they examine the upstream influence of policy on the effects of health and whether or not policies minimize or exacerbate gender disparities and inequities (Borrell et al., 2014). This upstream examination may inform researchers' knowledge about data collection and limitations in order to enhance the downstream focus of treatment.

The process of deinstitutionalization in the 1950s, which led to a crisis in outpatient care for patients with mental illnesses, illustrated the need for rethinking approaches to the provision of behavioral health care. The deinstitutionalization of behavioral health services, with the lack of community-based services, resulted in increased homelessness, involvement in the criminal justice system, risk of substance misuse and abuse, and use of local hospital psychiatric units for stabilizing acute disorders (Medford-Davis & Beall, 2017). Behavioral health services delivery systems should be concerned with problem-identification and problem-focused services for individuals with mental illnesses to reduce creating additional social and treatment problems.

However, gender-disaggregated data did not equal a female- or women-focused approach to intervention delivery or development. Research populations were primarily male until the 1993 National Institutes of Health Revitalization Act required the inclusion of women in all federally funded research studies. The consequences of deinstitutionalization, particularly on gender disparities and inequities, underscore the importance of incorporating gender-disaggregated data into behavioral health policy, practice, and research. Documenting service delivery challenges and changes across time provides us with a better understanding of how innovative data approaches can be used to address/minimize disparities in help-seeking behaviors and behavioral health services inequities.

Gender is a key social determinant of health, and the psychological and biological differences between women and men's help-seeking behaviors are well studied (Addis & Mahalik, 2003; Fleming & Agnew-Brune, 2015; Fleury et al., 2012; Galdas et al., 2005). However, applying a social constructionist perspective to services research may help to identify latent differences that lead to gaps in help-seeking behavior (Fleming & Agnew-Brune, 2015; Pattyn et al., 2015). In many cultures, gender norms stigmatize behavioral health help seeking for both mental and substance use disorders by limiting a woman's ability and agency to seek help (Fleming & Agnew-Brune, 2015). For example, women who are pregnant or have young children are more likely not to seek treatment or stop it prematurely due to a lack of childcare options or concerns about possible child custody issues (Grella, 2008). Although acknowledgment of these differences has informed policy initiatives and evolved treatment from generic (i.e., one-size-fits-all) to gender-specific approaches (Grella, 2008), it became evident that gender-specific treatment models were not sufficient and gender-responsive approaches were needed.

The evolution from gender-specific treatment models to gender-responsive approaches in behavioral health developed from pervasive mental health disparities among women, particularly with depression (Grella, 2008). Gender-responsive treatments are tailored to the unique needs and experiences of individuals beyond symptoms related to gender, such as trauma and other societal burdens. These treatments allow us to examine data on effectiveness, efficacy, and quality of life based on sociostructural elements to reduce the negative effects of social determinants on behavioral health outcomes using both big and small data. These data analyses may generate gender policy changes across countries with a better understanding of gender-based disparities, as well as to assess which policies are more effective in different regions (Borrell et al., 2014; World Health Organization, 2019).

However, gaps in access to care remain significant for women globally. Access to care for women is rooted in systemic inequities, such as educational attainment, political empowerment, economic participation and opportunity, gender wage gaps, and income (World Economic Forum, 2019, December 16). The lack of data and research to highlight gender gaps in areas, such as income and access to care, hamper efforts to foster accountability and promote policy reforms (WHO, 2019). Quality data is needed to develop evidence-based policies and interventions tailored to the unique needs and burdens of women in relation to their behavioral health.

Measuring Sex/Gender

Sex and gender are conceptually distinct complex, intersectoral constructs. However, measuring sex as a nonbinary construct requires consensus on definitions and characteristics of gender identity and sexual orientation before these concepts become foundations for such measures. This ensures sexually gender diverse (SGD) populations are counted and accurately represented in data collection instruments. The constructs of interest must be precisely defined, with no proxy constructs or "construct creep" allowed. However, sex, gender identity, and sexual orientation are not only complex constructs, but they are also "living" constructs, as people create new or crosswalk existing identities to represent themselves to the world (Davis, 2019; Glick et al., 2018; Jenkins & Short, 2017).

The National Academies of Science, Engineering, and Medicine (NASEM) defined sex, gender, and sexual orientation as multidimensional constructs. For each of these concepts, NASEM defined specific dimensions, characteristics, and identities (NASEM, 2022a, pp. 3–4). Sex is defined as "a multidimensional construct based on a cluster of anatomical and physiological traits (sex traits)" (NASEM, 2022a, pp. 3–4). Gender is defined as "a multidimensional construct that links gender identity, gender expression, and social and cultural expectations about status, characteristics, and behavior that are associated with sex traits." Sexual orientation is defined as "a multidimensional construct encompassing emotional, romantic, and sexual attraction, identity, and behavior" (NASEM, 2022a, pp. 3–4). NASEM (2022a) also acknowledged these concepts would need to be updated on an ongoing basis, as researchers, practitioners, or populations introduce new terms or change the scope of terms, which then become ubiquitous within the United States.

Recommending these measures becomes standard across research, clinical practice, and public health settings and processes. This ensures patient confidentiality and privacy. NASEM (2022a) also assessed each recommended measure for conceptual fit, populations involved in testing, any adjustments to previously included measures, and weaknesses and challenges. A goal of a measure is to identify populations most consistently at risk for differential treatment and outcomes. Measures of sex/gender identity/sexual orientation can help to establish equity across treatment, service delivery, and continuity of care for individuals who identify as SGD or cisgender.

Measuring Elements of Care

Measurement-based care is a significant issue in behavioral health care, especially when we look at specific populations and subgroups with expectations of specific outcomes. Measurement is a three-step process. One must define what is to be measured, select the right measure, and apply the metric correctly. Oftentimes, the biggest issue in collecting data and measuring care is examining the range of choices about which questions to ask. It depends on whether what we are measuring needs to be assessed from a structural, processual, or outcome-based perspective. In addition, two emerging issues in measuring elements of care for women: (1) small, hard to reach, or hidden populations and (2) developing core outcomes sets for patient-centered outcomes research.

Small, hard-to-reach, or hidden population research Hanson and Levin (2020, p. 360) define prevalence as "a proportion of persons in a population, in a given location and at a particular time." Prevalence data are used for many things, including providing the need for resources, establishing the scope of services, and determining workforce requirements. While reporting prevalence over a region can be problematic, it is exacerbated by the need for more specific, consistent, and disaggregated data required to address the challenges of increasingly diverse populations and subgroups of populations. The definitions of diversity go far beyond race and ethnicity to encompass gender identity, geographic location, homelessness, level of disability, migrant/immigrant/refugee status, sexual orientation, socioeconomic position, and more (for more rural populations, see Chap. 7 in this volume).

Increasing levels of population granularity (subgroups) requires researchers, practitioners, and policymakers, as well as the general public, to understand challenges with "small data." Srinivasan and colleagues (2015, p. 1) define small data as "the size, dispersion, or accessibility of the population of interest makes it difficult to obtain adequate sample sizes to test specific research questions." Small data presents its own challenges, as logistical costs for studying small populations are high and funding may be difficult to obtain. Additional challenges may include research design (e.g., qualitative, N-of-1, within group), statistical methodologies and analyses (aggregation, small area estimation, Bayesian), recruitment and retention, and intervention design and analytic approaches (Srinivasan et al., 2015), particularly as research design may affect level of evidence requirements for efficacy vs. effectiveness of clinical studies.

Patient-centered outcomes in comparative effectiveness research A major in comparative effectiveness research (CER) is the identification and prioritization of patient-centered outcomes. There is little consensus on the choice of outcomes across clinical settings. This lack of consensus affects study and/or trial design, as well as the conduct, analysis, and reporting of results. Patient characteristics should be associated with meaningful differences in outcomes regarding which outcomes are most important to patients and, hence, for investigators.

In behavioral health research, missing outcome data occur frequently. The research literature itself has noted the problems with inconsistencies in the outcomes reported in clinical trials and selective reporting of outcomes in published reports of studies (Clarke et al., 2007; Kahale et al., 2018; Kirkham et al., 2010). In their umbrella review of Cochrane systematic reviews (SRs) and meta-analyses, Spineli et al. (2015) found 92% of SRs did not explicitly report missing outcome data and 96% did not explain what was meant by the missing data. Meta-analyses did not fare much better than SRs. Although their study examined primary outcomes only, they suggest reporting, and the use of sensitivity analysis may be poorer for secondary outcomes (Spineli et al., 2015). Serious weaknesses in SRs and meta-analyses are in the description of missing outcome data and the statistical analysis used to address this data; however, it is incumbent upon researchers to effectively address these issues in their study design and reporting.

Core outcomes measures Different research studies may not measure the same outcomes. Researchers should not publish results on certain outcomes if the actual outcomes are not what they expected. Further, there is little to no evidence on the best way to engage with patient investigators and reviewers. Hence, study results are difficult to compare. One solution is the use of core outcomes sets (COS), which can address the difficulty in determining outcomes related to a specific health condition by associating possible outcomes with studies on diseases or interventions (Williamson & Clarke, 2012). A COS would be built on consensus, standard vocabulary, recommended instruments to measure specific outcomes, and improve the quality of measures used. It would also become a standard to measure and report a consistent set of outcomes in studies of a health condition and be supplemented with other outcomes of interest outside the core.

The COMET (Core Outcome Measures in Effectiveness Trials) Initiative collects and develops applied and methodological resources to develop COS as an international standard. There are reporting standards, protocols, guidelines, and checklists as well as a database of studies on the development of core outcome sets for use in clinical trials. As of May 2023, there were two ongoing COS studies on mental health, one on perimenopausal depressive disorder (PDD) and one on perinatal generalized anxiety disorder.

Developing COS is one approach to identifying and prioritizing outcomes for use in CER. However, developing a COS is difficult. The term "outcome" is comprised of five elements: (1) measure; (2) method of aggregation; (3) metric; (4) outcome domain; and (5) time point. Each outcome has its own elements; hence, an experimental study may have multiple outcomes for the same domain. The questions then become which outcome(s) show an intervention works and are the results meta-analyzable. In their systematic review on patient outcomes in quetiapine-bipolar depression RCTs, Mayo-Wilson et al. (2018) found significant differences across trials. Reports of RCTs with multiple and/or undefined outcomes, methodological problems, unclear statistical analyses, irreproducible meta-analyses, and ambiguity in handling missing data (within and across trials) made comparisons difficult (Mayo-Wilson et al., 2018).

Having evidence-based measures that can be used across public and private sectors for medical and specialty behavioral health care not only supports standardized assessment and clinical decision-making but also ensures more effective outcomes monitoring and better quality of care.

Implications for Women's Behavioral Health

Collecting, analyzing, and reporting robust comparable data is an essential step to develop sustainable intersectoral evidence-based interventions and programs and evidence-informed policies. However, factors, such as accessibility, dispersion, and size of a population, are significant challenges in acquiring relevant data and adequate sample sizes for small and hard-to-reach populations.

To develop evidence-based intersectoral interventions and programs for women requires robust and comparable data. However, nationally representative population-based surveys vary widely in quality. Inconsistency in definitions and types of measures makes study comparisons challenging, if not impossible. Adjusting for these variations is central for researchers, practitioners, policymakers, and the public. It allows us to more thoroughly comprehend the effects, nature, and prevalence of women's behavioral health disorders across the lifespan, ethnic and gender identities, and geographic areas.

While more research is needed to identify effective, scalable prevention behavioral health interventions for women, program and service evaluation must address comparability of clinical, administrative, and outcomes data (incidence) vis-à-vis accurately determined prevalence data. Causal analyses and better disaggregation of data are essential to create a better knowledge base for understanding women's behavioral health disorders.

Reliable and consistent data is critical to address effective treatment for subgroups of women. We know different factors affect the health of different groups of women. However, without solid data and transparency of data, it is difficult to understand which differences between subgroups of women may affect their behavioral health and their response to treatment. Hopefully, progress in the use of big and small data and new analytic techniques will provide new ways of understanding women's behavioral health needs and effective treatment solutions for an overall better quality of life.

References

Abresch, J., Hanson, A., & Reehling, P. J. (2008). Collection management issues with geospatial information. In J. Abresch, A. Hanson, S. J. Heron, & P. J. Reehling (Eds.), *Integrating geographic information systems into library services: A guide for academic libraries* (pp. 202–238). Information Science Pub.

Addis, M. E., & Mahalik, J. R. (2003). Men, masculinity, and the contexts of help seeking. *American Psychologist, 58*(1), 5–14. https://doi.org/10.1037/0003-066x.58.1.5

American Psychiatric Association. (2022). *Diagnostic and statistical manual of mental disorders, Fifth edition, Text revision (DSM-5-TR)*. Author.

Barra, M., Broqvist, M., Gustavsson, E., Henriksson, M., Juth, N., Sandman, L., & Solberg, C. T. (2020). Severity as a priority setting criterion: Setting a challenging research agenda. *Health Care Analysis, 28*(1), 25–44. https://doi.org/10.1007/s10728-019-00371-z

Black, S., Briggs, S., & Keogh, W. (2001). Service quality performance measurement in public/private sectors. *Managerial Auditing Journal, 16*(7), 400–405. https://doi.org/10.1108/EUM0000000005715

Borrell, C., Palència, L., Muntaner, C., Urquía, M., Malmusi, D., & O'Campo, P. (2014). Influence of macrosocial policies on women's health and gender inequalities in health. *Epidemiologic Reviews, 36*, 31–48. https://doi.org/10.1093/epirev/mxt002

Bradburn, N. M., Cartwright, N., & Fuller, J. (2016, September). *A theory of measurement* [CHESS Working Paper No. 2016-07]. Centre for Humanities Engaging Science and Society (CHESS). https://dro.dur.ac.uk/20087/1/

Castillo-Carandang, N. T., Buenaventura, R. D., Chia, Y. C., Do Van, D., Lee, C., Duong, N. L., Ng, C. H., Robles, Y. R., Santoso, A., Sigua, H. S., Sukonthasarn, A., Tan, R., Viora, E., Zakaria, H., Brizuela, G. E., Ratnasingham, P., Thomas, M., & Majumdar, A. (2020). Moving towards optimized noncommunicable disease management in the ASEAN region: Recommendations from a review and multidisciplinary expert panel. *Risk Management and Healthcare Policy, 13*, 803–819. https://doi.org/10.2147/rmhp.S256165

Clarke, L., Clarke, M., & Clarke, T. (2007). How useful are Cochrane reviews in identifying research needs? *Journal of Health Services Research & Policy, 12*(2), 101–103. https://doi.org/10.1258/135581907780279648

Coelho, A., de Bienassis, K., Klazinga, N., Santo, S., Frade, P., Costa, A., & Gaspar, T. (2022). Mental health patient-reported outcomes and experiences assessment in Portugal. *International Journal of Environmental Research and Public Health, 19*(18), 11153. https://doi.org/10.3390/ijerph191811153

Collins, P. Y., Patel, V., Joestl, S. S., March, D., Insel, T. R., Daar, A. S., Anderson, W., Dhansay, M. A., Phillips, A., Shurin, S., Walport, M., Ewart, W., Savill, S. J., Bordin, I. A., Costello, E. J., Durkin, M., Fairburn, C., Glass, R. I., Hall, W., Huang, Y., Hyman, S. E., Jamison, K., Kaaya, S., Kapur, S., Kleinman, A., Ogunniyi, A., Otero-Ojeda, A., Poo, M. M., Ravindranath, V., Sahakian, B. J., Saxena, S., Singer, P. A., & Stein, D. J. (2011). Grand challenges in global mental health. *Nature, 475*(7354), 27–30. https://doi.org/10.1038/475027a

Dalgleish, T., Black, M., Johnston, D., & Bevan, A. (2020). Transdiagnostic approaches to mental health problems: Current status and future directions. *Journal of Consulting and Clinical Psychology, 88*(3), 179–195. https://doi.org/10.1037/ccp0000482

Davidson, A. J., Xu, S., Oronce, C. I. A., Durfee, M. J., McCormick, E. V., Steiner, J. F., Havranek, E., & Beck, A. (2018). Monitoring depression rates in an urban community: Use of electronic health records. *Journal of Public Health Management and Practice, 24*(6), e6–e14. https://doi.org/10.1097/phh.0000000000000751

Davis, J. L. (2019). Refusing (mis)recognition: Navigating multiple marginalization in the U.S. two spirit movement. *Review of International American Studies, 12*(1), 65–86. https://doi.org/10.31261/rias.7328

Dhalla, S., & Kopec, J. A. (2007). The CAGE questionnaire for alcohol misuse: A review of reliability and validity studies. *Clinical and Investigative Medicine, 30*(1), 33–41. https://doi.org/10.25011/cim.v30i1.447

Fleming, P. J., & Agnew-Brune, C. (2015). Current trends in the study of gender norms and health behaviors. *Current Opinion in Psychology, 5*, 72–77. https://doi.org/10.1016/j.copsyc.2015.05.001

Fleury, M. J., Grenier, G., Bamvita, J. M., Perreault, M., & Caron, J. (2012). Determinants associated with the utilization of primary and specialized mental health services. *Psychiatric Quarterly, 83*(1), 41–51. https://doi.org/10.1007/s11126-011-9181-3

Galdas, P. M., Cheater, F., & Marshall, P. (2005). Men and health help-seeking behaviour: Literature review. *Journal of Advanced Nursing, 49*(6), 616–623. https://doi.org/10.1111/j.1365-2648.2004.03331.x

GBD 2019 Diseases and Injuries Collaborators. (2020). Global burden of 369 diseases and injuries in 204 countries and territories, 1990-2019: A systematic analysis for the Global Burden of Disease Study 2019. *Lancet, 396*(10258), 1204–1222. https://doi.org/10.1016/s0140-6736(20)30925-9

GBD 2019 Risk Factors Collaborators. (2020). Global burden of 87 risk factors in 204 countries and territories, 1990-2019: A systematic analysis for the Global Burden of Disease Study 2019. *The Lancet, 396*(10258), 1223–1249. https://doi.org/10.1016/S0140-6736(20)30752-2

Gelinas, L., Weissman, J. S., Lynch, H. F., Gupta, A., Rozenblum, R., Largent, E. A., & Cohen, I. G. (2018). Oversight of patient-centered outcomes research: Recommendations from a Delphi panel. *Annals of Internal Medicine, 169*(8), 559–563. https://doi.org/10.7326/m18-1334

Glick, J. L., Theall, K., Andrinopoulos, K., & Kendall, C. (2018). For data's sake: Dilemmas in the measurement of gender minorities. *Culture, Health & Sexuality, 20*(12), 1362–1377. https://doi.org/10.1080/13691058.2018.1437220

Graham, A. K., Lattie, E. G., Powell, B. J., Lyon, A. R., Smith, J. D., Schueller, S. M., Stadnick, N. A., Brown, C. H., & Mohr, D. C. (2020). Implementation strategies for digital mental health interventions in health care settings. *American Psychologist, 75*(8), 1080–1092. https://doi.org/10.1037/amp0000686

Grekin, E. R., Svikis, D. S., Lam, P., Connors, V., LeBreton, J. M., Streiner, D. L., Smith, C., & Ondersma, S. J. (2010). Drug use during pregnancy: Validating the drug abuse screening test against physiological measures. *Psychology of Addictive Behaviors, 24*(4), 719. https://doi.org/10.1037/a0021741

Grella, C. E. (2008). From generic to gender-responsive treatment: Changes in social policies, treatment services, and outcomes of women in substance abuse treatment. *Journal of Psychoactive Drugs, 40*(Suppl 5), 327–343. https://doi.org/10.1080/02791072.2008.10400661

Hanson, A., & Levin, B. L. (2020). Global services, systems, and policy. In B. L. Levin & A. Hanson (Eds.), *Foundations of behavioral health* (pp. 351–376). Springer Nature. https://doi.org/10.1007/978-3-030-18453_17

Institute for Health Metrics and Evaluation. (2022). *Global Burden of Disease (GBD)* [Database (GBD Results Tool)]. IHME, University of Washington School of Medicine. https://www.healthdata.org/gbd/2019 [Generated table. Data elements: GBD estimate: Cause of death or injury; Measure: DALYS; Metric: Number, Percent, Rate; Cause: All causes; Location: Global; Age: All; Sex: Both; Year: 2019].

Institute of Medicine. (2006). *Improving the quality of health care for mental and substance-use conditions*. The National Academies Press. https://doi.org/10.17226/11470

Jenkins, T. M., & Short, S. E. (2017). Negotiating intersex: A case for revising the theory of social diagnosis. *Social Science and Medicine, 175*, 91–98. https://doi.org/10.1016/j.socscimed.2016.12.047

Kahale, L. A., Diab, B., Brignardello-Petersen, R., Agarwal, A., Mustafa, R. A., Kwong, J., Neumann, I., Li, L., Lopes, L. C., Briel, M., Busse, J. W., Iorio, A., Vandvik, P. O., Alexander, P. E., Guyatt, G., & Akl, E. A. (2018). Systematic reviews do not adequately report or address missing outcome data in their analyses: A methodological survey. *Journal of Clinical Epidemiology, 99*, 14–23. https://doi.org/10.1016/j.jclinepi.2018.02.016

Kaiser Family Foundation. (2023a). *Medicaid Managed Care Tracker* [Web page; dataset]. KFF. https://www.kff.org/statedata/collection/medicaid-managed-care-tracker/

Kaiser Family Foundation. (2023b). *Women's health* [Web site]. KFF. https://www.kff.org/state-category/womens-health/

Keeley, J. W., Reed, G. M., Roberts, M. C., Evans, S. C., Medina-Mora, M. E., Robles, R., Rebello, T., Sharan, P., Gureje, O., First, M. B., Andrews, H. F., Ayuso-Mateos, J. L., Gaebel, W., Zielasek, J., & Saxena, S. (2016). Developing a science of clinical utility in diagnostic classification systems field study strategies for ICD-11 mental and behavioral disorders. *American Psychologist, 71*(1), 3–16. https://doi.org/10.1037/a0039972

Kirkham, J. J., Dwan, K. M., Altman, D. G., Gamble, C., Dodd, S., Smyth, R., & Williamson, P. R. (2010). The impact of outcome reporting bias in randomised controlled trials on a cohort of systematic reviews. *BMJ, 340*, c365. https://doi.org/10.1136/bmj.c365

Levin, M. E., MacLane, C., Daflos, S., Seeley, J., Hayes, S. C., Biglan, A., & Pistorello, J. (2014). Examining psychological inflexibility as a transdiagnostic process across psychological disorders. *Journal of Contextual Behavioral Science, 3*(3), 155–163. https://doi.org/10.1016/j.jcbs.2014.06.003

Mayo-Wilson, E., Golozar, A., Cowley, T., Fusco, N., Gresham, G., Haythornthwaite, J., Tolbert, E., Payne, J. L., Rosman, L., Hutfless, S., Canner, J. K., & Dickersin, K. (2018). Methods to identify and prioritize patient-centered outcomes for use in comparative effectiveness research. *Pilot and Feasibility Studies, 4*, 95. https://doi.org/10.1186/s40814-018-0284-6

McKenna, H., Treanor, C., O'Reilly, D., & Donnelly, M. (2018). Evaluation of the psychometric properties of self-reported measures of alcohol consumption: A COSMIN systematic review. *Substance Abuse Treatment, Prevention, and Policy, 13(1)*, 6. https://doi.org/10.1186/s13011-018-0143-8

Medford-Davis, L. N., & Beall, R. C. (2017). The changing health policy environment and behavioral health services delivery. *Psychiatric Clinics of North America, 40*(3), 533–540. https://doi.org/10.1016/j.psc.2017.05.013

Murray, C. J., & Lopez, A. D. (1994). Quantifying disability: Data, methods and results. *Bulletin of the World Health Organization, 72*(3), 481–494.

Murray, C. J. L., & Lopez, A. D. (1996). *The global burden of disease: A comprehensive assessment of mortality and disability from diseases, injuries, and risk factors in 1990 and projected to 2020.* Harvard School of Public Health on behalf of the World Health Organization and the World Bank. https://apps.who.int/iris/handle/10665/41864

National Academies of Sciences, Engineering, & Medicine. (2021). *Principles and practices for a federal statistical agency* (7th ed.). The National Academies Press. https://doi.org/10.17226/25885

National Academies of Sciences, Engineering, & Medicine. (2022a). *Measuring sex, gender identity, and sexual orientation* [Report]. The National Academies Press. https://doi.org/10.17226/26424

National Academies of Sciences, Engineering, & Medicine. (2022b). *Accelerating the use of findings from patient-centered outcomes research in clinical practice to improve health and health care: Proceedings of a workshop series.* The National Academies Press. https://doi.org/10.17226/26753

National Institute of Mental Health. (n.d.). *Grand challenges in global mental health initiative* [Web page]. https://www.nimh.nih.gov/about/organization/cgmhr/grandchallenges

National Institutes of Health Revitalization Act [Women and Minorities as Subjects in Clinical Research], Pub. L. No. 103-43. (1993). https://www.govinfo.gov/content/pkg/STATUTE-107/pdf/STATUTE-107-Pg122.pdf

National Research Council. (2011). *The importance of common metrics for advancing social science theory and research: A workshop summary.* The National Academies Press. https://doi.org/10.17226/13034

O'Campo, P., & Dunn, J. R. (2012). Are we producing the right kind of actionable evidence for the social determinants of health? *Journal of Urban Health, 89*(6), 881–893. https://doi.org/10.1007/s11524-012-9695-5

Pattyn, E., Verhaeghe, M., & Bracke, P. (2015). The gender gap in mental health service use. *Social Psychiatry and Psychiatric Epidemiology, 50*(7), 1089–1095. https://doi.org/10.1007/s00127-015-1038-x

Predmore, Z., Hatef, E., & Weiner, J. P. (2019). Integrating social and behavioral determinants of health into population health analytics: A conceptual framework and suggested road map. *Population Health Management, 22*(6), 488–494. https://doi.org/10.1089/pop.2018.0151

Reed, G. M., First, M. B., Kogan, C. S., Hyman, S. E., Gureje, O., Gaebel, W., Maj, M., Stein, D. J., Maercker, A., Tyrer, P., Claudino, A., Garralda, E., Salvador-Carulla, L., Ray, R., Saunders, J. B., Dua, T., Poznyak, V., Medina-Mora, M. E., Pike, K. M., Ayuso-Mateos, J. L., Kanba, S., Keeley, J. W., Khoury, B., Krasnov, V. N., Kulygina, M., Lovell, A. M., de Jesus Mari, J., Maruta, T., Matsumoto, C., Rebello, T. J., Roberts, M. C., Robles, R., Sharan, P., Zhao, M., Jablensky, A., Udomratn, P., Rahimi-Movaghar, A., Rydelius, P. A., Bahrer-Kohler, S., Watts, A. D., & Saxena, S. (2019). Innovations and changes in the ICD-11 classification of mental, behavioural and neurodevelopmental disorders. *World Psychiatry, 18*(1), 3–19. https://doi.org/10.1002/wps.20611

Ruisoto, P., Lopez-Guerra, V. M., Lopez-Nunez, C., Sanchez-Puertas, R., Paladines-Costa, M. B., & Pineda-Cabrera, N. J. (2022). Transdiagnostic model of psychological factors and sex differences in depression in a large sample of Ecuador [Article]. *International Journal of Clinical and Health Psychology, 22*(3), 8, Article 100322. https://doi.org/10.1016/j.ijchp.2022.100322

Sharp, C. (2022). New data toward fulfilling the promise of the ICD-11 severity criterion. *Personality and Mental Health, 16*(2), 93–98. https://doi.org/10.1002/pmh.1549

Sox, H. C., Helfand, M., Grimshaw, J., Dickersin, K., Tovey, D., Knottnerus, J. A., & Tugwell, P. (2010). Comparative effectiveness research: Challenges for medical journals. *Trials, 11*, 45. https://doi.org/10.1186/1745-6215-11-45

Spineli, L. M., Pandis, N., & Salanti, G. (2015). Reporting and handling missing outcome data in mental health: A systematic review of Cochrane systematic reviews and meta-analyses. *Research Synthesis Methods, 6*(2), 175–187. https://doi.org/10.1002/jrsm.1131

Srinivasan, S., Moser, R. P., Willis, G., Riley, W., Alexander, M., Berrigan, D., & Kobrin, S. (2015). Small is essential: Importance of subpopulation research in cancer control. *American Journal of Public Health, 105*(Suppl 3), S371–S373. https://doi.org/10.2105/ajph.2014.302267

Stevens, M. E., Parsons, J. A., Read, S. E., & Nixon, S. A. (2019). The conceptualization of stigma within a rehabilitation framework using HIV as an example. *Disability and Rehabilitation, 41*(2), 235–243. https://doi.org/10.1080/09638288.2017.1385099

Stevens, M. E., Parsons, J. A., Read, S. E., Bond, V., Solomon, P., & Nixon, S. A. (2021). The relationship between stigma and a rehabilitation framework [international classification of functioning, disability and health (ICF)]: Three case studies of women living with HIV in Lusaka, Zambia. *Disability and Rehabilitation, 43*(15), 2149–2156. https://doi.org/10.1080/0963828 8.2019.1693640

Study of Women Across the Nation. (2023). *About SWAN* [Website]. SWAN. https://www.swanstudy.org/about/about-swan/

Stuessy, M. M. (2022, March 31). *Access to government information: An overview* [Report; R47058]. Congressional Research Service. https://crsreports.congress.gov/product/pdf/R/R47058

The Lancet. (2022). *GBD cause and risk summaries* [Database]. Elsevier. https://www.thelancet.com/gbd/summaries

The State of the USA. (2023). *Health measures for the developed world* [Web page; dataset]. Author. http://www.stateoftheusa.org/content/health-measures-for-the-develo.php

Torous, J., Bucci, S., Bell, I. H., Kessing, L. V., Faurholt-Jepsen, M., Whelan, P., Carvalho, A. F., Keshavan, M., Linardon, J., & Firth, J. (2021). The growing field of digital psychiatry: Current evidence and the future of apps, social media, chatbots, and virtual reality. *World Psychiatry, 20*(3), 318–335. https://doi.org/10.1002/wps.20883

U.S. Office of the Surgeon General. (1999). *Mental health: A report of the Surgeon General* [Report]. U.S. Department of Health and Human Services, Substance Abuse and Mental Health Services Administration, Center for Mental Health Services, National Institutes of Health, National Institute of Mental Health. https://profiles.nlm.nih.gov/spotlight/nn/catalog/nlm:nlm uid-101584932X120-doc

Vigo, D., Thornicroft, G., & Atun, R. (2016). Estimating the true global burden of mental illness. *Lancet Psychiatry, 3*(2), 171–178. https://doi.org/10.1016/s2215-0366(15)00505-2

Williamson, P., & Clarke, M. (2012). The COMET (core outcome measures in effectiveness trials) initiative: Its role in improving. *Cochrane Reviews, 5*, ED000041. https://doi.org/10.1002/14651858.ED000041

World Economic Forum. (2019, December 16). *Global gender gap report 2020* [Report]. World Economic Forum. http://www3.weforum.org/docs/WEF_GGGR_2020.pdf

World Health Organization. (2001). *The world health report 2001: Mental health: New understanding, new hope.* WHO. https://www.who.int/whr/2001/en/whr01_en.pdf?ua=1

World Health Organization. (2017). *International classification of functioning, disability and health* [Interactive Online Web Site]. Author. http://apps.who.int/classifications/icfbrowser/Default.aspx

World Health Organization. (2018). *International classification of diseases and related health problems* [Interactive Online Web Site]. Author. https://icd.who.int/

World Health Organization. (2019). *Delivered by women, led by men: A gender and equity analysis of the global health and social workforce* (Author, Ed.) [Human Resources for Health Observer Series No. 24]. WHO. https://apps.who.int/iris/bitstream/handle/10665/311322/9789241515467-eng.pdf?ua=1

World Health Organization. (2020, December). *WHO methods and data sources for global burden of disease estimates 2000–2019* [Global Health Estimates Technical Paper WHO/DDI/DNA/GHE/2020.3]. WHO Department of Data and Analytics, Division of Data, Analytics and Delivery for Impact. https://cdn.who.int/media/docs/default-source/gho-documents/global-health-estimates/ghe2019_daly-methods.pdf?sfvrsn=31b25009_7

World Health Organization. (2022, June 16). *World mental health report: Transforming mental health for all* [Report]. Author [WHO]. https://apps.who.int/iris/rest/bitstreams/1433523/retrieve

World Health Organization, & Ministry of Social Affairs and Health. (2014). *Health in all policies: Helsinki statement. Framework for country action* [Report]. World Health Organization.

Yücel, M., Oldenhof, E., Ahmed, S. H., Belin, D., Billieux, J., Bowden-Jones, H., Carter, A., Chamberlain, S. R., Clark, L., Connor, J., Daglish, M., Dom, G., Dannon, P., Duka, T., Fernandez-Serrano, M. J., Field, M., Franken, I., Goldstein, R. Z., Gonzalez, R., Goudriaan, A. E., Grant, J. E., Gullo, M. J., Hester, R., Hodgins, D. C., Le Foll, B., Lee, R. S. C., Lingford-Hughes, A., Lorenzetti, V., Moeller, S. J., Munafò, M. R., Odlaug, B., Potenza, M. N., Segrave, R., Sjoerds, Z., Solowij, N., van den Brink, W., van Holst, R. J., Voon, V., Wiers, R., Fontenelle, L. F., & Verdejo-Garcia, A. (2019). A transdiagnostic dimensional approach towards a neuropsychological assessment for addiction: An international Delphi consensus study. *Addiction, 114*(6), 1095–1109. https://doi.org/10.1111/add.14424

Chapter 14
Policymaking Addressing Women and Behavioral Health

Ardis Hanson and Bruce Lubotsky Levin

Introduction

Women face numerous health and behavioral health issues across their lifespan. Women need access to care, care that addresses sex- and gender-specific behavioral health/health issues, and health outcomes that consider physiological, economic, and sociocultural issues. From a population health perspective, the underrepresentation of women in research studies that reflect promising and evidence-based treatments, the time lag in translating research into real-world practice, and the enactment of public health/behavioral health policies that affect them and their families remain problematic. If evidence influences practice, and evidence and practice influence policy, it follows that policy influences research and practice. That intersection of research, practice, and policy clearly affects access to and use of services, infrastructure design, continuity of care, and patient outcomes at both individual and population health levels and across private and public sectors. Hence, governmental responsibility and accountability for women's behavioral health are essential. This chapter will address two focal areas. First, it will examine the public health policymaking process with a focus on women's behavioral health. Second, it will make recommendations on how the process could be strengthened to improve the well-being of women with the provision of effective behavioral health services, treatment, and supports.

A. Hanson (✉)
USF Health Libraries and the College of Public Health, University of South Florida, Tampa, FL, USA
e-mail: hanson@usf.edu

B. L. Levin
College of Behavioral & Community Sciences, College of Public Health, University of South Florida, Tampa, FL, USA
e-mail: levin@usf.edu

Overview of Policymaking, Women, and Behavioral Health

Policymaking affects the design, receipt, and use of services, infrastructure development, direct and indirect costs of care, coverage of services, and payer-provider relationships. Policymaking also is affected by the implicit or explicit bias, discrimination, perceptions, and stigma attached to the receipt of or need for women's behavioral health services. The 4-A framework in Table 14.1 (availability, accessibility, affordability, and acceptability) drives the access and use of behavioral health services. Developed over 30 years ago, these four factors continue to be the foci for national (Bushy, 1997; Wilson et al., 2015) and global policy initiatives (Centers for Disease Control and Prevention (CDC), 2022; World Health Organization (WHO), 2017).

The upstream and downstream effects of policy development, implementation, and practice seldom address how gender equality policies influence gender inequities in women's health and behavioral health. However, available studies show a significant correlation between gender inequality, inequity, and disparity in behavioral health (Alvarenga et al., 2019; Borrell et al., 2014; Braveman et al., 2011; Yu, 2018). Further, the research and practice literature clearly show the relation between gender inequality, inequity, and disparity to availability, accessibility, affordability, and acceptability of behavioral health services.

Identifying and understanding potential trajectories and drivers of health and behavioral health are essential when determining long-term effects of policy implementation. The provision of effective health and behavioral health has become increasingly difficult as providers, health systems, and governments are faced with new or ongoing challenges. These challenges include aging populations, costs of care, shortages of providers and facilities, and increased morbidity and mortality due to the social determinants of health, natural and human orchestrated disasters, and/or global conflicts. A recent forecast by the Global Burden of Disease (GBD) Study Group for 2016–2040 shows an overall increase of years of life lived for both women and men but also an increase in the numbers of deaths from noncommunicable diseases, partially driven by population growth and aging (Foreman et al., 2018).

Mental and substance use disorders, which fall under noncommunicable diseases (NCDs), often co-occur and share many factors in common. These factors may be

Table 14.1 Availability, accessibility, affordability, and acceptability framework

Availability	Staffing or service shortages (professional, peer, lay workforce)
Accessibility	Coordination of services (public, private, peer, integrated)
Affordability	Costs of care (insurance, financing, indirect/direct costs)
Acceptability	Discrimination, perception, and stigma

Bushy (1997) and Wilson et al. (2015)

the results of the environment or societal conditions where persons live as well as exposure to other modifiable or non-modifiable risk factors. Health disparities and inequities arising from these factors are systemic and systematic but may be avoidable.

Globally, mental disorders ranked among the top three noncommunicable diseases as leading causes of disease burden (Wang et al., 2023). Disability-adjusted life years (DALYs) have been shown to increase dramatically with the onset of a women's reproductive years (Alvi et al., 2023). Women are more prone to experience more years of life lived with disabling physical and mental illnesses with fewer years of good health than men and up to twice as likely to have mental illnesses than men (Borrell et al., 2014; Ribeiro et al., 2008). Twenty-six percent of females (ages 16–24) experience mental health issues compared to 9% of males the same age (McManus et al., 2014). Women are three times more likely to be diagnosed with post-traumatic stress disorder, anxiety, or eating disorders compared to men (Newlove-Delgado et al., 2021).

A global 30-year trend analysis (1990–2019) conducted by Yang et al. (2023) using age-period-cohort (APC) modeling determined, on average, women showed worse depression status than men. The top five countries with increased incidence of depression incidence were Spain, Mexico, Malaysia, the United States, and Uruguay, and the incidence rates in areas with high sociodemographic indices are increasing, especially in the younger generations (Yang et al., 2023). Of more concern are reports that healthy life expectancy has decreased between 1990 and 2019 in 204 countries and territories with a corresponding rise in poor health (GBD 2019 Demographics Collaborators, 2020).

Behavioral health disorders are often not addressed when discussing NCDs, even though there are significant human and economic costs when these disorders are left untreated. The United Nations Generally Assembly (2018) estimates in developing countries, for example, the costs of ignoring NCDs are estimated to be more than seven trillion US dollars (USD) over the next 15 years. Globally, the economic burden of NCDs is estimated at 47 trillion USD from 2010 to 2030 (United Nations General Assembly, 2018). For policymakers, charting country-level trajectories is essential to address discrete geographic patterns of causes of years of life lost due to or compounded by poor mental health or increased substance use. Hence, from a policy perspective, it is reasonable for governments to address NCDs to improve population health, to reduce health inequities, and to reduce the consequences of the SDOHs, especially to address issues in women's behavioral health.

Global Influences on Women's Behavioral Health Policy

The WHO's *Comprehensive Mental Health Action Plan* (2021) mirrors its *World Mental Health Report* (WMHR, 2022) with its emphasis on leadership and governance for mental health. The *Action Plan* prioritizes health and equity as a core responsibility of governments; the *WMHR* focuses achieving health and equity, addressing universal health coverage, human rights, multisectoral frameworks, evidence-based practice, life-course approach, and addressing societal challenges, all essential elements for females to access and receive focused behavioral health services.

In the EU, several initiatives started in the mid-2000s, also using multi-sectoral, multipronged approaches to policymaking to address mental disorders. Starting in 2013 with *The Joint Action on Mental Health and Wellbeing* with 51 partners (all EU Member States and 11 European organizations), the EU created a formal process for structured collaborative work by its Member States to address mental health and well-being across the EU. The *EU Compass for Action on Mental Health and Wellbeing* initiative reported major developments in mental health legislation and policy frameworks, financing and funding, services delivery systems and quality, promotion and prevention, multisector governance engagement, and engagement by patient, families, and NGOs. The multi-year *Compass* project also focused on mental health surveillance (mental health and substance use disorders), monitoring mental health targets and health promotion strategies, and incorporation of the "Mental Health in All Policies" (MHiAP) framework in EU member States (EU-Compass for Action on Mental Health and Well-being, 2017, 2018; EU Joint Action on Mental Health and Wellbeing, 2016).

The *European Framework for Action on Mental Health and Wellbeing* acknowledged the need to make mental health one of the top public health priorities in Europe (EU Joint Action on Mental Health and Wellbeing, 2016). *Health at a Glance Europe* reported 12 countries had formal plans or policy documents in place to address promotion and prevention of mental disorders (OECD/EU, 2019). The *Recommendation of the Council on Integrated Mental Health, Skills and Work Policy* emphasized the importance of policies to establish frameworks to better identify and treat "mental ill health" across employment and education to improve health and social outcomes (OECD, 2022). More recently, the EU Health Policy Platform Thematic Network (2023) urged the EU and other European countries to expand the MHiAP multi-sectoral approach across local, regional, national, and European levels to incorporate mental health across and within all policy sectors.

In the United States, although mental health was not declared as an essential public health issue until 1999, once identified, the Surgeon General's *Report* formally recognized the important relationships between mental health (including substance use), physical health, and well-being (U.S. Office of the Surgeon General, 1999). Referring to behavioral health disorders as "syndemic" disorders allows the national *Health in All Policies'* (*HiAP*) initiative to incorporate behavioral health into the SDOH framework for policy and/or legislative initiatives. *HiAP* attempts to ensure public health policy and other social policies at the local, state, regional, and national levels have neutral or beneficial impacts on the social and/or behavioral determinants of health (Institute of Medicine, 2014; National Association of County and City Health Officials, 2019).

The SDOH approach is also a key focus for the US *Healthy People 2030*, which establishes national objectives to improve overall and/or selected population health and well-being over a 10-year period. *Healthy People 2030* has 359 core objectives, as well as a number of developmental and research objectives. The latter two objectives are high-priority public health issues that either do not have reliable baseline data or documented evidence-based interventions, respectively.

These documents and initiatives illustrate how governance is conceptualized and implemented at national, regional, and global levels. Governance should consider the distribution of power across public and private sectors and distinct types of authority (administrative, economic, political, and regulatory). However, it should also consider the explicit or implicit societal institutions and rules surrounding the provision of both health and behavioral health services across the majority, marginalized, or underserved populations, although there are a number of policy influences, universal health coverage, human rights, the use of a multisectoral approach, advocacy, and stigma.

Universal health coverage   Globally, millions of people lack access to behavioral health services. They also lack coverage for behavioral health services because these services may not be offered or are beyond the financial resources of persons who need services. Integrating mental health and substance use services into universal health coverage (UHC) is the first step to ensure equitable access to and use of behavioral health services regardless of identity, socioeconomic status, age, or gender. However, major barriers to UHC fall under regulation, accountability, oversight, and stewardship of national health systems.

Although health systems governance issues are complex when viewed across nations, the Asia-Pacific Region is using a number of strategies to accomplish UHC (Yeoh et al., 2019). Strategies range from incorporating UHC directly in existing national plans, increasing levels of coverage and out-of-pocket costs, decentralizing services, or creating integrated service delivery packages for differing levels across health systems. Health technology assessments, key performance indicators, and linkages across insurance claims and health utilization datasets are also used in the move toward UHC. Two major barriers to implementation, however, are the lack of electronic medical records systems and interoperability issues across heterogeneous health information systems. Additional barriers to UHC are workforce capacity, capability, and distribution, accountability (governance and financial) and responsibility, and comprehensive regulations (Yeoh et al., 2019).

Human rights   Addressing the needs of women with behavioral health disorders (regardless of sexual orientation or gender identity) requires a broader-based approach. Initiatives to address mental health services development and delivery should follow global and national human rights policies. Incorporating evidence-based practices and life-course approaches are central to ensure behavioral health services are acceptable, accessible, affordable, and available to everyone (Bushy, 1997). Health, as a fundamental human right, is more than physical health. The symbiotic relationship between physical and mental health must be acknowledged across health and behavioral health policies, plans, and services to accommodate behavioral health needs across all developmental stages of the life-course.

Multisectoral approach Partnerships with public and private sectors are necessary to develop comprehensive and coordinated responses for mental health. These partnerships may involve working with multiple agencies across health, education, employment, judicial, housing, and social and other relevant sectors, as appropriate to each individual country's needs and available resources. Empowering people with behavioral health disorders is essential to ensure active participation in daily life activities and with their communities. Such empowerment includes engagement in advocacy and research, informing legislation and policymaking, planning services and infrastructure, and monitoring and evaluation.

Advocacy An important aspect of advocacy is a shared understanding and congruence that mental health is an essential element of the health policy frame. This requires overarching global and national policy documents, such as the *WMHR*, *MHiAP*, or Presidential documents, to reiterate consumer, family, and community advocacy positions and implementing advocacy positions into actionable policy. The WHO's *Quality Rights Guidance Manual* (2019) created actionable items using a multipronged approach that crosswalks and integrates issues common to mental health, disability, and human rights. It begins by building capacity to fight stigma and discrimination, using a human rights and recovery framework. Recovery is an important concept in crafting the delivery of mental health and social services to improve patient-focused/patient-oriented outcomes. Mental health, as a basic human right, encompasses the right to least restrictive, recovery-based services delivered in community-based settings. Social movements have been and remain an important vehicle to strengthen advocacy for persons with behavioral health disorders and to influence policymaking. Finally, the *Manual* calls for actual policy and legislative reform to ensure services to persons with mental illnesses and other disabilities are part of both international and national human rights standards.

Stigma The continued stigma and discrimination toward individuals with behavioral health disorders, their family members, and even behavioral health workforce staff are societal factors in the increase of mental and addictive disorders. Other factors include lack of buy-in by policymakers, little or no systematic services infrastructure, and no leadership, as behavioral health disorders are often considered as "forgotten diseases" (Lopez et al., 2014). Although there are broad-based documents that emphasize the need to address stigma, with actionable items, there is no single blueprint action plan or coherent, detailed strategy for implementation that fits all countries. However, countries are at various stages in developing and implementing appropriate and comprehensive responses. (For more information on stigma, see Chap. 9 in this text.)

All these factors contribute to the affordability of care. In the EU, *Health at a Glance Europe 2018* estimated the costs of behavioral health disorders, which affect approximately 84 million Europeans, exceeding 4% of the 28 EU countries' GDP (>EUR 600 billion) when looking at health systems, social programs, and individual/societal outcomes.

Framing Women's Behavioral Health as a Public Policy Issue

Even though gender is shown to be a strong determinant of many health outcomes, gender inequities still play a major role in the delivery of women's health and behavioral health services (Krieger, 2003; Sen & Ostlin, 2008). Gender roles and stereotypes, which start in childhood, continue throughout the life-course, and contribute to the social and behavioral determinants of health (e.g., societal behaviors and beliefs, public policies, and legislation). Since closing the treatment gap for women with behavioral health disorders remains a global policy focus, these upstream and downstream determinants of health (DOH) affect both the implementation of gender equity policies and their effects on health (Östlin et al., 2011).

The incremental evidence on diminishing gender inequalities in health suggests that policies designed to explicitly support women show improved health outcomes for women as well as their families. European and US data, for example, show that women have better mental health when policies address women's concerns around economic security, family planning, and violence against women (Borrell et al., 2014). While dual-earner models in Nordic countries show better mental health outcomes for women (McAllister et al., 2018), market-oriented models show worse mental health outcomes for women (Lund et al., 2018; McAllister et al., 2018). Labor market support, such as family-focused benefits, for women may improve mental health outcomes but may not address socioeconomic inequities (Shah et al., 2021). A comparative study on cross-national variation in Europe examined clusters of family-related, mental health, and socioeconomic factors to determine cross-national differences between countries on the relationships of these determinants on gender differences in the use of mental health services (Buffel et al., 2014). Substantial cross-national variation was found in the relationships between gender differences and mental health-care seeking. This finding suggests that improvement in mental health care-seeking and utilization of services by women would be improved by the expansion of gendered, family-focused, and labor market policies (Buffel et al., 2014).

These studies and others show that there is some evidence which supports the causal effects of structural determinants on inequities in mental health access, treatment, and utilization (McAllister et al., 2018; Shah et al., 2021). However, building an evidence-informed case to justify public policies to address the financing, delivery, and provision of behavioral health services is difficult. As a group, behavioral health disorders are heterogenous and have varying levels of acuity, disability, and chronicity. Case-mix classifications and cost weights often are used as predictive measures for resource utilization for mental health and substance use disorder services based on type and severity of disorder. Further, looking at financing behavioral health systems and services delivery from only a diagnostic or a cost-effectiveness perspective is not the best way to establish a rationale for a service need. A broader "public good" perspective is needed to effectively determine the potential and improved population outcomes for public intervention in behavioral health. Challenges must be addressed including (but not limited) to resource scarcity, improving equity, efficient allocation of resources, and efficient delivery of services. The intent of policy should be to improve population health.

Informing Gendered Policy

Demonstrating the complex relationship between gender, behavioral health, socio-economic, family, and other determinants of health characteristics can help bridge the gap in unmet need in behavioral health care. Initiatives, such as Mapping NCD, an EU project, provide information on what research is conducted across disorders and at-risk populations, such as women, in the EU's 28 Member States and Iceland, Norway, and Switzerland (Berg Brigham et al., 2016).

However, these types of projects are difficult due to the nature and typology of behavioral health disorders as well as other factors, including comorbidity, variations in diagnostic criteria, differences in reporting/data collection, financing of care, structures of healthcare systems, differences in benefits/reimbursement practices, and the social and economic heterogeneity across countries. We are reminded "not everything that counts can be counted, and not everything that can be counted counts" (Berg Brigham et al., 2016, p. 6). One way to connect research to policy is by linking specific gender policy instruments to the study designs, typologies, and models used to examine women's health, and behavioral health (Borrell et al., 2014). For example, comparability across study designs, data, and variables may be problematic. Ecological study designs, which are correlational, are useful for generating hypotheses as to how or why a policy worked. Multi-level study designs, which use secondary data, link policies and health outcomes in their analytical models. Longitudinal designs, which examine data before the implementation of a policy and data post-implementation, offer an idea of the time lag before the effects of a policy can be truly assessed.

Hence, gender policy instruments must encompass tools that not only describe social inequities that exacerbate women's behavioral health disorders but also address problem-solving or provide solutions. Creating hypotheses to map trajectories of influential factors for different types of policies is a first step toward strengthening the evidence for behavioral health policy. One example is the framework developed by Diderichsen et al. (2001), which examines the intersections of policy entry points to social contexts related to health outcomes. Social context is defined as the social and policy environments which inform and shape mechanisms that lead to exposures detrimental to health and which create health inequities. Mechanisms that generate gender inequalities in health include differential exposure, differential vulnerability, differential consequences, and social stratification. Policy entry points are those elements influencing stratification, reducing harmful exposures, reducing vulnerability, and preventing unequal consequences. Diderichsen et al.'s framework has been used successfully in a cross-national study looking at the health of women in Italy, Sweden, and Britain by Burstrom et al. (2010), who determined that the type of policy regime did matter in the differences between countries, specifically when it came to the health of single mothers.

Addressing intersectionality of policy with other axes of inequality can illuminate stress points created by policy and its implementation, such as the lag time of the effects of macrolevel polices. Looking at the long-term effects of income inequality on health at a national level, Zheng (2012) created a new discrete-time hazard model to address the effects of policy changes when determining income inequality on individual mortality risk. The discrete-time hazard model treats lags of income inequality as two variables (person-specific and time-variance). Using this model, Zheng determined that the effects of policy changes were shown at 5 years, were highest at 7 years, and diminished around 12 years. This kind of analysis supplies insights into long-term consequences of policy implementation, which could provide significant insights into the intersection of other sectors and behavioral health services design and provision, especially for women.

Policy cannot address what it does not know about. Unmet needs due to hidden populations, such as no formal recognition of place (recognized vs. non-recognized villages) or people (such as girls' births not added to a birth registry), affect the ability of research and practice to inform policy. Gendered perspectives for behavioral health policy and service provisions continue to be essential to reduce health inequalities, inequities, and disparities that may be ascribed to historical, political, economic, and sociocultural factors.

Pilgrim and Rogers' (1999) three-tiered analytical framework examines issues from the micro-, meso-, and macro-level perspectives. Micro-level addresses local and personal factors; meso-level addresses cultural and national factors; and macro-level addresses global and transhistorical factors. This type of assessment is particularly good at addressing patterns of (dis)continuity and periodicity. However, determining boundaries/intersections of societal and policy language used in or over a given time and domain must explicitly analyze gender disparities in risk and societal/population outcomes.

Gathering that evidence comes with its own challenges, especially as evidence may be socially constructed, (re)entextualized, or (re)contextualized (Hanson, 2014). Entextualization is when excerpts of a text or a paper are bound into another document or work. Recontextualization, defined as the reframing or reorganization of a text, allows a second author to substantiate new, and possibly different, claims that are different from the claims made by the original author. Evidence excerpted and added to a policy analysis or used in legislative or regulatory documents is open to more (re)interpretation or (re)entextualization as that language is excerpted and recirculated by other policymakers or stakeholders. If we accept Austin's (1962) maxim that we "do things with words," then it is important to remember that words (language) "implement service provision, afford protections, regulate societal and individual behaviors, provide accountings of actions, and contextualize issues for diverse audiences" (Hanson, 2014, p. 17).

Brooks et al. (2023) found the term "evidence" was often defined further based upon its intended or possible use, through the addition of modifiers, such as "conceptual," "direct," "tactical," "political," "imposed," or "procedural." Knowing how language is to be used may affect its effectiveness and how evidence is communicated through language may result in unintended consequences pre- and post-implementation. The use of consistent evidence across networks of users can strengthen the use of evidence in policymaking and inform the development of legislation, such as Mental Health Acts, to address the gendered challenges found in behavioral health services delivery, financing, and service utilization.

An Overview of Mental Health Acts

In their review of the literature, Ayano (2018) found mental health legislation covered 36% of individuals in low-income countries compared to 92% or persons living in high-income countries. However, in high-income countries, such as the U. S., coverage of mental health services may be limited to a specific number of visits over a defined period, resulting in out-of-pocket payments for these services or having no services. Employer coverage may also be limited based upon the size of the company. Limitations like these which circumvent the intent of legislation are common but often go unnoticed in the debate and passage of legislation. It behooves us to carefully read what is in legislation, how it is framed, and the claims that substantiate mental health acts from both a national and international lens as shown in these examples: Beck et al. (2021); Becker & Fangerau (2018); Bhugra et al. (2018); and Bikker et al. (2021).

"Unfragmenting" Mental Health Systems and Policies

There is a significant burden of disease regarding behavioral health disorders throughout the world. In addition, there continues to be variation in the funding for research, services delivery, and policy for physical and behavioral health services in countries throughout the world. Bhugra et al. (2018) surveyed 52 member countries of the Commonwealth to examine the existence of mental health policies and the degree of equal funding between physical and mental health services. Results showed that fewer than 50% of surveyed countries had a mental health policy and there was no existing equity for the funding of physical and mental health services. Furthermore, gender plays a role in the consequences of health and behavioral health. For example, women suffer from physical and behavioral health disorders more than men despite having a longer life expectancy (Glei & Horiuchi, 2007; Wang et al., 2012).

In the examination of health care delivery system reform, the WHO first proposed several basic foundations for health policy systems reform (Saltman & Figueras, 1997). These reforms included the integration of health and behavioral health services, addressing resource scarcity, improving equity of services, supporting efficient allocation of resources, and effectively delivering health and mental health services to at-risk populations (Saltman & Figueras, 1997). These same health care delivery system concerns still exist today.

When countries do offer behavioral health services, there remains substantial fragmentation of health and mental health services. The fragmentation inhibits the access, utilization, and effectiveness of health and behavioral health programs and services which, in turn, challenges the implementation of health-related Sustainable Development Goals (Agyepong et al., 2021; Spicer et al., 2020). Spicer et al. (2020) identified five problems affecting services fragmentation, including (1) proliferation of health organizations, (2) problems in health leadership, (3) divergent health interests, (4) problems of accountability, and (5) problems related to power relationships as opposed to initiating more intersectoral approaches to services integration. These five problems affect upstream and downstream policy actions. Policy (laws, policies, and regulations) is upstream action, screening and supported social and human services are midstream actions, and services delivery activities are downstream actions (patient level) (National Academies of Sciences et al., 2022). All three should be considered in how we can best "marry" health system efforts and community-based infrastructures to address behavioral health and the SDOH, particularly the social-behavioral determinants of health. There are indications this approach is happening, especially in the areas of health promotion, health security, and universal health coverage, as shown by recent work in Ethiopia and Rwanda (Rudasingwa et al., 2022; Tadesse et al., 2021).

Implications for Women's Behavioral Health

Throughout this chapter, we have emphasized the development and implementation of effective policymaking to help address the well-being of women through the design of more effective behavioral health access, treatment, and support services. Among the many challenges facing women of all ages in seeking and accessing behavioral health services, five issues are paramount to address: (1) the ability to collect, analyze, and report comparable epidemiologic data concerning the incidence and prevalence of women's behavioral health problems from a population perspective, (2) the differences between women and men in how they access and use behavioral health services, (3) the lack of policies and legislation for women's behavioral health services in low- and middle-income countries, (4) the continued stigmatization of individuals who suffer from mental and substance use disorders, and (5) prioritizing behavioral health as NCDs.

Behavioral health data In the twenty-first century, there are major gaps in data collected that inform the need for women's behavioral health services. For many countries, data simply is either incomplete, inaccurate, or not collected. Policy cannot address the unknown. For example, mental health legislation covers approximately one-third of the population living in low-income countries and varies across middle- and high-income countries. The legislation is informed by data, or its lack thereof.

Access to and use of behavioral health services Globally, millions of people have little or no access to needed mental and substance use services. They lack insurance coverage because they lack the financial resources to pay for needed services. When countries do offer behavioral health services, significant fragmentation of behavioral health services still occurs, particularly between integrated health and behavioral health services. The fragmentation inhibits the access, utilization, and effectiveness of these services and programs, particularly for women.

Policies and legislation for women's behavioral health services in developing countries Integrating mental and substance use services into some form of universal health coverage is an initial step to encourage equitable access to and use of behavioral health services, regardless of identity, socioeconomic status, age, or gender. Addressing women's behavioral health can improve overall health, reduce health inequities, and reduce the consequences of the SDOHs.

Stigma of individuals who suffer from a mental and/or substance use disorder The continued stigmatization and discrimination toward people who suffer from mental and substance use disorders remains a critical issue in behavioral health. While the research and policy literature addresses stigma, currently no strategy, plan, or legislation provides detailed guidance or offers a national or global strategy for implementation.

Noncommunicable diseases (NCDs) Globally, mental and substance use disorders rank among the top three NCDs as leading causes of disease burden (Wang et al., 2023). Nevertheless, behavioral health disorders are often not addressed when discussing NCDs, even though there are significant human, societal, and economic costs when these disorders are left untreated. The authors of this chapter have suggested that governments/countries address NCDs to advance population health, particularly for women, thereby reducing health inequities and their consequences. One option to achieve this is to develop and use more robust modeling scenarios. As illustrated above, these models show potential outcome trajectories among policy options that can more effectively address consequences of policymaking, SDOHs, and NCDs.

To effectively address these issues, women need access to care, care that addresses sex- and gender-specific behavioral health/health issues, and health outcomes that consider physiological, economic, and sociocultural issues. That intersection of research, practice, and policy clearly affects access to and use of services, continuity of care, infrastructure design, and patient outcomes at both individual and population health levels and across private and public sectors. Therefore, governmental accountability for women's behavioral health is essential. Accountability can be shown through the adoption and implementation of policies that address and mitigate these issues for the benefit of women across the lifespan and of society as a while. In conclusion, effective and thoughtful policymaking can help to address the sociostructural or social determinants of health that adversely affect women and their behavioral health.

References

Agyepong, I. A., M'Cormack-Hale, F. A. O., Brown Amoakoh, H., Derkyi-Kwarteng, A. N. C., Darkwa, T. E., & Odiko-Ollennu, W. (2021). Synergies and fragmentation in country level policy and program agenda setting, formulation and implementation for Global Health agendas: A case study of health security, universal health coverage, and health promotion in Ghana and Sierra Leone. *BMC Health Services Research, 21*(1), 476. https://doi.org/10.1186/s12913-021-06500-6

Alvarenga, A., Bana, E. C. C. A., Borrell, C., Ferreira, P. L., Freitas, Â., Freitas, L., Oliveira, M. D., Rodrigues, T. C., Santana, P., Lopes Santos, M., & Vieira, A. C. L. (2019). Scenarios for population health inequalities in 2030 in Europe: The EURO-HEALTHY project experience. *International Journal for Equity in Health, 18*(1), 100. https://doi.org/10.1186/s12939-019-1000-8

Alvi, M. H., Ashraf, T., Naz, F., Sardar, A., Ullah, A., Patel, A., Kiran, T., Gumber, A., & Husain, N. (2023). Burden of mental disorders by gender in Pakistan: Analysis of Global Burden of Disease Study data for 1990–2019. *BJPsych Bulletin*, 1–8. https://doi.org/10.1192/bjb.2023.76

Austin, J. L. (1962). *How to do things with words: The William James Lectures delivered at Harvard University in 1955*. Clarendon Press.

Ayano, G. (2018). Significance of mental health legislation for successful primary care for mental health and community mental health services: A review. *African Journal of Primary Health Care & Family Medicine, 10*(1), e1–e4. https://doi.org/10.4102/phcfm.v10i1.1429

Beck, A., Farmer, P., & Wykes, T. (2021). Proposed reforms of the Mental Health Act. *BMJ, 372*, n727. https://doi.org/10.1136/bmj.n727

Becker, T., & Fangerau, H. (2018). 40th birthday of the Italian Mental Health Law 180 – Perception and reputation abroad, and a personal suggestion. *Epidemiology & Psychiatric Sciences, 27*(4), 314–318. https://doi.org/10.1017/s2045796017000658

Berg Brigham, K., Darlington, M., Wright, J. S., Lewison, G., Kanavos, P., & Durand-Zaleski, I. (2016). Mapping research activity on mental health disorders in Europe: Study protocol for the Mapping_NCD project. *Health Research Policy and Systems, 14*(1), 39. https://doi.org/10.1186/s12961-016-0111-6

Bhugra, D., Pathare, S., Joshi, R., Kalra, G., Torales, J., & Ventriglio, A. (2018). A review of mental health policies from Commonwealth countries. *International Journal of Social Psychiatry, 64*(1), 3–8. https://doi.org/10.1177/0020764017745108

Bikker, A. P., Lesmana, C. B. J., & Tiliopoulos, N. (2021). The Indonesian Mental Health Act: Psychiatrists' views on the act and its implementation. *Health Policy and Planning, 36*(2), 196–204. https://doi.org/10.1093/heapol/czaa139

Borrell, C., Palència, L., Muntaner, C., Urquía, M., Malmusi, D., & O'Campo, P. (2014). Influence of macrosocial policies on women's health and gender inequalities in health. *Epidemiologic Reviews, 36*, 31–48. https://doi.org/10.1093/epirev/mxt002

Braveman, P. A., Kumanyika, S., Fielding, J., Laveist, T., Borrell, L. N., Manderscheid, R., & Troutman, A. (2011). Health disparities and health equity: The issue is justice. *American Journal of Public Health, 101*, S149–S155. https://doi.org/10.2105/ajph.2010.300062

Brooks, C., Mirzoev, T., Chowdhury, D., Deuri, S. P., & Madill, A. (2023). Using evidence in mental health policy agenda-setting in low- and middle-income countries: A conceptual meta-framework from a scoping umbrella review. *Health Policy and Planning, 38*(7), 876–893. https://doi.org/10.1093/heapol/czad038

Buffel, V., Van de Velde, S., & Bracke, P. (2014). Professional care seeking for mental health problems among women and men in Europe: The role of socioeconomic, family-related and mental health status factors in explaining gender differences. *Social Psychiatry and Psychiatric Epidemiology, 49*(10), 1641–1653. https://doi.org/10.1007/s00127-014-0879-z

Burstrom, B., Whitehead, M., Clayton, S., Fritzell, S., Vannoni, F., & Costa, G. (2010). Health inequalities between lone and couple mothers and policy under different welfare regimes – The example of Italy, Sweden and Britain. *Social Science and Medicine, 70*(6), 912–920. https://doi.org/10.1016/j.socscimed.2009.11.014

Bushy, A. (1997). Mental health and substance abuse: Challenges in providing services to rural clients. In Center for Substance Abuse Treatment (Ed.), *Bringing excellence to substance abuse services in rural and frontier America* (pp. 45–54). HHS Publication No. [SMA] 97–3134; TAP Series 20. U.S. Department of Health and Human Services, Rural Information Center Health Service. http://adaiclearinghouse.net/downloads/TAP-20-Bringing-Excellence-to-Substance-Abuse-Services-in-Rural-and-Frontier-America-110.pdf

Centers for Disease Control and Prevention. (2022, December 2). *Global health equity strategy 2022–2027* [Web Report (multiple pages)]. CDC. https://www.cdc.gov/globalhealth/equity/index.html

Diderichsen, F., Evans, T., & Whitehead, M. (2001). The social basis of disparities in health. In T. Evans, M. Whitehead, F. Diderichsen, A. Bhuiya, & M. Wirth (Eds.), *Challenging inequities in health. From ethics to action* (pp. 12–23). Oxford University Press.

EU Health Policy Platform Thematic Network. (2023). *Mental health in all policies* [Joint Statement]. Author. https://www.mhe-sme.org/wp-content/uploads/2023/05/Joint-Statement-with-endorsements.pdf

EU Joint Action on Mental Health and Wellbeing. (2016). *European framework for action on mental health and wellbeing: Final conference – Brussels, 21–22 January 2016* [Report]. Author. https://ec.europa.eu/research/participants/data/ref/h2020/other/guides_for_applicants/h2020-SC1-BHC-22-2019-framework-for-action_en.pdf

EU-Compass for Action on Mental Health and Well-being. (2017). *Annual activity reports of Member States and stakeholders* [Report]. Author. https://health.ec.europa.eu/system/files/2018-03/2017_compass_activityreport_en_0.pdf

EU-Compass for Action on Mental Health and Well-being. (2018). *Annual activity reports of member states and stakeholders* [Report]. Author. https://health.ec.europa.eu/system/files/2019-02/2018_compass_activityreport_en_0.pdf

Foreman, K. J., Marquez, N., Dolgert, A., Fukutaki, K., Fullman, N., McGaughey, M., Pletcher, M. A., Smith, A. E., Tang, K., Yuan, C. W., Brown, J. C., Friedman, J., He, J., Heuton, K. R., Holmberg, M., Patel, D. J., Reidy, P., Carter, A., Cercy, K., Chapin, A., Douwes-Schultz, D., Frank, T., Goettsch, F., Liu, P. Y., Nandakumar, V., Reitsma, M. B., Reuter, V., Sadat, N., Sorensen, R. J. D., Srinivasan, V., Updike, R. L., York, H., Lopez, A. D., Lozano, R., Lim, S. S., Mokdad, A. H., Vollset, S. E., & Murray, C. J. L. (2018). Forecasting life expectancy, years of life lost, and all-cause and cause-specific mortality for 250 causes of death: Reference and alternative scenarios for 2016–40 for 195 countries and territories. *Lancet, 392*(10159), 2052–2090. https://doi.org/10.1016/s0140-6736(18)31694-5

GBD 2019 Demographics Collaborators. (2020). Global age-sex-specific fertility, mortality, healthy life expectancy (HALE), and population estimates in 204 countries and territories, 1950–2019: A comprehensive demographic analysis for the Global Burden of Disease Study 2019. *Lancet, 396*(10258), 1160–1203. https://doi.org/10.1016/s0140-6736(20)30977-6

Glei, D. A., & Horiuchi, S. (2007). The narrowing sex differential in life expectancy in high-income populations: Effects of differences in the age pattern of mortality. *Population Studies (Camb), 61*(2), 141–159. https://doi.org/10.1080/00324720701331433

Hanson, A. (2014). Illuminating the invisible voices in mental health policymaking. *Journal of Medicine and the Person, 12*(1), 13–18. https://doi.org/10.1007/s12682-014-0170-9

Institute of Medicine. (2014). *Applying a health lens to decision making in non-health sectors: Workshop summary.* The National Academies Press. https://doi.org/10.17226/18659

Krieger, N. (2003). Genders, sexes, and health: What are the connections – And why does it matter? *International Journal of Epidemiology, 32*(4), 652–657. https://doi.org/10.1093/ije/dyg156

Lopez, A. D., Williams, T. N., Levin, A., Tonelli, M., Singh, J. A., Burney, P. G., Rehm, J., Volkow, N. D., Koob, G., & Ferri, C. P. (2014). Remembering the forgotten non-communicable diseases. BMC Medicine, 12(1), Article 200.

Lund, C., Brooke-Sumner, C., Baingana, F., Baron, E. C., Breuer, E., Chandra, P., Haushofer, J., Herrman, H., Jordans, M., Kieling, C., Medina-Mora, M. E., Morgan, E., Omigbodun, O., Tol, W., Patel, V., & Saxena, S. (2018). Social determinants of mental disorders and the Sustainable Development Goals: A systematic review of reviews. *Lancet Psychiatry, 5*(4), 357–369. https://doi.org/10.1016/s2215-0366(18)30060-9

McAllister, A., Fritzell, S., Almroth, M., Harber-Aschan, L., Larsson, S., & Burström, B. (2018). How do macro-level structural determinants affect inequalities in mental health? – A systematic review of the literature. *International Journal for Equity in Health, 17*(1), 180. https://doi.org/10.1186/s12939-018-0879-9

McManus, S., Bebbington, P., Jenkins, R., & Brugha, T. (2014). *Mental health and wellbeing in England: Adult psychiatric morbidity survey.* NHS Digital. https://webarchive.nationalarchives.gov.uk/ukgwa/20180328140249/http:/digital.nhs.uk/catalogue/PUB21748

National Academies of Sciences, Engineering, & Medicine. (2022). *Models for population health improvement by health care systems and partners: Tensions and promise on the path upstream: Proceedings of a workshop.* The National Academies Press. https://doi.org/10.17226/26059

National Association of County and City Health Officials. (2019, March). *Statement of policy: Health in All Policies* [Policy 12-01]. NACCHO. https://www.naccho.org/uploads/downloadable-resources/12-01-Health-in-All-Policies.pdf

Newlove-Delgado, T., Williams, T., Robertson, K., McManus, S., Sadler, K., Vizard, T., Cartwright, C., Mathews, F., Norman, S., Marcheselli, F., & Ford, T. (2021). *Mental health of children and young people in England, 2021: Wave 2 follow up to the 2017 survey* [Report]. NHS Digital. https://digital.nhs.uk/data-and-information/publications/statistical/mental-health-of-children-and-young-people-in-england/2021-follow-up-to-the-2017-survey#

OECD. (2022). *Recommendation of the Council on OECD Integrated Mental Health, Skills and Work Policy* [Report]. OECD/LEGAL. https://legalinstruments.oecd.org/public/doc/334/334.en.pdf

OECD/EU. (2019, February). *Health at a Glance Europe: 2018: State of health in the EU cycle* [Report; EW-01-18-697-EN-N]. OECD Publishing. https://health.ec.europa.eu/system/files/2020-02/2018_healthatglance_rep_en_0.pdf

Östlin, P., Schrecker, T., Sadana, R., Bonnefoy, J., Gilson, L., Hertzman, C., Kelly, M. P., Kjellstrom, T., Labonté, R., Lundberg, O., Muntaner, C., Popay, J., Sen, G., & Vaghri, Z. (2011). Priorities for research on equity and health: Towards an equity-focused health research agenda. *PLoS Medicine, 8*(11), e1001115. https://doi.org/10.1371/journal.pmed.1001115

Pilgrim, D., & Rogers, A. (1999). Mental health policy and the politics of mental health: A three tier analytical framework. *Policy & Politics, 27*(1), 13–24. https://doi.org/10.1332/030557399782019570

Ribeiro, P. S., Jacobsen, K. H., Mathers, C. D., & Garcia-Moreno, C. (2008). Priorities for women's health from the Global Burden of Disease study. *International Journal of Gynaecology and Obstetrics, 102*(1), 82–90. https://doi.org/10.1016/j.ijgo.2008.01.025

Rudasingwa, M., Jahn, A., Uwitonze, A. M., & Hennig, L. (2022). Increasing health system synergies in low-income settings: Lessons learned from a qualitative case study of Rwanda. *Global Public Health, 17*(12), 3303–3321. https://doi.org/10.1080/17441692.2022.2129726

Saltman, R. B., & Figueras, J. (1997). *European health care reform: Analysis of current strategies.* Regional Office for Europe of the World Health Organization. https://eurohealthobservatory.who.int/publications/i/european-health-care-reform-analysis-of-current-strategies-study

Sen, G., & Ostlin, P. (2008). Gender inequity in health: Why it exists and how we can change it. *Global Public Health, 3*(Suppl 1), 1–12. https://doi.org/10.1080/17441690801900795

Shah, N., Walker, I. F., Naik, Y., Rajan, S., O'Hagan, K., Black, M., Cartwright, C., Tillmann, T., Pearce-Smith, N., & Stansfield, J. (2021). National or population level interventions addressing the social determinants of mental health – An umbrella review. *BMC Public Health, 21*(1), 2118. https://doi.org/10.1186/s12889-021-12145-1

Spicer, N., Agyepong, I., Ottersen, T., Jahn, A., & Ooms, G. (2020). 'It's far too complicated': Why fragmentation persists in global health. *Globalization and Health, 16*(1), 60. https://doi.org/10.1186/s12992-020-00592-1

Tadesse, A. W., Gurmu, K. K., Kebede, S. T., & Habtemariam, M. K. (2021). Analyzing efforts to synergize the global health agenda of universal health coverage, health security and health promotion: A case-study from Ethiopia. *Globalization and Health, 17*(1), 53. https://doi.org/10.1186/s12992-021-00702-7

U.S. Office of the Surgeon General. (1999). *Mental health: A report of the Surgeon General* [Report]. U.S. Department of Health and Human Services, Substance Abuse and Mental Health Services Administration, Center for Mental Health Services, National Institutes of Health, National Institute of Mental Health. https://profiles.nlm.nih.gov/spotlight/nn/catalog/nlm:nlm uid-101584932X120-doc

United Nations General Assembly. (2018, October 17). *Political declaration of the third high-level meeting of the General Assembly on the prevention and control of non-communicable diseases* [Report; A/RES/73/2]. United Nations. https://digitallibrary.un.org/record/1648984?ln=en [Select language for download].

Wang, H., Dwyer-Lindgren, L., Lofgren, K. T., Rajaratnam, J. K., Marcus, J. R., Levin-Rector, A., Levitz, C. E., Lopez, A. D., & Murray, C. J. (2012). Age-specific and sex-specific mortality in 187 countries, 1970–2010: A systematic analysis for the Global Burden of Disease Study 2010. *Lancet, 380*(9859), 2071–2094. https://doi.org/10.1016/s0140-6736(12)61719-x

Wang, H., Song, Y., Ma, J., Ma, S., Shen, L., Huang, Y., Thangaraju, P., Basharat, Z., Hu, Y., Lin, Y., Peden, A. E., Sawyer, S. M., Zhang, H., & Zou, Z. (2023). Burden of non-communicable diseases among adolescents and young adults aged 10–24 years in the South-East Asia and Western Pacific regions, 1990–2019: A systematic analysis for the Global Burden of Disease Study 2019. *Lancet Child & Adolescent Health, 7*(9), 621–635. https://doi.org/10.1016/s2352-4642(23)00148-7

Wilson, W., Bangs, A., & Hatting, T. (2015, February). *Future of rural behavioral health (National Rural Health Association Policy Brief)*. National Rural Health Association. https://www.ruralhealthweb.org/NRHA/media/Emerge_NRHA/Advocacy/Policy%20documents/The-Future-of-Rural-Behavioral-Health_Feb-2015.pdf

World Health Organization. (2017, December 29). *Human rights and health*. [Web page]. WHO. https://www.who.int/news-room/fact-sheets/detail/human-rights-and-health

World Health Organization. (2019). *Advocacy for mental health, disability and human rights: WHO QualityRights guidance module* [Report]. WHO. https://apps.who.int/iris/handle/10665/329587

World Health Organization. (2021). *Comprehensive mental health action plan 2013–2030* [Report]. WHO. https://apps.who.int/iris/handle/10665/345301

World Health Organization. (2022, June 16). *World mental health report: Transforming mental health for all* [Report]. Author [WHO]. https://apps.who.int/iris/rest/bitstreams/1433523/retrieve

Yang, F., Lodder, P., Huang, N., Liu, X., Fu, M., & Guo, J. (2023). Thirty-year trends of depressive disorders in 204 countries and territories from 1990 to 2019: An age-period-cohort analysis. *Psychiatry Research, 328*, 115433. https://doi.org/10.1016/j.psychres.2023.115433

Yeoh, E. K., Johnston, C., Chau, P. Y. K., Kiang, N., Tin, P., & Tang, J. (2019). Governance functions to accelerate progress toward universal health coverage (UHC) in the Asia-Pacific Region. *Health System and Reform, 5*(1), 48–58. https://doi.org/10.1080/23288604.2018.1543521

Yu, S. (2018). Uncovering the hidden impacts of inequality on mental health: A global study. *Translational Psychiatry, 8*(1), 98. https://doi.org/10.1038/s41398-018-0148-0

Zheng, H. (2012). Do people die from income inequality of a decade ago? *Social Science and Medicine, 75*(1), 36–45. https://doi.org/10.1016/j.socscimed.2012.02.042

Index

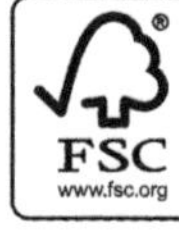